Musculoskeletal Examination
for Undergraduates

Musculoskeletal Examination
for Undergraduates

Chief Editor

Vivek Pandey MBBS MS (Orthopaedics)
Professor, Unit Head
Trauma, Joint Replacement, Sports Medicine, and
Arthroscopy Division
Department of Orthopaedic Surgery
Kasturba Medical College, Manipal
Manipal Academy of Higher Education
Manipal, Karnataka, India

Co-editor

Saktthi Shanmuganathan
Assistant Professor
Department of Orthopaedic Surgery
Kasturba Medical College, Manipal
Manipal Academy of Higher Education
Manipal, Karnataka, India

Foreword

Sharath K Rao

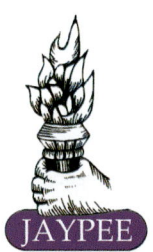

JAYPEE BROTHERS MEDICAL PUBLISHERS
The Health Sciences Publisher
New Delhi | London

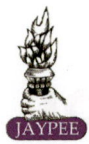

Jaypee Brothers Medical Publishers (P) Ltd

Headquarters
Jaypee Brothers Medical Publishers (P) Ltd
EMCA House, 23/23-B
Ansari Road, Daryaganj
New Delhi 110 002, India
Landline: +91-11-23272143, +91-11-23272703
+91-11-23282021, +91-11-23245672
Email: jaypee@jaypeebrothers.com

Corporate Office
Jaypee Brothers Medical Publishers (P) Ltd
4838/24, Ansari Road, Daryaganj
New Delhi 110 002, India
Phone: +91-11-43574357
Fax: +91-11-43574314
Email: jaypee@jaypeebrothers.com

Overseas Office
J.P. Medical Ltd
83 Victoria Street, London
SW1H 0HW (UK)
Phone: +44 20 3170 8910
Fax: +44 (0)20 3008 6180
Email: info@jpmedpub.com

Website: www.jaypeebrothers.com
Website: www.jaypeedigital.com

© 2023, Jaypee Brothers Medical Publishers

The views and opinions expressed in this book are solely those of the original contributor(s)/author(s) and do not necessarily represent those of editor(s) and publisher of the book.

All rights reserved. No part of this publication may be reproduced, stored or transmitted in any form or by any means, electronic, mechanical, photocopying, recording or otherwise, without the prior permission in writing of the publishers.

All brand names and product names used in this book are trade names, service marks, trademarks or registered trademarks of their respective owners. the publisher is not associated with any product or vendor mentioned in this book.

Medical knowledge and practice change constantly. This book is designed to provide accurate, authoritative information about the subject matter in question. However, readers are advised to check the most current information available on procedures included and check information from the manufacturer of each product to be administered, to verify the recommended dose, formula, method and duration of administration, adverse effects and contraindications. It is the responsibility of the practitioner to take all appropriate safety precautions. Neither the publisher nor the author(s)/editor(s) assume any liability for any injury and/or damage to persons or property arising from or related to use of material in this book.

This book is sold on the understanding that the publisher is not engaged in providing professional medical services. If such advice or services are required, the services of a competent medical professional should be sought.

Every effort has been made where necessary to contact holders of copyright to obtain permission to reproduce copyright material. If any have been inadvertently overlooked, the publisher will be pleased to make the necessary arrangements at the first opportunity.

Inquiries for bulk sales may be solicited at: jaypee@jaypeebrothers.com

Musculoskeletal Examination for Undergraduates

First Edition: **2023**

ISBN: 978-93-5465-979-9

Printed at Nutech Print Services - India

Dedicated to

My Parents
Kuldip Narain Pandey and Manju Pandey

My wife
Deeksha

and son
Krish

My brother and his family
Abhishek, Susanne, Demira and Maya

My Teachers and Students!

Foreword

As a teacher and clinician in orthopaedics, I am pleased to write the foreword for this valuable book on musculoskeletal examination for undergraduates.

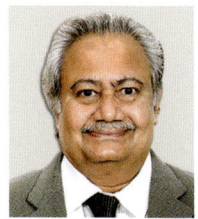

In the two decades, there have been immense developments in the field of orthopaedics, and more and more young doctors are opting for orthopaedics as their speciality. However, their undergraduate orthopaedic skills remain raw as no book has been dedicated solely to musculoskeletal examinations for undergraduate medical students. With our population's increasing burden of musculoskeletal conditions, it is crucial to equip our undergraduates with the knowledge and skills to diagnose and manage these conditions effectively.

This book thoroughly introduces musculoskeletal examination, addressing the essentials of history taking, physical examination, and finding interpretation. The authors have presented the examination approaches straightforwardly and succinctly, making them simple for readers to comprehend and use professionally. The inclusion of clinical examination videos is one of this book's most advantageous features because it will significantly aid students in honing their examination techniques.

Furthermore, students can quickly diagnose a problem in an outpatient department environment with the help of this book's clinical snippets, in which authors provide a hint regarding the most probable clinical condition with one or more standard presentations.

This book also briefly discusses common musculoskeletal conditions and their management, a valuable resource for medical students.

The author of this book, Professor Vivek Pandey, is not only a reputed clinician but also an excellent teacher. His effort in imparting clinical skills to undergraduates through this book goes well with the vision and mission of the Kasturba Medical College, Manipal, Karnataka, India. Undoubtedly, this book will be the most sought-after among undergraduates.

Overall, this book is an excellent resource for any undergraduate students seeking to develop their musculoskeletal examination skills. I highly recommend it as a must-read for all medical students and healthcare practitioners managing musculoskeletal conditions.

Sharath K Rao MBBS D Ortho MS (Ortho)
Pro-Vice-Chancellor–Health Sciences
Manipal Academy of Higher Education
Professor of Orthopaedics
Kasturba Medical College
Manipal, Karnataka, India

Preface

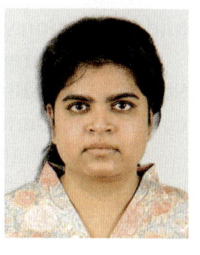

The musculoskeletal examination is a crucial clinical practice component; all healthcare providers must be proficient in it. Making an accurate diagnosis, creating a treatment plan, and offering patients the best care depend on your ability to conduct a complete musculoskeletal examination.

For all these years, we have believed that a book should exist that strives to give undergraduate students in healthcare fields including medicine, nursing, physiotherapy, and occupational therapy a complete introduction to musculoskeletal evaluation. This book is intended to serve as a valuable tool to help undergraduate students of healthcare discipline learn and comprehend the concepts and procedures involved in musculoskeletal assessment.

It is difficult to comprehend the ideas of a bone and joint assessment without having a basic understanding of anatomy and biomechanics. So, before describing a step-by-step process for musculoskeletal assessment, this book provides an introduction to the anatomy and physiology of the musculoskeletal system. The fundamentals of inspection, palpation, range-of-motion testing, and specific tests for each joint are covered in the book. Chapters on gait analysis, amputation stump assessment, and the evaluation of swelling, sinus-scar are also included in this book.

The book is easy to read and includes multiple pictures and images to help the reader grasp the subject. To help reinforce the subject presented, almost all important clinical examination videos have been included.

In conclusion, this is our humble attempt to simplify musculoskeletal testing for undergraduate medical students without sacrificing the subject's integrity.

In order to improvise the further editions, we would humbly request you all to provide a feedback and suggestions on *vivekortho@yahoo.co.in*.

Vivek Pandey
Saktthi Shanmuganathan

Acknowledgments

Guru Devo Brahma!

May this book be a tribute to all our mentors.

We would like to begin by thanking our teachers and mentors, Profs Varghese Chacko, Bhaskaranand Kumar, Benjamin Joseph, Sripathi Rao, SP Mohanty and Sharath Rao, whose shoulders we stood on to see the orthopaedic world.

We also want to convey our sincere gratitude to our families for their unflagging support and inspiration while we worked on finishing this academic assignment.

In an expression of gratitude, we wish to acknowledge our senior colleagues Profs Shyamsunder Bhat, Kiran Acharya, Monappa Naik, Hitesh Shah, and Anil Bhat and for all the constant academic guidance and support.

We also thank Prof Ashwath Acharya, without whom we could not have tailored the examination of the peripheral nerve chapter neatly to maintain adequacy regarding content. We also thank Dr Navaneeth Kamath (Musculoskeletal Oncologist, Mangalore) for helping improvise the examination of bone tumors.

Although it is the hard work of the author and several reviewers, this edition would not have existed if M/s Jaypee Brothers Medical Publishers (P) Ltd, New Delhi, India, and their staff had not assisted. I appreciate the hard work put forward by Shri Jitendar P Vij (Group Chairman), Mr Ankit Vij (Managing Director), Mr MS Mani (Group President), Dr Madhu Choudhary (Director-Educational Publishing), Ms Pooja Bhandari [Director-Production (Books and Journals)] and Dr Aditya Tayal (Team Lead–UG Publishing) in delivering the revised version.

Brevity in writing is the best insurance for its perusal." ~ Rudolf Virchow

This book has constantly been evolving to always be within the current orthopaedic trend, and we owe it to all students for inspiring and encouraging us to improve.

Contents

1. **Basics of History Taking and Examination in Orthopaedics** — 1
   - History Assessment in Orthopaedics — 1
   - Examination — 10

2. **Clinical Evaluation of Polytrauma and Acute Injury of Bones and Joints** — 18
   - Polytrauma — 18
   - History — 20
   - General Assessment — 22
   - Local Examination — 23
   - Trauma-related Orthopaedic Emergencies — 28

3. **Clinical Evaluation of Diseased Long Bones and Joints** — 30
   - History Taking in Long Bone Disease — 30
   - General and Systemic Examination — 32
   - Local Examination — 32
   - Differential Diagnosis — 34
   - Clinical Evaluation of Pathological Joints — 39

4. **Clinical Evaluation of the Shoulder Joint** — 50
   - Surgical Anatomy and its Clinical Significance — 50
   - History and its Evaluation — 51
   - Examination — 55
   - Shoulder Examination Proforma — 71
   - Common Conditions Affecting Shoulder and their Salient Features — 71

5. **Clinical Evaluation of the Elbow Joint** — 76
   - Relevant Surgical Anatomy and its Clinical Significance — 76
   - History and its Evaluation — 79
   - Examination — 81
   - Elbow Examination Proforma — 92
   - Common Conditions Affecting Elbow and their Salient Features — 92

6. **Clinical Evaluation of the Wrist and Hand** — 95
   - Surgical Anatomy of the Wrist Joint and its Clinical Significance — 95
   - Surgical Anatomy of the Hand and its Clinical Significance — 97
   - History and its Evaluation — 98
   - Examination — 103
   - Wrist and Hand Examination Proforma — 114
   - Common Conditions Affecting Wrist-hand and their Salient Features — 115

7. Clinical Evaluation of the Hip Joint — 120
- Surgical Anatomy and its Clinical Significance — 120
- History and its Evaluation — 120
- Examination — 125
- A Note on Abductor Mechanism and Trendelenburg Test — 140
- Use of Cane in Hip Diseases — 141
- Hip Examination Proforma — 142
- Common Conditions Affecting Hip and their Salient Features — 143

8. Clinical Evaluation of the Knee Joint — 146
- Surgical Anatomy and Function of the Knee Joint — 146
- History and its Evaluation — 152
- Examination — 155
- Knee Examination Proforma — 173
- Common Conditions Affecting Knee and their Salient Features — 174

9. Clinical Evaluation of the Foot and Ankle Joint — 178
- Surgical Anatomy of Foot-ankle and its Clinical Significance — 178
- History and its Evaluation — 180
- Examination — 184
- Foot-ankle Examination Proforma — 196
- Common Conditions Affecting Foot-ankle and their Salient Features — 197

10. Clinical Evaluation of the Spine — 200
- Surgical Anatomy of Spine-spinal Cord and its Clinical Significance — 200
- History and its Evaluation — 205
- Examination — 209
- Spine Examination Proforma — 229
- Common Conditions Affecting Spine and their Salient Features — 230

11. Clinical Evaluation of the Peripheral Nerves — 236
- Surgical Anatomy of the Peripheral Nerve and its Clinical Significance — 236
- History and its Evaluation — 239
- Examination — 241
- Peripheral Nerve Examination Proforma — 270
- Common Deformities following Specific Nerve Injuries and Other Conditions — 270

12. Clinical Evaluation of the Bone Tumors — 272
- Classification of Bone Tumors — 272
- History Taking in Bone Tumors — 272
- Examination — 276
- Bone Tumor Examination Proforma — 279
- Important Bone Tumors (in Brief) — 280

13. Clinical Evaluation of the Amputation Stump	**283**
• Indications for Amputation	283
• The Scheme of History Taking in a Patient with Amputation Stump	283
• Examination	285
• Amputation Stump Examination Proforma	289
14. Clinical Evaluation of Gait and Various Patterns of Gait	**290**
• Definition of Gait	290
• Phases of Gait	290
• Etiology of Gait Disturbance	290
• Commonly Encountered Gait Patterns	292
15. Clinical Evaluation of the Swelling, Scar, Sinus, and Ulcer	**296**
• History and Examination of a Swelling	296
• Examination	298
• History and Examination of a Scar	305
• History and Examination of a Sinus	307
• History and Examination of an Ulcer	309
Index	*315*

CHAPTER 1

Basics of History Taking and Examination in Orthopaedics

HISTORY ASSESSMENT IN ORTHOPAEDICS

Basic rule of thumb: Before history taking and examination, it is essential that the clinician greets the patient and introduces himself/herself to the patient, which helps build confidence by creating a rapport with the patient.

The art of extracting relevant history and eliciting positive examination findings to clinch a diagnosis during orthopedic case presentations is taught with modifications from the other subjects.

The evaluation of the patient starts with basic demographic details mentioned below.
- Name
- Age
- Gender
- Occupation
- Address
- Hand dominance

Initial demographic details and chief complaints are informed as Miss PY, a 26-year-old female from Mumbai, left-hand dominant, a software professional, presents with chief complaints of pain in her right shoulder for 3 months, difficulty in elevating arm and reaching overhead objects for 20 days.

The importance of various demographic factors is discussed below.
1. **Age:** Typically, most orthopedic conditions have a predilection for a particular age group. Several examples are mentioned below:
   a. *At birth*: Developmental dysplasia of the hip (DDH)
   b. *6–36 months*: Rickets
   c. *5–10 years*: Perthes' disease, Ewing's sarcoma
   d. *10–15 years*: Slipped capital femoral epiphysis (SCFE), osteosarcoma
   e. *18–40 years*: Giant cell tumor, patella/shoulder dislocation, sports injuries
   f. *20–40 years*: Inflammatory arthritis (Rheumatoid)
   g. *>40 years*: Various degenerative conditions such as osteoarthritis, tendinopathy, osteoporosis, and rotator cuff tear; malignancies such as multiple myeloma and secondaries.

Note that trauma-induced maladies can happen at any age.

2. **Gender:** Certain conditions have gender predilection, such as:
   a. *Females*: DDH, connective tissue disorders, giant cell tumor, rheumatoid arthritis
   b. *Males*: Perthes' disease, and ankylosing spondylitis.
3. **Occupation:** Various occupations may pose a hazard for different orthopedic conditions. For example, painters, heavy manual workers, and those who participate in overhead sports are

more prone to shoulder pathologies. Pneumatic tool drillers, chain saw workers are more prone for carpal tunnel syndrome. Further, the treatment plan can be altered or tailored according to various occupations.
4. **Address:** The residence may play a significant role in the development of certain diseases in a person, especially if the person has been staying in that place for long or since birth to have enough exposure to environmental factors. For example, natives of places high fluoride content in the water, are more prone to early-onset secondary osteoarthritis of joints and spinal canal stenosis.
5. **Hand dominance:** Considering hand dominance is an essential aspect while treating or rehabilitating a patient. For example, a minor deformity and/or less than optimal function following a "left sided" malunited Colles' fracture is more acceptable in a right-hand dominant person than a left-hand dominant person.

Chief Complaints (In Chronological Order)

One must always present chief complaints in chronological order. For example,
- Pain in the right shoulder for six months
- Difficulty in elevating and reaching overhead objects for three months
- Swelling over the right shoulder for two weeks.

The common chief complaints in orthopedic patients are:
- Pain
- Swelling
- Inability or difficulty in bearing weight
- Limp
- Inability or difficulty in moving a joint
- Discharging sinus, nonhealing wound
- Deformity
- Shortening or lengthening of a limb
- Instability of the joint
- Locking
- Clicks, crepitus
- Altered sensations
- Constitutional symptoms and other systemic features
- Effect on activities of daily living and occupation: Routinely, it may not be part of chief complaints. However, it must be included at the end of the history of the present illness to understand the effect of the disease process on one's daily activities and occupation.

History of Present Illness (HOPI)

The fundamental idea of HOPI assessment is that each chief complaint must be extracted and described in detail regarding onset, duration, progression, aggravating, relieving factors, and other specific points, if any. Once all the chief complaints are well described, the relevant positive and negative history is taken. ***The aim of detailing HOPI with positive and negative history is to narrow down to the probable etiology and pathology of the symptoms in question.***

Of note: Typically, the HOPI starts by stating, patient was apparently all right … days/weeks/ months back after which he/she started to develop complaints of...
The clinician must ask the patient when he/she was all right before the onset of the complaint(s). Often, patients may not disclose the chronicity of the complaint as they would have adjusted to the problem and worry only about the acute exacerbation of the said complaint. A symptom with acute or chronic duration may have a different etiology. Missing this one aspect during HOPI assessment can change the entire diagnosis.
Next, one must always ask, "How did it start"? It means what changed to trigger that complaint or symptom. Was it a traumatic event (minor or major), or was it insidious in onset? The complaints are further elaborated in standard fashion.

Pain

Pain is the most common complaint in orthopedic conditions. Pain should be probed on several parameters such as site, duration, onset, timing, progression, quality, radiation, relieving-aggravating factors, severity, and timing.
- **Site:** Often, identifying the site of pain can localize the structures involved in producing/causing pain.
- **Onset:** Sudden or insidious. What triggered the pain, must be probed.
- **Severity:** The pain could be mild, moderate, severe or excruciating.
  - *Mild pain:* Easily ignored
  - *Moderate pain:* Cannot be ignored, interferes with function, and needs time-to-time intervention/medication
  - *Severe:* Cannot be ignored, interferes with function, and demands constant attention and intervention
  - *Excruciating:* Incapacitating pain.
- **Timing of pain:** Apart from elaborating the pain on the above-mentioned factors, it is crucial to understand the timing or nature of pain, which could be *"mechanical"* pain, *"rest"* pain, or pain of *"neurological origin"*.
  - *Mechanical pain* results from loading the joint (standing, walking, turning, running, jumping, etc.). Typically, mechanical pain is due to degenerative pathologies such as osteoarthritis, spondylosis, tendinopathies, and fasciitis, and characteristically resolves upon adequate rest.
  - *Rest pain* happens during periods of rest even without loading the joint, and might be associated with morning stiffness. It is usually due to inflammatory, infective, or tumorous disorders such as rheumatoid arthritis, ankylosing spondylitis, tuberculosis (TB) of the joint, and malignant tumors. Night cries are a special type of rest pain, which are described in tuberculosis of the joints, especially in children. These so-called night cries are due to decreased voluntary muscle tone during sleep, permitting the diseased joint surfaces to rub against each other more than when the child is awake when the muscle spasm does not allow gross movement.
    However, there are a *few exceptions* to the general rule about rest pain, e.g., shoulder and cervical spine degenerative pathologies (cervical disc prolapse, rotator cuff pathologies, frozen shoulder) are painful at night. However, they may not be infective/inflammatory/tumorous in origin. So, although these conditions are painful at night, they do not indicate any sinister pathology.

- **Progression:** The assessment of progression is important to ascertain whether it is constant/worsening/improving/is it intermittent.
  - *Trauma:* Initially more (at the time of the injury) followed by a decrease in severity
  - *Neoplasia:* Constant or gradually worsening pain
  - *Acute inflammation:* Sudden increase followed by a gradual decrease
  - *Chronic inflammation:* Remissions and exacerbation of pain
  - *New origin pain in a painless condition:* Malignant change or pathological fracture.
- **Character** could be throbbing, burning, or dull aching type.
  - *Throbbing*: Abscess
  - *Burning or with tingling*: Neuralgic origin
  - *Dull aching:* Mechanical pain of degenerative conditions (osteoarthritis, spondylitis, tendinopathies)
- **Radiation:** Ask about the site of radiation of pain, if any. The radiation site may give a clue of pathology. For example, the cervical intervertebral disc prolapse (IVDP) pain radiates along the shoulder, arm, and forearm up to the lateral three fingers indicating the level of IVDP as C5, 6, and 7.
- **Aggravating and relieving factors:**
  - Ask about aggravating and relieving factors with direct and indirect questions such as what happens when you move your joint, run, jump, squat, etc., whether pain relieves with analgesic or rest.
  - Its relation to food, e.g., pain due to gout increases after eating red meat, organ meat, or cabbage.

Swelling

The symptom of swelling must be thoroughly probed on the following parameters: Site, onset, duration, progression, painful/painless, and number (single/multiple). The swelling could be intra-articular (effusion/synovial swelling) or arising from extra-articular structures. The swelling from an extra-articular structures should be evaluated as per the standard assessment *(Refer to Chapter 15 on Swelling)*. The Onset of swelling with the event of trauma can give some clue towards the diagnosis, such as:

- **If the intra-articular swelling appears immediately after or within a few hours of trauma**, it indicates *hemarthrosis*. The hemarthrosis results either from intra-articular fractures or injury to any intra-articular structure which has a rich blood supply, e.g., peripheral meniscal tear, cruciate ligament tear, synovial or capsular tears.
- **If the intra-articular swelling appears 12–24 hours after the injury**, it indicates *excess synovial fluid* production in the joint following synovial irritation. Synovial irritation could result from cartilage injury, meniscal tear, or a foreign body reaction.
- **A nontraumatic origin intra-articular swelling** could be due *to synovial hypertrophy, excess synovial fluid, a combination of synovial hypertrophy and fluid, or pus.* It can occur in infections (TB), inflammation (rheumatoid), degenerative conditions (osteoarthritis, meniscal, or cartilage damage), synovial chondromatosis, etc.

Inability or Difficulty in Bearing Weight (Lower Limb)

Typically, normal weight-bearing is possible due to the normal linkage between *"normally innervated painless bone-joint-ligament-muscle-tendon-capsule complexes."* Any *disturbance in this linkage could lead to inability or difficulty in bearing weight.* Several examples are discussed below to understand how normal weight-bearing is affected or compensated.

- Inability to bear weight after acute trauma indicates a significant bone or joint injury (fracture or dislocation), nerve palsy, complete ligament injury, complete muscle-tendon tear, or significant capsular disruption.
- If the patient can bear weight immediately or soon after (within few hours or a day) the first acute injury, it "fairly well rules out" any significant bony or soft tissue injury. Nevertheless, in impacted fractures or cases of partial soft tissue injuries (muscle, tendon, and ligament), one can still bear weight, albeit with pain!
- A chronic history of inability to bear weight on the lower limb with a fracture indicates a nonunion of a fracture.

Limp

Limp is frequently observed in affections of the lower limb. It could be painful or painless. The various causes of limp could be *painful conditions of bones and joints*, weakness in muscles or *paralysis*, or *limb length discrepancy*.

Inability or Difficulty in Moving a Joint

The typical sequence to move a joint is completed by a **"normal neuromuscular–tendinous–ligamentous–capsular–bone and joint-soft tissue pathway." Figure 1.1** shows the normal pathway required for joint movement and **Table 1.1** mentions various abnormal conditions, which can affect the working of the normal pathway for joint movement. A detailed history and examination would ascertain the cause of inability or difficulty in moving a joint.

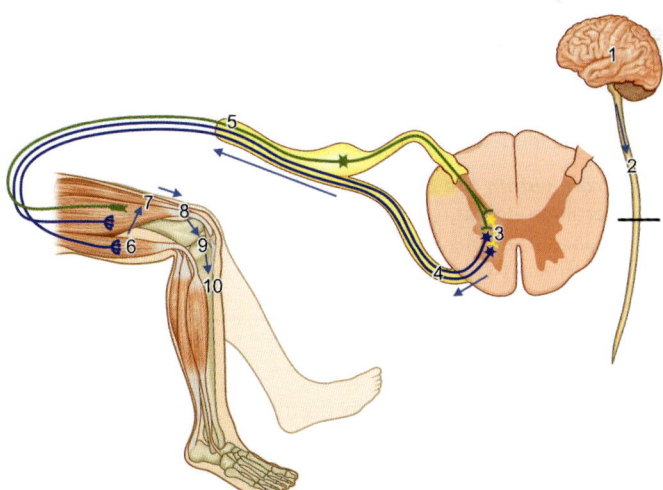

Fig. 1.1: Illustrative neuromusculoskeletal pathway required for a normal joint movement. Horizontal line in the spinal cord depicts cross-section of spinal cord. 1. Brain, 2. Spinal cord, 3. Anterior horn cell, 4. Nerve roots, 5. Peripheral nerve, 6. Neuromuscular junction, 7. Muscle, 8. Tendon, 9. Joint and bones, 10. Ligaments, capsule and other soft tissue.

TABLE 1.1: Normal pathway required for joint movement and conditions which can affect its function.

Normal component for joint movement	Pathology(ies) affecting joint movement
1. Normal central nervous system (CNS) where the patient can hear, comprehend, and send the motor command to the spinal cord	Hemiplegia, Parkinson's, or any other brain disorder affecting its function
2. Normal spinal cord and nerve roots	Spinal cord injury, poliomyelitis, nerve plexus (brachial or lumbar) affection, nerve root compression, intervertebral disc prolapse
3. Normal peripheral nerve	Nerve injury, neuropathy, Hansen's disease
4. Normal neuromuscular junction	Myasthenia gravis
5. Normally functioning muscle	Muscular dystrophy, myopathies, muscle contracture (post-traumatic, infective)
6. Normal tendon to transmit the muscle power	Tendinopathy, tendon tear, contractures
7. Normal articulation of joint	Dislocation or subluxation, arthritis, osteophytes
8. Normal bone	Acute fracture, non- or malunion
9. Normal ligaments	Ligament tear, ligament contracture
10. Normal capsule and soft tissue (skin and subcutaneous tissue) to stretch while joint is moving	Post-traumatic capsular contracture, frozen shoulder, postburn scar, scleroderma, etc.

One of the major causes of difficulty in moving a joint is 'joint stiffness, which could be due to various intra- or extra-articular causes. **Box 1.1** briefly discusses the differences between the two types of stiffness.

BOX 1.1: A note on a stiff joint.

A joint becomes stiff due to *extrinsic, intrinsic,* or both causes.

Extrinsic causes arise outside the joint capsule such as ectopic bone (myositis ossificans), contracture of muscle, tendon, ligament, fascia, subcutaneous tissue and skin. It also involves adherence of muscle/other soft tissue over the fracture site away from the joint. There is no history of intra-articular fracture(s). Clinically, there is no joint line tenderness, and the movement is painless.

Intrinsic causes arise from within the confines of the capsule (inside the joint) such as capsular contracture, articular cartilage damage, arthritis, prominent intra-articular osteophytes, malunited or nonunited intra-articular surface resulting in articular incongruity, internal hardware, and bony or fibrous ankylosis. Clinically, there is a history of intra-articular fracture. Presence of a joint-line tenderness indicates arthritis or cartilage damage.

Discharging Sinus

Chronic osteomyelitis is the most common condition in a orthopedic patient causing a discharging sinus. One must probe regarding the condition, which led to the onset of sinus (postsurgical or spontaneous after a swelling suggestive of hematogenous osteomyelitis), progression, number, remissions and exacerbation, and type of discharge (serous/seropurulent/purulent).

Of note: If there is a discharge of a bony spicule from the sinus, it is a confirmatory sign of chronic osteomyelitis.

However, one must remember that the mere presence of a discharging sinus in an "orthopedic case" does not confirm underlying osteomyelitis. Any dead and infected material [natural (bone) or foreign (nonabsorbable suture material, foreign body, etc.)] could result in a discharging sinus. Unless the sinus is fixed to the underlying bone, it cannot arise from a bone infection.

Deformity

A deformity is defined as a permanent deviation from the normal shape or contour of a bone or a joint which is not correctable by any active or passive maneuver by the patient or clinician (c.f. attitude, which is either position of ease of a limb or a temporary deviation from anatomical position, which can be corrected). Deformity could be *structural or spasmodic*. Structural deformities are passively not correctable. In contrast, spasmodic (due to pain) deformity resolves after subsidence of the pain.

- **Structural deformities** could be arising from:
  - *Bone:* Congenital malformation (scoliosis), malunion/nonunion of fracture, and growth plate damage (traumatic, infective, metabolic, or iatrogenic)
  - *Joint:* Dislocated or subluxated, ankylosed
  - *Muscle–tendon contractures:* Volkmann's ischemic contracture, poliomyelitis
  - *Fascial contractures:* Dupuytren's contracture, poliomyelitis
  - *Capsular or ligament contractures*
  - *Skin or scar contractures:* Postburn contracture, scleroderma
- **Spasmodic deformities** are observed in acute painful musculoskeletal conditions due to muscle spasms, e.g., paraspinal muscle spasm after acute IVDP leading to postural scoliosis or list. These deformities improve as the spasm decreases.

Shortening or Lengthening of a Limb

The limb of the patient may be short or long due to a congenital, traumatic, infective, or a metabolic cause.

Instability of a Joint

Before we understand the instability of a joint, it is essential to understand what imparts stability to a joint. A stable joint is formed by two "morphologically normal" articulating surfaces that are normally linked and stabilized by various soft tissues such as ligament, capsular, and muscle-tendon complex innervated by a nerve. *Any deformation or disruption in one or more structures that form and stabilize a joint could result in an unstable joint.* The joint instability could arise from *complete tear in ligament,* muscle, *paralysed muscles* or even from *deformed articulating surfaces.*

Locking

Locking implies a sudden inability to complete a particular movement. Locking of a joint is an intermittent phenomenon, which may last from several minutes to hours.

Locking is of two types: True locking and pseudo locking. True locking is a structural phenomenon, whereas pseudo locking is a spasmodic phenomenon due to pain.

True locking: Typically, the joint movement is smooth without getting "stuck or fixed" in a particular position because nothing gets in between the two mobile articulating surfaces. Therefore, if something loose (structural) comes between the two articulating surfaces and gets entrapped, it prevents smooth gliding of articulating surfaces, resulting in a locked joint. Once the loose fragment moves out between the articulating surfaces, the joint gets unlocked.

Some common causes of locking are:
- *Meniscal tear in the knee joint:* Bucket handle tears of the meniscus
- *Loose body in any joint:* Single (osteochondral fracture fragment, osteochondritis dessecans) or multiple (synovial chondromatosis).

Clicks, Crepitus

Click is a short, often single sound, whereas crepitus is longer lasting sound, often multiple.

Typically, crepitus occurs when two rough surfaces rub against each other during movement, e.g., arthritic joint. Clicks often happen when a tendon/fascia slips over a bony prominence or slip in-and-out of a groove.

Altered Sensation

Many patients complain of altered sensations (tingling, numbness, burning, less or no sensations over the skin) resulting from affections of the brain, spinal cord, or nerves.

Constitutional Symptoms

Many symptoms such as fever, malaise, weight loss, or loss of appetite are part of the chief complaint. It is essential to ask about constitutional symptoms during history evaluation as it almost always indicates a sinister pathology such as infection, inflammation, or tumor, and it helps in ruling out differentials.

Effect on Activities of Daily Living or Activities

One of the essential parts of the complaint assessment is to evaluate the effect of the disease process on the activities of daily living and occupation such as walking, squatting, ability to clean back, tie hair, overhead activities, and sports.

> **Note: A common mistake while taking the history of present illness!**
>
> Often students start with HOPI and then abruptly include treatment history with HOPI, resulting in dilution of assessment of the chief complaints. It could lead to a wrong diagnosis, especially if the diagnosis established by the previous treatment provider were inaccurate or incomplete. The student may get carried away by "**diagnosis at arrival**" and may stop his efforts to assess the complaints further and establish an accurate diagnosis.

Past History

One must confirm past history about:
- A similar history on the same or contralateral limb
- Other orthopedic diagnosis such as underlying osteoporosis, gout, etc.
- Medical history of diabetes, hypertension, thyroid disorder or other medical illness
- Relevant surgical history such as hysterectomy, thyroidectomy, etc.

Personal History

Personal history comprise smoking, alcohol intake, tobacco-chewing, sleep, diet (vegetarian, mixed), bowel–bladder habit, education, and marital status. Specific examples of the importance of personal history are: Patients who are chronic smokers and tobacco-chewers are at risk of poor wound healing, delayed or nonunion, while chronic alcoholics are at higher risk of avascular necrosis of the hip. Alcohol and meat consumption can increase the level of uric acid in body resulting in gout.

Treatment History

One can get vital clues about diagnosis with treatment history. For example, a patient who underwent multiple debridements for chronic osteomyelitis of the tibia can have shortening of the leg, which can be explained by bone loss during multiple debridements. However, one must assess treatment separately and avoid mixing it with HOPI. An exception where treatment history is a part of HOPI is a case of trauma wherein discussing the treatment history in a sequence (open fracture → debridement, external fixator → re-debridement → intramedullary nailing → discharging sinus) helps understand the evolution of the current status of the problem.

Family History

It is essential to confirm the family history of disorders such as congenital disorders (congenital talipes equinus varus, developmental dysplasia of the hip), hemophilia, sickle cell anemia, rheumatoid arthritis, ankylosing spondylitis, tumors, etc.

Menstrual History

Postmenopausal women are prone to osteoporosis and resulting complications such as chronic back pain and fragility fractures. Also, chronic menstrual disorder and pelvic inflammatory diseases (PIDs) are related to chronic low back pain, exacerbating during cyclical menstruation changes.

History of Allergies and Drug Intake

Documenting the history of drug allergies is crucial as inadvertent administration could be life-threatening and have medicolegal implications. Eliciting the history of any other drug intake is essential as many of them are implicated in disease causation or fitness for the surgery. For example,
- Chronic steroid therapy may result in avascular necrosis of the hip.
- Chronic phenytoin therapy is implicated in the etiology of Dupuytren's contracture. Also, long-term treatment with phenytoin and carbamazepine (antiepileptics) inhibit resorption of calcium and vitamin D from the intestine resulting in rickets/osteomalacia.
- Long-term bisphosphonates (for osteoporosis) can result in pathological fractures in the subtrochanteric region of the femur, which are quite challenging to treat.
- Pyrazinamide, which is an ATT, is known to cause hyperuricemia and can precipitate acute gout in a patient.

Perinatal and Birth History

Important in congenital conditions, such as DDH or the conditions which are peripartum related (cerebral palsy, obstetrics brachial plexus palsy).

Developmental Milestone History

It is essential to elicit the developmental history (gross motor, fine motor, speech and language, and social) in pediatric patients with congenital disorders.

Immunization History

It is important in disorders such as poliomyelitis.

At the end of the complete history assessment, the clinician must arrive at a possible conclusion about the etiopathology of the condition. The possible etiologies are mentioned in **Box 1.2**. After thorough history evaluation, one must proceed towards examining the patient.

BOX 1.2: Possible etiopathologies in orthopaedics with characteristic history pointer.

- **Congenital:** Present from birth/late presentation of the congenital pathology
- **Traumatic:** History of (h/o) trauma
- **Inflammatory:** H/o multiple joint/area involvement, morning stiffness, malaise, seasonal variation, and multisystem affection
- **Infective:** H/o fever, chills, night cries, purulent discharge from the bone/joint
- **Neoplastic:** H/o slowly or rapidly growing swelling, pain, loss of weight, and loss of appetite
- **Metabolic:** Nutritional, aging, and other—osteoporosis, gout, and pseudogout
- **Degenerative:** Mostly age-related osteoarthrosis, spondylosis, tendinosis, or tendon tear. Such conditions often present with H/o mechanical pain
- **Hematologic:** Hemophilia (H/o repeated hemarthrosis, deformity, arthritis, contractures); sickle cell anemia (avascular necrosis, bone infarct, osteomyelitis, septic arthritis)
- **Neurological:** H/o tingling, numbness, weakness, and burning sensation
- **Others:** Avascular necrosis

EXAMINATION

The examination involves general, systemic, and local examinations, which are discussed below. The crucial prerequisites for examination are mentioned in **Box 1.3**.

The examination always starts with a general and systemic examination, whether it is a short or long case. *The general and systemic examination is mandatory as per the standard protocol. It would be improper to say that "I have not done the general and systemic examinations".*

A. General Examination

The general examination must start with assessment of consciousness, orientation to time, place and person, built, and nutritional status of the patient. It is followed by assessment of vital parameters (blood pressure, pulse, respiratory rate, and temperature), pallor, icterus, clubbing, cyanosis, lymph nodes, and pedal edema. Note that one must report the relevant findings and avoid nonstandard abbreviations such as "PICCLE" in examination.

- Other essential parameters such as height, weight, and body mass index (BMI) should be assessed in relevant patients.

BOX 1.3: Prerequisites for clinical examination.

A: Acquaintance with the patient and make him/her comfortable
B: Bright/optimal light
C: Consent to examination, comfortable couch or chair
D: Devices (measuring tape, knee hammer, goniometer, etc.)
E: Expose the part adequately, explain the examination process and methods to the patient
F: Female attendant for a female patient, another adult for vulnerable adults, kids, and adolescents (chaperoning)

- A general survey from head-to-toe can give a lot of clue to the underlying disease. For example,
  i. Black discoloration of pinna is observed in patients with ochronosis, who can have back pain due to disc calcification and osteoporosis.
  ii. Neurocutaneous markers such as Cafe-au-lait spots and neurofibromatosis are associated with scoliosis and congenital pseudoarthrosis of tibia.

B. Systemic Examination

A quick and relevant examination of the *central nervous system (CNS), cardiovascular system (CVS), respiratory system (RS), abdomen, and pelvis should be done.*

> **Tips for Presenting General and Systemic Examination Findings**
> - **If the general and systemic examination findings are normal**, it can be summarized as "general and systemic examination findings are normal". The student can proceed to local examination rather than typically repeating pallor, icterus, etc.
> - **If the general and systemic examination findings are abnormal,** the student can summarize the relevant findings such as "pallor is present, the patient is hypertensive," etc., rather than narrating the entire systemic examination findings routinely.

C. Local Examination

The standard order of examination in orthopedic cases is as follows:
- **Gait:** It must be evaluated in patients with lower limb or spine affections. However, it can be avoided, if the patient refuses to walk due to severe pain or an unstable spine condition that may potentially induce or exacerbate neurological deficit.
- **Hand dominance (in an upper extremity case), inspection of footwear, orthosis, prosthesis, if applicable**
- **Attitude:** It is described as the position of ease assumed by joint and bone at rest, which is comfortable to the patient.
- **Inspection (look)**
- **Palpation (feel)**
- **Movements (move)**
- **Measurement**
- **Neurovascular (NV) examination:** It should be done before special tests as adequate power is required for most special tests.
- **Special tests** for individual pathology/region
- **Examination of joint above and below**
- **Lymph node examination**

Pearls and Pitfalls while Performing Local Examination

General rules while presenting the examination findings:
- *Adjectives must be avoided unless it has been standardized in the literature*, e.g., "severe" tenderness. One's "severe tenderness" could be someone else's "moderate"! Tenderness is either present or absent. Further, no such grading is discussed in the literature.
- Unless specifically asked, the *methodology of examination should not be mentioned or discussed* during the presentation. One must present the clinical finding and avoid its methodology during the examination.
- *Avoid discussing the etiology of the finding* while presenting the finding. It must be left for discussion.

Inspection (Look)

The affected part must be inspected from all the sides. The position for inspection (standing/sitting/supine/prone) depends upon the region. There are many important findings to be observed on inspection such as deformity, muscle wasting, limb length discrepancy, swelling, scar, sinus, ulcer, condition of skin, etc. Assessment of many of these findings are already well known to students due to their previous clinical experiences. Other important findings are discussed below.

A. **Deformities:** Specific standard terms that are used to describe deformity in limbs and spine are described below.
   i. ***Varus:*** It implies "part of the body moving closer to the midline." Genu varum implies that "genu" or "knee" is the referencing point and the "part," i.e., the leg has moved closer to the midline **(Fig. 1.2A)**.
   ii. ***Valgus:*** It implies "part of the body moving away from the midline." Genu valgum means that "genu" or "knee" is the referencing point, and the "part," i.e., the leg, has moved away from the midline **(Fig. 1.2B)**. Another example, cubitus valgus means that "cubitus," i.e., the elbow is the referencing point, and the forearm has moved away from the midline.
   iii. ***Recurvatum:*** It implies hyperextension and is observed in the elbow and knee joints. It is known as genu recurvatum in the knee. When a patient is observed from the side, the axis of the lower limb passes through the center of the hip, knee, and ankle in an erect standing patient. However, in genu recurvatum, the axis passes anterior to the knee **(Figs. 1.2C to E)**.
   iv. ***Flexion deformity:*** It implies that the affected joint cannot be brought into complete extension, passively or actively.
   v. ***Scoliosis, kyphosis, torticollis, and other deformities:*** These important deformities will be discussed in their relevant chapters.

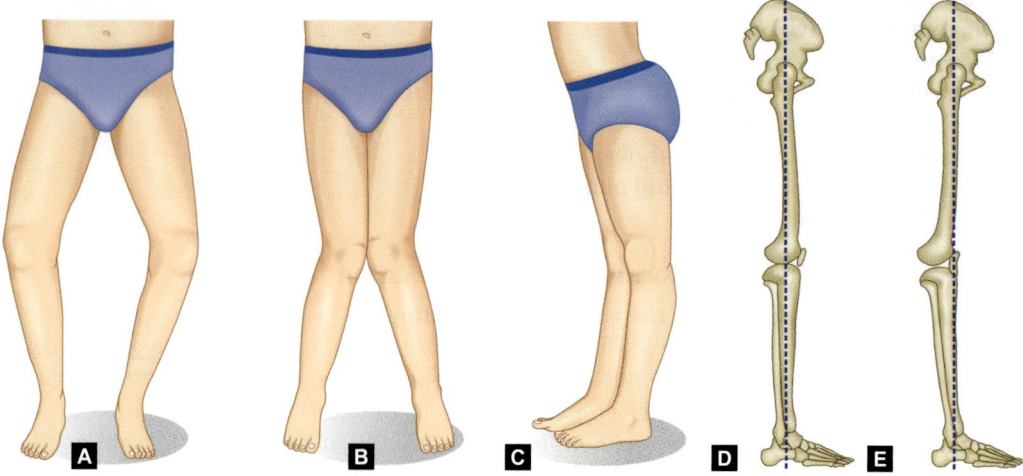

Figs. 1.2A to E: Images demonstrate varus (A), valgus (B), and recurvatum (C) deformities of the knee joint. (D and E) Illustrative images show the weight-bearing axis (hip-knee-ankle) passing 'through the knee' in a normal knee and 'in front of the knee' in a genu recurvatum, respectively.

CHAPTER 1 ♦ Basics of History Taking and Examination in Orthopaedics

> **Note: Principles of Deformity Assessment**
> **Always stand in the plane perpendicular to the plane of deformity.** Several examples are mentioned below.
> - **To assess coronal plane deformities of the knee, i.e., varus and valgus at the knee,** the clinician must stand in the sagittal plane of the patient (in front of the patient) to assess the deformity.
> - **Scoliosis is a coronal plane deformity:** So, stand in the sagittal plane, i.e., behind the patient, to observe scoliosis.
> - **Kyphosis is a sagittal plane deformity:** So, stand in the coronal plane, i.e., on the side of the patient, to observe kyphosis.

B. **Limb length discrepancy:** It could be shortening or lengthening. The shortening could be true or apparent.

C. **Muscle wasting:** Any chronic disuse of the limb results in muscle wasting.

> Note: Special terms for joints: Elbow-cubitus; Wrist-manus; Hip-coxa; and Knee-genu

Palpation (Feel)

During palpation, one must confirm the findings observed during the inspection. Key palpatory findings include *local rise in temperature*, palpation of important *bony-soft tissue landmarks*, *joint-line tenderness* and *other specific findings*, if any, such as synovial hypertrophy, paraspinal muscle spasm. Specific rules must be followed during palpation such as:

- Always start palpation with assessment of **local rise in temperature** using dorsum of the hand, and compare with a normal area or opposite side. A rise in local temperature suggests increased local vascularity due to underlying infection, inflammation, tumor, and trauma.
- Before assessing local tenderness, **always ask the patient to mention the exact site of tenderness with one finger** as it helps localize the site of the pathology. Further, it helps the clinician to remain cautious while palpating the tender area in order to avoid hurting the patient inadvertently. The palpation must be done with **utmost gentleness using thumb or finger pulp,** especially in tender areas. A hasty and jerky palpation could result in increased pain followed by guarding. Afterward, the patient may not cooperate with the rest of the examination. *The tenderness could be superficial or deep*. Once the superficial tenderness is ruled out, the clinician should gently increase the pressure to elicit the deep tenderness.
- In order to avoid missing crucial areas or landmarks, the palpation must follow a sequence of eliciting tenderness over important bony prominences, soft tissues, and joint lines.

Movement (Move)

There are essential rules to be followed while assessing the movements at a joint—assess deformities, active ROM followed by passive, and crepitus.

> First and foremost principle of movement assessment is to 'start movement assessment of contralateral normal side' followed by assessment of index side.

1. Always **assess the deformities** before commenting on the range of movement (ROM). An example of how deformity is included in ROM. If a patient has 20° flexion deformity in the right elbow and further flexion up to 105° is possible, then elbow flexion ROM is 20–105°. Further, it is important to note that the movement in direction opposite to the deformity is not possible. For example, in a patient with palmar flexion deformity of the wrist, dorsiflexion would not be possible.

2. Always assess **active ROM followed by passive ROM**, and the rationale behind that is:
   - If active movement is full, then there is no need to perform passive ROM.
   - An actively mobile joint indicates possibly an intact neural innervation and intact bony-musculotendinous connections. However, it may not rule out partial or recovering nerve injuries or other partial soft injuries.
   - If the patient's active movement stops at a particular point due to pain, one must not force passive ROM beyond that point to avoid exacerbating the pain.
3. The ***ROM should be measured with a goniometer***.
4. While recording the movement, mention the ***total "ROM" with starting and an endpoint***, e.g., elbow flexion is 0–160°.
5. The range of motion should have ***adjectives of painless or painful***, e.g., the total knee flexion is 110°. The first 0–100° of flexion is painless, and the remaining 10° of flexion is painful.
6. ***Assess associated crepitus with passive ROM, if any***: It is essential to conclude that whether crepitus is fixed or mobile. Fixed crepitus is present in an arthritic joint with fixed rough areas over the cartilage, while mobile crepitus is observed in other conditions where one of the structures is mobile and not fixed.

> **Note:** How to Mention the Range of Movement along with other Characteristics?
> 1. **Elbow flexion movement:** The range of elbow flexion is 0–120°. The first 0–100° is painless, and the remaining 20° is painful, and further flexion is not possible. Both active and passive movements are the same, and there is no associated crepitus.

Important terminologies regarding joint movement pathologies are as follows:
i. **Stiff joint:** Stiff joint implies a joint which has lost movement in one or more directions.
ii. **Ankylosed joint:** A joint with total or near-total loss of movements due to an underlying pathological process. Ankylosis could be either intra-articular (true ankylosis) or extra-articular (false ankylosis).
A. **True ankylosis:** It is also known as intrinsic cause of joint stiffness and implies involvement of intra-articular structures such as cartilage, bone, articular surface, capsule, synovium, intra-articular adhesions, intra-articular ligaments and intra-articular hardware. True ankylosis is of two types—bony and fibrous.
   - **Bony ankylosis:** A condition wherein a complete loss of joint movement occurs *due to bony fusion between the two joint surfaces*. Clinically, there is absolutely *no movement across the joint, and there is no pain* if the clinician attempts to elicit the movement. Radiologically, the bony trabeculae are seen crossing the joint with obliteration of joint space **(Fig. 1.3)**. *Typically, bony ankylosis is seen after septic arthritis of an axial joint and between the vertebrae in the TB of the spine.*
   - **Fibrous ankylosis:** A condition wherein there is near-total loss of movement across the joint *due to thick fibrous intra-articular adhesions*. Clinically, there is a *jog of movement elicited, and there is pain if clinician attempts to elicit the movement*. Radiologically, the joint space is preserved. However, there may be other features such as reduced irregular joint space due to arthritis, or articular incongruity. *Typically, fibrous ankylosis is seen after TB of peripheral joints, rheumatoid arthritis, and gonococcal arthritis.*
B. **False/Pseudo-ankylosis:** It is also known as extrinsic cause of joint stiffness, and implies involvement of extra-articular structures such as:

- **Skin and subcutaneous tissue:** Contracture following trauma, surgery, burns.
- **Muscle tendon complex:** Contracture of muscle tendon complex after trauma or surgery, Volkmann ischemic contracture or adherence to the fracture site.
- **Deep fascia:** Dupuytren's contracture.
- **Extra-articular ligaments:** Collateral ligaments of the knee. For example, medial collateral ligament is contracted in OA knee with severe varus deformity.
- **Bony blocks:** Bony block of myositis ossificans, callus, displaced fracture fragments, and exostosis.

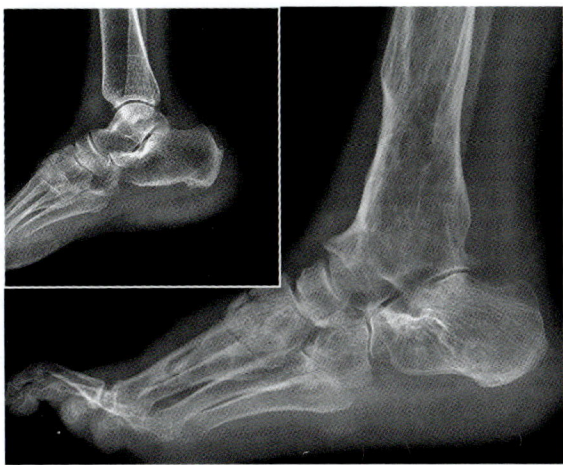

Fig. 1.3: X-ray showing bony ankylosis of the ankle joint with trabaculae crossing the joint. Inset picture shows normal ankle joint space.

Sound and unsound ankylosis: Sound ankylosis is a condition wherein a joint is ankylosed in a functional position, whereas a joint ankylosed in a nonfunctional position is unsound ankylosis, e.g., a knee ankylosed in extension is sound ankylosis, whereas a knee ankylosed in flexion is unsound.

Measurement

During measurement, limb length, muscle girth, or other region specific measurements (three bony point relation, Bryant's triangle, etc.) are performed. The measurements are always compared with the normal side.

The objective of limb length measurement is to analyze the discrepancy in limb length, if any, and to identify the segment of discrepancy (arm and forearm/thigh and leg).

Certain guidelines must be followed during the measurement of the limb length.
1. A **pre-existing deformity in the limb must be checked and corrected,** such as squaring the pelvis. A pre-existing limb length discrepancy must be asked for, if any.
2. The **limb measurement is performed between the two predesignated bony landmarks,** marked with a skin marking pencil.
3. The **two limbs must be kept in identical positions** for measurement.
4. The **segmental length** of the limb must be measured.
5. While measuring the length of the lower limbs, there is a concept of true and apparent length. This concept is important while measuring lower limb length in spine, pelvis and hip pathologies as there is compensation due to pelvic tilt.
   - A **true discrepancy** in the limb length is due to "the lengthening or shortening of the bone" due to traumatic (fracture/dislocation), infective, or metabolic pathology truly altering the length of the bone.
   - An **apparent discrepancy** in the limb length is due to a *"deformity or posture,"* but there is no actual deficit in the limb length when measured. *It appears short or long; however, not truly long or short!*

❑ Finally, while mentioning the limb length assessment, the student should inform the discrepancy/normalcy of limb length rather than narrating the individual bone length measurements. **Box 1.4** mentions the correct way of describing the limb length discrepancy.

Note: During the case presentation, the examiner is not interested in the individual measurements of bone length unless asked! However, the segmental length must be recorded in the examination sheet.

BOX 1.4: Description of limb length discrepancy.

- ***The incorrect method of informing the limb length discrepancy:*** "The right femur is 48 cm long, and the right tibia is 32 cm long. The left femur is 48 cm long, and the left tibia is 31 cm long." After this statement, many students think that the job is over. However, after measuring segmental lengths of the limb, the *goal* is to measure the "limb length discrepancy," if any. Therefore, one must calculate the discrepancy, if any, and report accordingly.
- ***The correct way of describing limb length discrepancy is*** "The left lower limb is 1 cm shorter than the right, and the shortening is in the tibia."
- ***If the limbs (total and segmental) are equal in length,*** it is sufficient to inform that "there is no limb length discrepancy.

Neurovascular Examination

It should be performed as per the standard NV assessment of the limb:
- **If the NV examination of the limb/part is normal,** it should be summarized as *"neurovascular examination is normal."*
- **If the NV examination is abnormal,** then *individual pathological findings should be mentioned,* e.g., if the posterior tibial pulse is feeble on the right side and neurological examination is normal, then it is appropriate to state that "neurological examination is normal. However, the posterior tibial artery is feeble on the right side."

Special Tests

One or more special tests are performed to confirm the diagnosis. The clinician must be well versed with the correct technique and interpretation of each test. The key to the special tests is **"explain–demonstrate–interpret–compare."**

"Explain (to the patient)–demonstrate (on normal side/on self)–interpret (finding)–compare (with normal side)."

Examination of Joint Above and Below

It should be performed as per standard examination practice.

Clinical assessment of the joints above and below is essential as the disease or affection of the proximal or distal joint may affect the functioning of the index joint in various ways, e.g., radiation of pain to the knee joint in patients with hip pathology is quite frequent. Another example is bilateral flat foot could result in knee pain due to altered mechanical loading.

While reporting the finding of 'normal' neighboring joints, it can be summarized as "joints above and below are normal." However, if there is an abnormal finding in the neighboring joint, it should be mentioned in standard fashion.

Lymph Node Examination

It should always be done, especially in a suspected case of infective, inflammatory, and tumorous conditions.
- **In upper limb:** Epitrochlear, axillary and supraclavicular
- **In lower limb:** Popliteal and inguinal.

Final Diagnosis

The final diagnosis should have the following components:
- Duration
- Anatomical site
- Side (right/left)
- Pathology
- Etiology
- Complication, if any

> **An example of a complete diagnosis:** An 11-month-old, right femur shaft nonunion due to road traffic accident with 3-cm shortening of the femur with **knee stiffness.**
>
> **Description:** An **11-month-old** (duration) **right** (side) **femur shaft** (anatomical site) **nonunion** (pathology) due **to road traffic accident** (etiology) with **shortening** of femur and stiffness of knee (complications).

Certain guidelines are to be followed while mentioning the diagnosis which are as follows:
1. The primary diagnosis should be based upon points favoring the diagnosis from history and examination. The diagnosis must not be based upon negative points (points against primary diagnosis); the negative pointers from history and examination are for differential diagnosis.
2. The presence of points against the primary diagnosis must stimulate the student to think about the differential diagnosis.
3. Unless there are several pointers against primary diagnosis, giving a differential diagnosis is not always essential. For example, there will not be any differential diagnosis for fracture femur nonunion. However, tuberculosis of the knee is a possible differential diagnosis in patients with monoarticular rheumatoid arthritis of the knee.

Plan the Investigations Relevant to "Your Patient" and Not a Hypothetical Case

Avoid the statement "routine investigations" as no investigation is asked as a routine. Every investigation has a specific goal that could help either corroborate-confirm-refute the diagnosis or further help decide the patient's surgical management.

The Final Plan of the Treatment

It could be conservative or operative. Discuss the plan of treatment, which is relevant for the patient's diagnosis and expectation.

CHAPTER 2

Clinical Evaluation of Polytrauma and Acute Injury of Bones and Joints

INTRODUCTION

Trauma is the leading cause of death and disability in the first four decades and the third most common cause of death overall. This chapter will briefly focus on the concepts of polytrauma, triaging, advanced trauma life support (ATLS) protocol followed by assessment of acute injury of bone and joint in a stable patient.

POLYTRAUMA

Polytrauma does not merely imply fracture of multiple bones. These patients have involvement of multiple systems and are hemodynamically unstable.

Definition of Polytrauma

There are multiple definitions of polytrauma, such as:
1. When injury severity score is >18
2. There is hemodynamic instability or coagulopathy on admission
3. Involvement of more than one systems of the body

Polytrauma is both a surgical and a medical emergency. Not only will the patient require surgical interventions to stabilize the traumatized systems, but also a close monitoring of the general conditions to counter the systemic effects of trauma. The management of a polytrauma patient requires a holistic multidisciplinary approach. The orthopedic surgeons carry the responsibility of stabilizing the musculoskeletal system, using principles of either damage control orthopaedics (external fixator application) or early total care (emergency internal fixation). The management is dictated by various pathophysiological factors and scoring systems that have been developed to aid in decision-making. These scoring systems help the team to communicate better and provide prognosis for a given patient. The ISS is an anatomical scoring system that utilizes the abbreviated injury scale (AIS)—a standardized system of classification for the severity of individual injuries. The ISS is calculated from the sum of the squares of the three worst regional values and ranges from 1 to 75. ISS>15 carries a mortality of more than 10%.

Importance of Time in a Polytrauma Patient

Time is of utmost importance in a polytrauma patient. Mortality and morbidity can be significantly reduced if that patient is given due attention within the "**golden hour**," which is the **1st hour** after the injury. **Figure 2.1** summarizes the quick timeline in a polytrauma patient right from the site of accident to the medical intervention.

The management of a patient with trauma should begin at the field of injury and should include:
- Immediate call for help
- In-line immobilization of the cervical spine

- Jaw-thrust and chin lift to clear the airway
- Splinting the limb with a firm, linear object such as an umbrella, folded newspaper, stick, etc.
- Applying compression over an actively bleeding injury
- Arranging for safe transport to a trauma center at the earliest.

Triaging in Trauma

- Triaging in trauma refers to the process by which emergency medical personnel *sort and prioritize victims of mass casualty incidents at the scene.* It is intended to *identify those victims most in need of immediate care,* in order to make the best use of limited treatment and transport resources. In the descending order for priority of attention, the patients are triaged into four categories: RED, YELLOW, GREEN, and BLACK, respectively.
- Triaging in trauma center of the hospital also refers to the process used in the *emergency departments* to determine the order in which the presenting patients will be seen. **Table 2.1** describes the triaging sequence and examples.

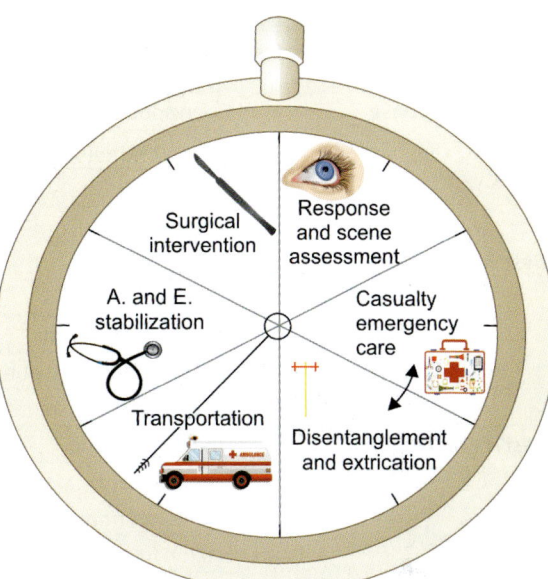

Fig. 2.1: Timeline in a polytrauma patient.

Once in the hospital, triaged, the patient should be managed according to the principles laid down by ATLS. The detailed workflow of ATLS is beyond the scope of this chapter. Nevertheless, each patient must be quickly assessed for ***Airway, Breathing, Circulation, Disability*** (to assess neurological status of patient), and ***Exposure*** (bearing the dignity of patient in mind,

TABLE 2.1: Triaging of patient in trauma.

Color	Triage priority	Type of injury	Examples
Red	**Red—Immediate**	Life threatening	• Tension hemopneumothorax • Fracture pelvis with uncontrolled bleeding and hypotension • Convulsions
Yellow	**Yellow—Urgent**	Serious, but stable patient and not in any danger Requires observation	• Fracture femur • Stable liver laceration
Green	**Green—Minor**	Patient who will require treatment at some point	Fracture distal radius
Black	**Black—Deceased/Un-survivable**	Deceased or patients with extensive injuries that they will not be able to survive given the care available	• Massive open head injury with GCS 3 • 95% third degree burns

TABLE 2.2: Glasgow come scale.

Feature	Response	Score
Best eye response	Open spontaneously	4
	Open to verbal command	3
	Open to pain	2
	No eye opening	1
Best verbal response	Oriented	5
	Confused	4
	Inappropriate words	3
	Incomprehensible sound	2
	No verbal response	1
Best motor response	Obeys command	6
	Localizes pain	5
	Withdraws from pain	4
	Flexion from pain	3
	Extension to pain	2
	No motor response	1

completely undress to assess other injuries especially spine, chest, abdomen, and pelvis) approach. Glasgow coma scale helps in assessing the conscious level in a patient with a head injury **(Table 2.2)**. After a quick primary survey, a brief history is taken along with AMPLE **(Box 2.1)**. Other adjuncts are relevant investigations like X-rays (trauma series [spine, pelvis, chest] and other limb X-ray, if applicable), FAST (Focused Assessment with Sonography in Trauma) abdominal four quadrant scan to look for free fluid/blood in abdomen, blood tests [hemoglobin, packed cell volume (PCV), renal and liver function tests], pulse oximetry, arterial blood gas analysis, and electrocardiogram (ECG).

> **BOX 2.1:** AMPLE history.
>
> **A:** Allergies
> **M:** Medications
> **P:** Past medical history
> **L:** Time since last meal
> **E:** Events surrounding the injury

Once the patient is hemodynamically stable, secondary survey can be conducted. **Flowchart 2.1** summarizes the management of a polytrauma patient.

This chapter will focus only on a stable patient with orthopedic injuries.

HISTORY

The appropriate relevant history must be directly taken from the patient who is hemodynamically stable, conscious and oriented. In a situation where patient is unable to provide history, it should be taken from bystanders. However, it should be corroborated once patient is stable, conscious and oriented.

Age

- **Pediatric age group:** Common injuries seen in young children are greenstick fracture, epiphyseal injury or a pulled elbow. One must always keep a note of battered baby syndrome in kids where history and pattern of fracture(s) do not match.

Flowchart 2.1: Summary of polytrauma—advanced trauma life support (ATLS) care.

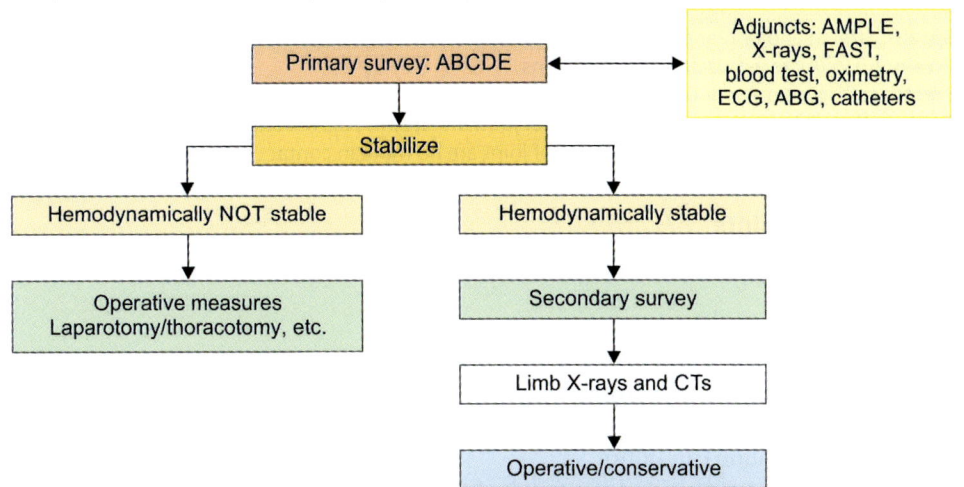

(ABG: arterial blood gas; CT: computed tomography; ECG: electrocardiogram; FAST: focused assessment with sonography in trauma)

- **Young adults:** Young adult patients are more prone to high-velocity road traffic accidents.
- **Elderly:** Elderly patients are more prone to falls and subsequent fragility fractures (fracture distal radius, proximal humerus, neck of femur, intertrochanteric femur fracture, or vertebral fracture) due to osteoporosis.

Mechanism and Force of Trauma

- The **mechanism of trauma** entails how the patient sustained the injury. This can give a clue to the structures injured. For example, a fall from a height can cause a fracture of the calcaneum, tibia, pelvis, and spine, whereas a fall from a bike onto the tip of the shoulder with facial abrasions could result in brachial plexus injury.

    In a setting of acute trauma, the mechanism of injury could be *direct or indirect*. Direct injury means fracture/dislocation at the site of impact, whereas indirect trauma results in fracture/dislocation at a site away from the point of impact. Indirect injury can also result from a forceful muscle contraction resulting in a fracture of the bone onto which it is attached. Further, the type of fracture varies in both mechanisms. Several examples of both mechanisms are mentioned below.
    - *Direct injury:* It could result in transverse fracture, comminuted fracture, open fracture, or a crush injury of the limb.
    - *Indirect injury:* Spiral/oblique fracture due to twisting force distal to the site of fracture; dashboard injury to the knee can cause posterior dislocation of the hip; forceful quadriceps contraction over a flexed knee results in a transverse fracture patella, whereas peroneus brevis contraction over an inverted foot results in fracture of the base of the fifth metatarsal.
- The **force/velocity of trauma** must be probed as significant trauma or force can undoubtedly cause a fracture. However, if an insignificant force results in the fracture, this indicates that the bone was diseased before the trauma (osteoporosis, infection, and tumor), and such fractures are known as *pathological fractures*.

Certain common terminologies used in an injured patient are mentioned in **Box 2.2**.

> **BOX 2.2:** Pertinent terminologies in an injured patient.
> - **Sprain:** Stretch and or tear of a ligament
> - **Strain:** An injury to a muscle and/or tendons
> - **Fracture:** Discontinuity or break in the anatomical continuity of the bone
> - **Subluxation:** When two articular surfaces of joint are only in partial contact with each other
> - **Dislocation:** When two articular surfaces of joint are no more in contact with each other

Presenting Complaints

An injured patient will have one or more complaints such as:
1. **Pain**
2. **Swelling**
3. **Deformity:** A deformed limb indicates fracture or dislocation.
4. **Inability or difficulty to use limb/weight bear:** Any such difficulty or inability to use the limb indicates severe soft tissue injury (ligament/muscle/nerve or combination), bony injury (fracture or dislocation), or both.
5. **Open wound:** Any open wound around the fracture site must be considered "open fracture" unless proved otherwise. In open fractures, enquiring specific history is mentioned in **Box 2.3**.

> **BOX 2.3:** In case of an open fracture, specific history has to be taken.
> - *Time since injury:* Time is of utmost importance in the management of open injuries. The longer the duration of the open wound which remained unclosed/not debrided (>8 hours), the higher is the chance of local infection and morbidity! Another important aspect of time is impending damage to the limb if there is an injury to neurovascular structure, which should be attended as early as possible to salvage the limb as the warm ischemia time is considered to be less than 8 hours.
> - *High- or low-velocity of trauma accidents:* High-velocity injuries could lead to severe bone and soft tissue damage.
> - *Site of the accident:* To understand the possible type of contamination. Organic contamination is more detrimental than industrial contamination because *farm accidents where there is* contamination with mud, grass or organic fertilizers could lead to anaerobic infection due to *Clostridium welchii*.

Other History

Relevant (past, personal, family, and treatment) history should be taken in standard fashion. Occupation of the patient is quite important in deciding the treatment and rehabilitation.

GENERAL ASSESSMENT

Apart from the history to evaluate the local injuries, one must assess the rest of the body's other systems (head and maxillofacial, chest, spine and spinal cord, abdomen, and pelvis) as per ATLS protocol. Glasgow coma scale helps in assessing the conscious level in a patient with a head injury **(Table 2.2)**. A polytrauma patient or patient with multiple long bone fracture and/or pelvis fracture may be hemodynamically unstable due to profound blood loss. Quick assessment of vital parameters and appropriate resuscitative measures should be initiated in form of oxygen supplement (nasal prongs/intubation), catheterization, intravenous fluid (normal saline/ringer lactate) via a 16- or 18-gauge cannula followed by blood transfusion. One must also keep **"massive transfusion protocol" (MTP)** in mind if transfusion of multiple packed red blood cells (PRBC) in a short period is foreseeable (>4 units of PRBC in one hour) due to significant blood loss. MTP involves transfusion of PRBC, plasma, and platelets in a ratio of 1:1:1 to avoid the perils of mere PRBC transfusion (hypothermia, acidosis, and coagulopathy).

After the quick general and systemic evaluation, focus is shifted to the local examination. ***This chapter will refrain from the detailed systemic evaluation of a trauma patient as that is out of the scope of this chapter.*** However, it is imperative to note that while the injured limb is being examined, the cervical spine should be immobilized with a Philadelphia collar until a suspected cervical spine injury is ruled out with adequate imaging.

LOCAL EXAMINATION

Attitude

The presenting attitude of the injured limb may suggest a specific diagnosis. For example, a patient presenting with posterior hip dislocation, the index hip assumes flexion, adduction, and internal rotation. In patients with fracture neck of the femur or intertrochanteric femur, the lower limb appears short and externally rotated.

However, in most cases, making a diagnosis merely by the attitude of the limb is not possible. An abnormal attitude merely indicates that the limb is injured.

Inspection

1. **Swelling:** It is a sign of an injury either to a bone/joint/soft tissue.
2. **Deformity:** A deformity always suggests displaced fracture or a dislocation.
3. **Limb length discrepancy:** Typically, a displaced fracture with over-riding of fracture ends or a dislocated joint presents as a shortening of the limb. However, in certain situations, the injured limb may appear longer, e.g., anterior dislocation of the hip.
4. **Condition of overlying skin and the presence of a wound (if any):** The skin may look stretched and shiny in case of compartment syndrome. The overlying skin at the site of injury must be thoroughly inspected for any of the following:
    i. *Fracture blisters:* It indicates severe injury to the soft tissue envelope and possibly compromised circulation to the soft tissue **(Fig. 2.2)**. The presence of blisters is a contraindication to "acute" open reduction and internal fixation (ORIF).
    ii. *Ecchymosis/bruise/contusion:* It is characterized by discoloured intact skin (bluish or red) which indicates bleeding under the skin **(Fig. 2.3)**.
    iii. *Abrasion:* Abrasions are superficial injuries of the skin resulting in a break in the continuity of epidermal tissue **(Fig. 2.4)**. As abrasions are confined to the epidermis, they result in minimal bleeding and heal uneventfully without permanent scar.
    iv. *Laceration:* Both skin and underlying tissues are cut with irregular wound margins **(Fig. 2.5A)**. It heals by scarring. One must always examine the integrity of structures which are lying deep to the lacerated wound such as nerves, tendons, and vessels. For example, a laceration over cubital fossa **(Fig. 2.5B)** may result in injury to median nerve, brachial vessels, and underlying muscle tendon.
    v. *Puncture wound:* A small wound that occurs due to a sharp, penetrating object either from outside or inside **(Fig. 2.6)**. A puncture wound associated with a fracture should never be taken lightly as these 'innocuous-looking' puncture wounds almost always occur due to sharp ends of fracture, making it an inside-out open fracture. Hence, a puncture wound must be adequately explored and debrided.

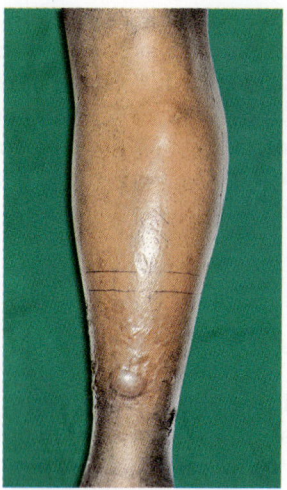

Fig. 2.2: Fracture blisters.

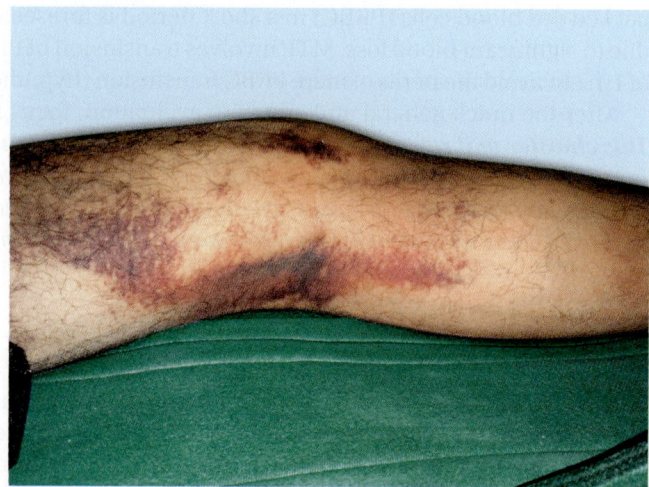

Fig. 2.3: Ecchymotic contuse skin over medial aspect of the knee.

vi. ***Degloving injury:*** It is a type of soft tissue injury wherein skin and underlying soft tissues are ripped off the underlying muscle/fascia/bone secondary to a sudden shearing force applied to the skin surface. Degloving could be open and closed. *Open degloving injuries* are associated with a large irregular wound with the degloved skin like a flap, which is detached from underlying fascia and muscle, and can be everted **(Fig. 2.7A)**. A *closed degloving injury* is identified by a large fluctuant swelling under an intact skin. However, the overlying skin might be contused **(Fig. 2.7B)**. It is known as *Morel-Lavallée lesion* in the hip and thigh.

vii. ***Skin loss:*** There may be a skin loss around the site of injury **(Fig. 2.8)**.

viii. ***Mangled extremity:*** A mangled extremity is defined as an injury to a limb resulting from a high-energy or crush mechanism involving at least three out of four structures (soft tissue, bone, nerves, and vessels) **(Fig. 2.9)**. Dr Johansen (1990) developed the mangled extremity severity score (MESS) with components of skeletel/soft tissue injury, limb ischemia,

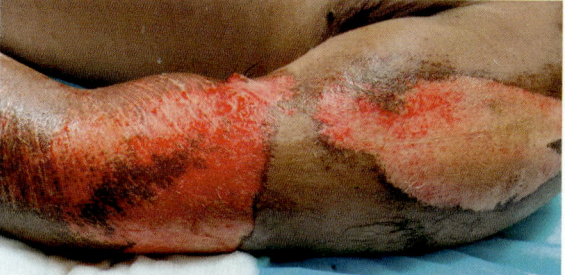

Fig. 2.4: Multiple abrasions over arm and forearm.

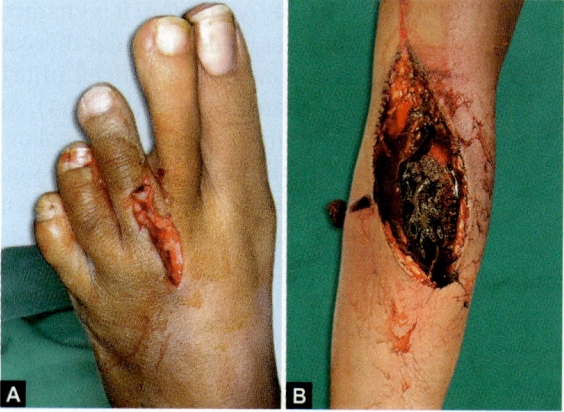

Figs. 2.5A and B: (A) Lacerated wound over forefoot; (B) Lacerated wound over the cubital fossa and proximal forearm.

shock and age to predict the viability of a limb. MESS score ≥ 7 indicates almost 100% possibility of amputation. However, modern orthopedic techniques have given a possibility of limb survival even up to MESS scores of 8 or 9.

ix. **Total or near-total amputation:** Total amputation refers to a complete detachment of a body part (surgical/traumatic) with separation of all structures with no connection between the two parts. Near-total (subtotal) amputation is defined as an incomplete detachment of a body part with a definite separation of the blood vessels with a tag of soft tissue (skin, tendon, or muscle) still remains intact and attached **(Fig. 2.10)**.

Various soft tissue injuries can be graded according to the Tscherne classification. However, details of Tscherne classification are out of the scope of the chapter.

5. **Open fracture:** An open fracture is defined as an injury where the fracture fragment/bone/fracture hematoma are communicating with the external environment through the soft tissue injury. Open fracture are classified based on Gustilo–Anderson classification **(Table 2.3)**.

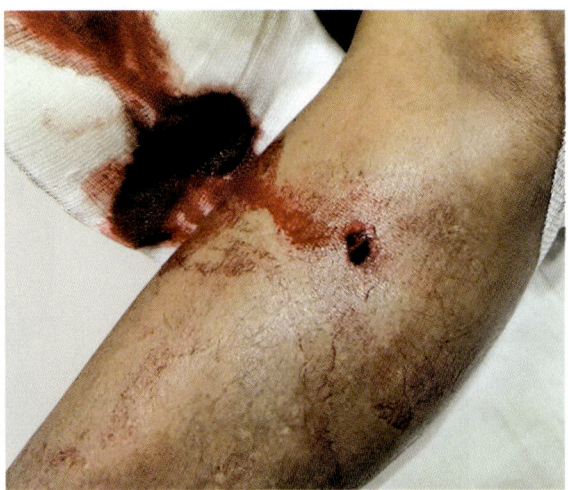

Fig. 2.6: Puncture wound.

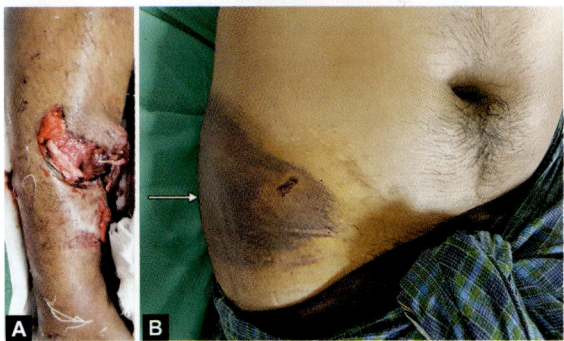

Figs. 2.7A and B: (A) Open degloving with skin loss; (B) Morel-Lavallée lesion (Closed degloving injury) in a patient with pelvis fracture.

Palpation

Before the palpation is initiated, the clinician should ask the patient about the site of maximum tenderness. *The traumatized limb should be palpated and moved with utmost care* as it causes severe pain.

A limb with fracture has certain specific signs:
1. **Bony tenderness:** The fracture site is tender when palpated through the overlying soft tissue.
2. **Bony crepitus:** A grating sensation is felt when the two ends of the fractured bone are moved. *However, bony crepitus is a very painful maneuver; hence, it is never deliberately elicited*. Note that the bony crepitus is absent in undisplaced fractures.
3. **Palpation of a gap** between two ends of the fracture is a certain sign of a fracture.
4. **Abnormal mobility:** When two ends of the fracture are held together, the abnormal mobility at the fracture site can be elicited. *However, abnormal mobility is not deliberately elicited as it is quite a painful maneuver.*

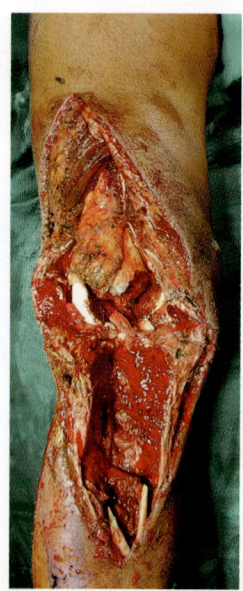 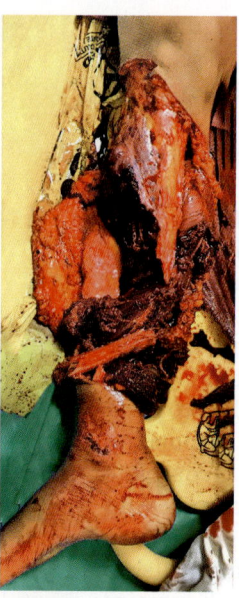 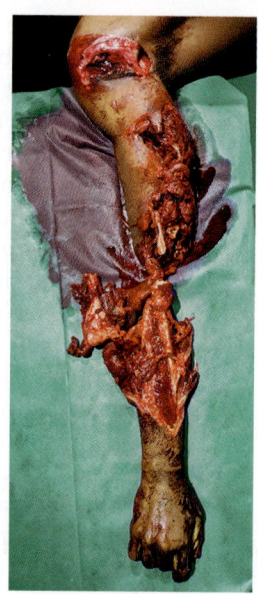

Fig. 2.8: Skin loss over the lower end of thigh, knee and upper end of tibia with associated fracture of distal femur and proximal tibia.

Fig. 2.9: Mangled lower limb.

Fig. 2.10: Near-total upper amputation of right limb at the level of mid-forearm.

> **Note about penetrating injury with offending object in situ:** It is crucial to understand that if there is a penetrating injury to any part of the body with penetrating object in situ (rod/pin/knife/bullet, etc.), one must never remove these objects either at the place of accident or in triage/casualty. These objects should be removed only in an operation room as these objects may lie next to a vessel, and sudden removal might result in dislodgement of the hematoma/clot causing torrential bleeding and hypotension. In operation room, bleeding can be controlled and vessel can be immediately repaired. However, outside the operating room, there might be no facility to effectively control the bleeding and repair the vessel resulting in potential complications. Moreover, the fingerprints over these object might be of medicolegal value which needs be preserved in standard fashion to aid the legal system.

TABLE 2.3: Gustilo–Anderson classification of open fracture.	
Type	Description
1	An open fracture with wound <1 cm long, simple fracture (#) pattern
2	An open fracture with a wound 1–10 cm long without extensive soft tissue damage, flaps or avulsion, simple # pattern
3	High-energy injury involving extensive soft tissue damage OR multifragmentary # OR bone loss irrespective of wound size OR severe crush injuries OR severe farmland contamination. Usually wound size >10 cm
3A	Adequate soft tissue coverage of a fractured bone is possible without any additional procedure despite extensive soft tissue laceration or flaps, or high-energy trauma (multifragmentary or segmental #) irrespective of the size of the wound
3B	Extensive soft tissue injury with periosteal stripping and bony exposure with massive contamination, *requiring additional soft tissue reconstructive procedure to cover the wound*
3C	Open fracture with *arterial injury* requiring a repair

5. **Compression test:** This is an indirect tenderness test wherein the pressure is exerted over a group of normal bone(s), leading to tenderness over the fracture. Compression or squeeze elsewhere along the length of the bone other than injured site would result in the force of compression to propagate via bones rather than soft tissue and would cause pain at the fracture site.

   This test is performed where there is a suspicion of a fracture in a region with two or more parallel bones (ribs, metatarsal or metacarpals, forearm, and leg). For example, if the ribs are fractured (one or more), gentle pressure over the sternum with one hand and other hand over the dorsal spine or gentle side-to-side squeezing the rib cage in the axilla with both hands causes pain over the fractured rib. Another example, gentle side- to-side squeezing of the forearm, hand, leg or foot causes a painful response in radius-ulna, metacarpal, tibia-fibula or metatarsal fracture.
6. **Loss of transmitted movements:** The fractured limb fails to transmit the movements performed at the distal segment. For example, if the ankle is manually rotated in a patient with a tibia shaft fracture, the proximal tibia will not rotate as there is a break in the continuity of the bone.
7. **Passive stretch pain, a red flag sign!** Severe pain on a passive stretch of fingers and toes in injury to forearm or leg respectively could indicate underlying compartment syndrome. One must suspect compartment syndrome, if there is unrelenting pain in body parts, especially in the forearm, leg, hand, and foot, which fails to subside with appropriate analgesics and splintage.
8. **Soft tissue crepitus in case of gas in soft tissue planes:** Surgical emphysema in case of fracture ribs and gas gangrene.
9. **Palpation of all other bones, contralateral limb, spine and pelvis**.

Movements
It is always difficult to assess the movement at the joint near the fracture site due to pain and discontinuity in the lever (fracture). Nevertheless, after stabilizing the limb in a splint, one should ask the patient to move adjacent joints actively, especially the ones which are free and distal to the injured area to get an idea of integrity of nerves and tendon.

Measurement
- *Measurement of the limb length is not performed in acute fractures, as maneuvering would be very painful.* A mere visual assessment of the limb length is fair enough! However, sequential girth assessment may be of some value in patients with impending compartment syndrome who are kept under observation. Any sequential increase in the girth with unrelenting pain may require urgent fasciotomy.
- Muscle wasting is not a feature of acute trauma unless there were a pre-existing one such as pre-existing poliomyelitis in the limb.

Auscultation
It is relevant in patients with fractured ribs. One must try to record the breath sounds on both sides of the chest.

Neurovascular Examination
A thorough systematic neurovascular examination of the extremity is mandatory to rule out any neurovascular deficit. *A handheld Doppler may be used to supplement the examination of*

peripheral pulses, especially if there is a significant limb edema obscuring the palpation of artery. If a detailed neurological assessment is not possible in the presence of multiple injuries or an uncooperative patient, it should be recorded to avoid litigation. Later, neurological examination must be performed once the patient is conscious and cooperative.

Joint Above and Below

Careful assessment of the joint above and below is essential to rule out any transmitted injury to the neighboring joints. For example, after a fall from height, the foot, knee, hip, pelvis, and spine should be examined as axial force can be transmitted from the 'lower' point of impact (calcaneum) to higher levels (ankle, knee, pelvis, spine).

Special Tests

The special tests especially pertaining to the ligament injury are often difficult to perform in primary survey due to other priorities and painful local conditions (fracture, dislocation, wounds). Hence, it should be preformed with care only when patient is stable as a part of secondary or tertiary survey.

A Note on Relevant Investigations in Stable Trauma Patients

- **X-rays:** Plain radiograph with relevant views must be asked for to *assess or rule out bony injuries*. Trauma series X-rays (chest, spine, and pelvis) are asked for patients with polytrauma.
- **FAST scan:** It is a rapid bedside ultrasound examination performed by emergency physicians, surgeons, or paramedics as a *screening test for blood around the heart* (pericardial effusion) and *abdominal organs* (hemoperitoneum) after trauma. The four classic areas that are examined for free fluid are the perihepatic space (including Morison's pouch or the hepatorenal recess), perisplenic space, pericardium, and the pelvis. The presence of free fluid will usually be due to bleeding.
- **Computed tomography (CT) scan:** It is requested in patients with specific situations such as:
  - *Intra-articular or periarticular fractures.*
  - *Areas where the anatomy is complex*: Spine, pelvis, scapula, or joints.
- **Arterial Doppler:** It is requested to *rule out any arterial injury* if there is a vascular injury (arterial). For example, pulse is not palpable/feeble/pulse not palpable due to swelling, cold extremity, poor capillary filling.
- **CT angiogram:** It is requested when there is *suspicion of vascular injury* to the limb. It is superior to Doppler imaging in terms of sensitivity and specificity.
- **Magnetic resonance imaging (MRI):** It is usually requested *if there is suspicion of soft tissue injury involving ligament, muscle–tendon, or nerves*. It is also valuable for *undisplaced fractures wherein one can visualize fractures and associated bone marrow edema*. However, unless really required for an emergency management of a patient, MRI is conducted once patient has been completely stable for a day or two and all other major emergency managements are over.

TRAUMA-RELATED ORTHOPEDIC EMERGENCIES

Open Fractures

The wound of open fracture can vary from a puncture wound at the fracture site to composite soft tissue loss along with severe contamination. These fractures require emergency intervention in the form of thorough debridement preferably within 8 hours, empirical antibiotics to minimize the risk of infection followed by stabilization of fracture with appropriate method (external/internal).

Compartment Syndrome

Compartment syndrome is defined as an increase in the pressure of a closed osteomyofascial compartment to levels high enough to cause ischemia. Compartment syndrome is usually seen in the leg and forearm, where there are two long bones connected by an interosseous membrane and surrounded by different groups of muscles enclosed in tight fascial structures. Compartment syndrome may also happen in the hand, foot, and thigh. Stretched shiny skin, unrelenting pain after fracture that fails to subside with regular analgesics, and pain on the passive stretch of the finger/toes are clinical signs of compartment syndrome. A quick clinical assessment may help to establish the diagnosis and may require urgent fasciotomy and fracture fixation.

Dislocations

A dislocation is an emergency as dislocated part often lies next to the neurovascular bundle, which can compress the neurovascular bundle. For example, in anterior dislocation of the shoulder, the head lies next to the axillary nerve/brachial plexus. Further, the vascularity of the dislocated part is under stress, which may result in avascular necrosis if the part is not reduced early. For example, dislocation of the hip tents the retinacular vessels. Therefore, a dislocation must be reduced as early as possible.

Major Vascular Injury of the Limb/Traumatic Amputation of a Limb

The *re-implantation of a traumatically amputated part or repair of a major vascular injury of the limb* compromising the circulation must be tackled as an utmost priority. Both (re-implantation/re-vascularization) should be undertaken within 8–12 hours of the injury as the warm ischemia time of the limb is less than 12 hours. Associated fracture/dislocation should be managed on standard lines.

Absolute contraindications for re-implantation include severely crushed or mangled parts, amputations at multiple levels, and prolonged warm ischemia more than 12 hours. The amputated limb/part should not transported from the site of accident to the hospital with direct contact of ice. It should be kept in a plastic bag and this bag should be kept in another plastic bag with ice so that the limb/part is not in the direct contact with the ice. This will aid in retaining the viability of the limb when re-vascularization is attempted.

Notes

CHAPTER 3

Clinical Evaluation of Diseased Long Bones and Joints

INTRODUCTION

Although the history and examination pattern of the skeletal system follows a standard protocol, the clinical evaluation of the diseased or pathological bone is different from acutely traumatized bones and joints. The clinical evaluation of a traumatized limb has been discussed in Chapter 2. The current chapter will discuss pathological bone diseases and some chronic sequels of trauma.

HISTORY TAKING IN LONG BONE DISEASE

In evaluation of chronic bone diseases, several important parameters such as age and onset of complaints/disease may give important clues to the current pathology.

Certain examples of *relevance of age* are mentioned below.
- **Young children:** Acute osteomyelitis, Ewing's sarcoma, osteosarcoma
- **Adolescence and young adults:** Most benign bone tumors
- **Elderly:** Osteoporosis

Regarding *onset of complaints*, one must always probe whether the present complaint is insidious in onset or did it start after an episode of trauma. In certain situations like bone tumors, which are atraumatic in origin, it is quite likely that trauma draws attention towards the tumor swelling, that has been pre-existing. Sometimes, patients with hematogenous osteomyelitis also give a history of trauma (without any open wound) followed by pain, swelling and discharge from the bone. Although, it is hard to explain a hematogenous bone infection due to a local trauma, it is a rare possibility that the local hematoma may get infected due to bacteremia, possibly arising out of a covert or overt source of infection elsewhere in the body.

The common presenting complaints in patients with diseased bone and joint are mentioned in **Box 3.1**.

BOX 3.1: Common presenting complaints in diseased bones.

- Pain
- Swelling
- Inability or difficulty to bear weight
- Sinus
- Deformity
- Joint stiffness
- Limp
- Joint instability
- Limb length discrepancy
- Weakness
- Pathological fractures

Most of these complaints have been discussed in detail in Chapter 1. Therefore, this chapter will discuss these complaints briefly.

Chief Complaints and History of Present Illness

1. **Pain:** Bone pain without significant trauma is indicative of atraumatic pathology. Infection and tumors are common atraumatic pathologies.
   - *The onset of pain:*
     - *Acute onset:* Infection (acute osteomyelitis), malignant change in a benign tumor, pathological fracture
     - *Insidious onset:* Benign tumors, subacute osteomyelitis (Brodie's abscess).
   - *The character of pain:*
     - *Dull aching pain:* Mechanical pathology such as degenerative arthritis
     - *Throbbing pain:* Acute inflammation, acute intramedullary stage of osteomyelitis
     - *Shooting pain along with tingling, numbness:* Pain of neural origin.
   - *Activities causing pain:*
     - *Pain while load-bearing/mechanical pain:* Degenerative arthritis
     - *Pain at rest:* Inflammatory (rheumatoid, gout), infective (osteomyelitis), or malignant tumors (osteosarcoma)
     - *Typical night cries:* Tuberculosis of joint.
2. **Swelling:**
   - *Insidious onset, chronic swelling:* Benign tumors of bone, tubercular or other low-grade pyogenic infection of bone, others such as osteochondritis (Osgood–Schlatter)
   - *Acute-onset pain with sudden swelling of the bone:* Acute osteomyelitis, malignant change in benign bone tumor
   - *Similar swellings elsewhere in the body:* Neurofibromatosis, multiple exostosis.
3. **Inability or difficulty to bear weight:** Inability/difficulty in weight-bearing is observed in painful bone or a joint, nonunion of a fracture, chronically subluxated or a dislocated joint, and neuromuscular disorder.
4. **Sinus:** The presence of a sinus indicates a focus of dead material inside the soft tissue or bone. It could be a sequestrum, suture material, or any other foreign body. A pus-discharging sinus associated with the discharge of bony spicules suggests chronic osteomyelitis. If associated with fracture, one must ask history of open fracture.
5. **Deformity:** It could be in the axial/coronal/sagittal plane. One must probe regarding the onset of deformity that whether it is congenital or acquired. It could happen after trauma, infection, or metabolic (rickets) conditions.
6. **Pathological fractures:** Pathological fractures happen in metabolic disorders (osteoporosis, osteomalacia), underlying tumors, infection, or others (osteogenesis imperfecta).
   In a patient with pathological fracture, one must probe into details of history to ascertain the plausible etiology.
7. **Limb length discrepancy:** It is observed in nonunion or malunion of fracture or dislocated/subluxated joint.
8. **Weakness:** It could arise out of associated neuromuscular disorders such as poliomyelitis, muscular dystrophy or nerve palsies.
9. **Stiffness of joints:** In a bone disease, there is possibility of joint stiffness due to surgeries, infection, and immobilization.
10. **Abnormal gait pattern**

11. **Feeling of instability:** Occurs in associated ligament injury of the joint or malformed articulating bones.

History of Constitutional and Other Systemic Symptoms
One must elicit history of fever, malaise, weight loss and appetite in patients with bone diseases, as that may indicate underlying infection, inflammation, or tumor.

Past History
All diseases/ailments suffered by the patient excluding the present one must be probed as it may have influence on the current problem.

Family History
Family history of similar disorders may be present due to genetic predispositions, such as multiple exostosis, osteogenesis imperfecta.

Drug History
Relevant drug history is important in many cases. For example, avascular necrosis of the femoral head can occur due to prolonged steroid intake.

Personal, Treatment, Menstrual and Other Relevant History
- *Personal history:* History of smoking, alcohol intake, diet (vegetarian, mixed), marital status, allergies, immunization, surgical and medical history.
- *Treatment history* (of current complaint): It may give insight to how the current complaint may have evolved over last few weeks to month after several rounds of treatment.
- *Menstrual history:* Hormonal imbalance in a post-menopausal status is one of the predisposing risk factors for osteoporosis.

GENERAL AND SYSTEMIC EXAMINATION
A detailed systemic and general examination is essential as it forms an integral part of the examination in nontraumatic conditions such as tumors, inflammatory, metabolic, and infective conditions of the bone.

LOCAL EXAMINATION

Gait
Gait assessment is important in lower limb pathologies. *For details, refer to Chapter 14.*

Attitude
It should be described in a standard fashion.

Inspection
- **Alignment of the limb and deformity, if any:**
  - Sagittal, coronal, and rotation malalignment of the limb must be noted **(Fig. 3.1A)**.
  - The site, side, and anatomical area of the deformity must be recorded.

CHAPTER 3 ♦ Clinical Evaluation of Diseased Long Bones and Joints

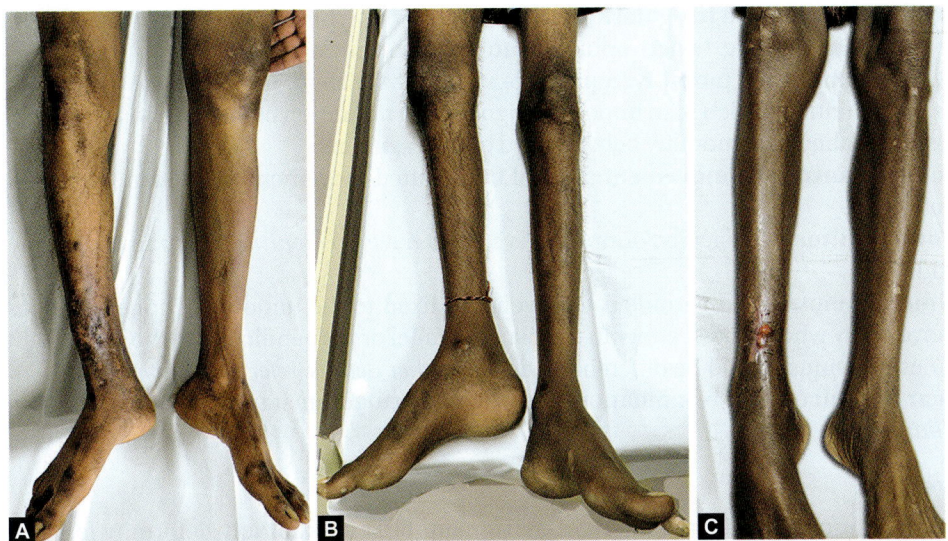

Figs. 3.1A to C: (A) Varus deformity of the right tibia; (B) Short and externally rotated right lower limb; (C) Sinus over the distal tibia with pouting granulation tissue.

- **Muscle wasting:** Wasting should be noted and compared with contralateral limb. Presence of wasting is suggestive of chronic disuse of the limb due to a chronic underlying pathology.
- **Limb length discrepancy:** Check the comparative length of the limb—whether short, long, equal. A short limb may be seen following a chronic sequel of trauma due to deformity, bone loss, and growth plate damage **(Fig. 3.1B)**.
- **Swelling:** Note whether the swelling is single or multiple (neurofibromatosis, multiple exostosis). *For further details of swelling examination, refer to Chapter 15.*
- **Skin overlying the limb:** The skin around the affected bone and neighboring joints must be visualized for any scar, sinus, or ulcer. Look for any exposed bone or underlying implant via the chronic ulcer or sinus. Note any trophic skin changes distal to the injured site due to complex regional pain syndrome. *For further description of scar, sinus and ulcer, refer to Chapter 15.*
- **Presence of a sinus, ulcer:** Note the location, number, active/quiescent, type of discharge, bony spicules, and presence of pouting granulation tissue at the sinus. A pouting granulation tissue indicates underlying dead material such as sequestrum, suture material, or a foreign body **(Fig. 3.1C)**.

Palpation

One must palpate the diseased bone for local temperature, bony tenderness, irregularity, and thickening. Feel for any abnormal mobility between proximal and distal ends of bone, step and crepitus assess loss of transmitted movement.

- **Temperature:** An increase in local temperature around the affected site must raise suspicion of infection/inflammation/tumor of underlying bone. *A rise in local temperature is absent in cold abscess.*
- **Tenderness:** Apart from bony tenderness, assess tenderness over important soft tissue landmarks and joint lines. While bony tenderness may be present in osteomyelitis and malignant tumor, it may be absent in malunion, nonunion.

- **Bony thickening and irregularity:** Localized abnormal thickening of the bone is suggestive of old healed fracture, hypertrophic nonunion or chronic osteomyelitis.
- **Step and abnormal mobility:** A palpable step over the shaft of a long bone is suggestive of its discontinuity, which is an important sign for gap nonunion of the long bone. A nonunion results in abnormal mobility between two bone fragments.
- **Loss of transmitted movement:** Loss of transmitted movement is noted in nonunion of a fracture.
- **Bony crepitus:** Classically, nonunion is said to have *no crepitus* due to rounded fracture ends.
- **Sinus:** A sinus due to chronic osteomyelitis is fixed to the underlying bone and does not move freely when moved either in the plane parallel or perpendicular to the bone. Active or quiescent sinus should be differentiated. *For further details, refer to Chapter 15.*
- **Scar and ulcer:** The examination must be performed on standard principles *(Refer to Chapter 15).*

Movement

Follow the principles of assessment of movement. First look for any deformity followed by active and passive movements. Stiffness of adjacent joint may be present in long-standing nonunion, malunion, or chronic infection.

Measurement

Bone length and **muscle girth** is assessed. Bone length must be assessed on standard principles (Refer Chapter 1), and compare with contralateral side. The length of the bone/limb can be normal, increased, or decreased compared to the opposite side. Limb shortening may be present in nonunion, malunion, chronic osteomyelitis or a pathological fracture. *Muscle girth* may reveal wasting on the diseased side.

Examination of Neurovascular Structures, Lymph Node, Joint Above and Below, and Distal Part of the Limb

It is necessary to examine the distal neurovascular structures, joints above and below, lymph nodes, and swelling of the extremity distal to the diseased area of the bone. Typically, local limb disorders causes unilateral swelling of the limb, whereas bilateral swelling of the lower limb is usually due to systemic causes (cardiac, renal, hepatic, cor pulmonale, low albumin levels, etc.). The unilateral **swelling of the distal limb** may be present deep vein thrombosis, pressure effect over the venous system (tumor pressing veins), infection, inflammation, or post-traumatic conditions. Multiple surgeries can scar the lymphatic and venous system of the limb leading to distal swelling.

DIFFERENTIAL DIAGNOSIS

There are many common bony disorders which present as pain, swelling, deformity and pathological fractures in a bone, which are categorized under:

A. **Congenital, genetic and developmental disorder:** Cleidocranial dysostosis, Marfan's syndrome, osteogenesis imperfecta, achondroplasia, congenital pseudoarthrosis, Paget's disease
B. **Traumatic:** Malunion, nonunion, delayed union, myositis ossificans
C. **Infective:** Chronic osteomyelitis, Brodie's abscess

D. **Neoplastic:** Benign and malignant tumors *(Refer to Chapter 12)*
E. **Metabolic:** Rickets, osteomalacia, osteoporosis
F. **Others:** Pathological fractures.

Various Important Long Bone Affections

1. Malunion

- History of trauma followed by fracture. A history of inadequate treatment might be present in many cases.
- **Clinical features:**
  - Typically, it is characterized by a *nonprogressive, painless deformity*. However, the deformity can be progressive, if it involves growth plate in a growing child. Furthermore, malunion could be painful if there is involvement of the joint surface or abnormal loading of the adjacent joint due to deformity.
  - *Bony thickening* is present at the fracture site. There is absence of bony tenderness, gap, crepitus and abnormal mobility. There may be alteration in various adjacent bony point relations.
  - *Associated shortening* of the limb may be present and the adjacent joint may be stiff.
  - *Functional loss* due to malunion may vary from none to severe. There may be *cosmetic concerns* regarding the deformity.
- **Management:** X-rays establish the diagnosis. No treatment is offered, if there is no functional deficit. Symptomatic cases may require corrective osteotomy.

2. Nonunion

- History of trauma followed by a fracture.
- **Presents with:** Typically, the patient may present with loss of function and not able to bear weight (in case of lower limb fracture nonunion) or use the limb adequately.
- **Etiology:** Infection, inadequate blood supply, interposed soft tissue, inadequate treatment, intact fellow bone, bone loss, and systemic causes, such as diabetes, smoking.
- **Clinical features:** Classically, *there is "painless abnormal mobility" at the nonunion site*. There is no tenderness/crepitus at the nonunion site, and *gap is felt at the nonunion site*. The limb may be shortened and deformed. Adjacent joint may be stiff.
- **Diagnosis:** X-rays show atrophic/hypertrophic type of nonunion.
- **Treatment:** Asymptomatic patients with no functional deficit may not require any treatment. Symptomatic ones need Open reduction, freshening of bone ends, opening of medullary canal, fixation of fracture and bone grafting.

3. Delayed Union

- History of trauma followed by fracture.
- **Etiology:** Tantamount to nonunion
- **Clinical features:** Typically, the patient presents with loss of function and inability to bear weight (in case of lower limb fracture delayed union) or use the limb adequately. Tenderness and gap is felt at the fracture site. Minimal abnormal mobility may be felt at the fracture site along with mild tenderness (as the fracture has not yet united).
- **Management:** X-rays establish the diagnosis.
- **Treatment:** Observation, ultrasound stimulation of fracture site bone marrow injection, and bone grafting.

4. Chronic Osteomyelitis

- In case of hematogenous osteomyelitis, there may be history of infection at another site prior to the onset of bone infection (respiratory/urinary/gastrointestinal tract infection). In a post-traumatic osteomyelitis, past history of open fracture may be present. Occasionally, it could be postoperative with an implant *in situ*.
- **Location:** Hematogenous osteomyelitis is common in metaphysis, whereas post-traumatic can occur anywhere.
- **Bacteriology:** *Staph. aureus* is the most common organism.
- **Clinical features:**
  - History of pus-discharging sinus. *Discharge of bony spicules, if any, is quite diagnostic of chronic osteomyelitis*. Pain (tenderness) may be present or absent.
  - Bony tenderness, thickening and irregularity are present around the sinus. Sinus is always fixed to the underlying bone.
  - Absence of gap and abnormal mobility unless there is associated pathological fracture. There may be associated shortening and deformity of the bone. Adjacent joint may be stiff.
  - Overlying skin is usually hyperpigmented and scarred.
- **Investigations:** Blood test (CBC, ESR, CRP), pus culture, X-rays, CT scan and MRI.
- **Treatment:** Sinus tract excision, saucerization, sequestrectomy, curettage of the cavity, local antibiotic beads, IV followed by oral antibiotics. Later, filling of the saucerized cavity may require bone grafting and/or a flap coverage.

> **Tubercular osteomyelitis:** Ends of long bone and short bones of hand and foot are commonly affected. Insidious in onset, pain and swelling of the affected bone. *Formation of cold abscess and sinus with undermined edge are the typical hallmarks.*

5. Brodie's Abscess

- Common localized bone infection in the age group of 10–20 years, due to *low virulence Staph. aureus infection*. Typically observed in long bone metaphysis—upper and lower end of tibia, upper end of femur and humerus.
- **Clinical features:** Chronic, recurrent low-grade boring pain, and occasional fever. Mild swelling and bony tenderness during recurrent episodes.

6. Achondroplasia

- One of the common condition of dwarfism. It is an autosomal dominant disease
- **Clinical features:** While these patients have normal intelligence, it is characterized by **Rhizomelic dwarfism** where trunk is normal in size and short height is more in proximal segment of the limb **(Fig. 3.2)**.

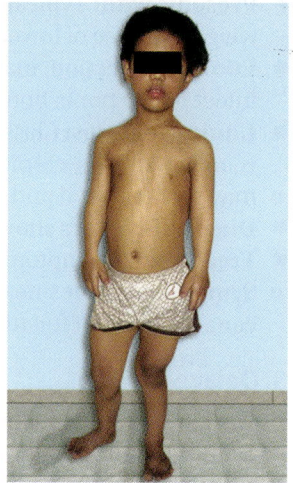

Fig. 3.2: Rhizomelic dwarfism in achondroplasia.

7. Osteogenesis Imperfecta/Brittle Bone Disease/Lobstien Syndrome/Vrolik Disease

- Osteogenesis imperfecta (OI) occurs due to decrease in amount of normal type I collagen in bones resulting in a brittle bone. (*Note: Type I collagen is seen in skin, bone, ligaments, teeth and sclera*).

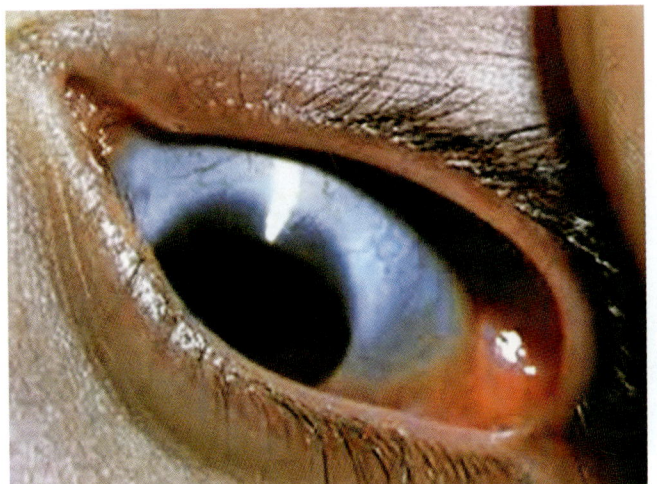

Fig. 3.3: Blue sclera in osteogenesis imperfecta.

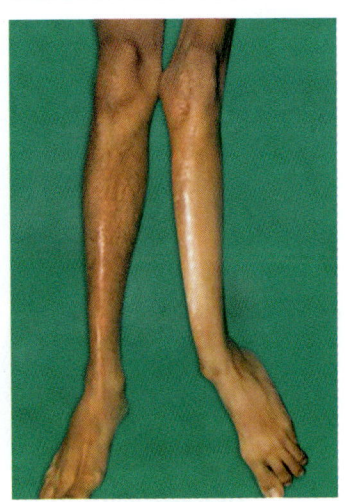

Fig. 3.4: Anterolateral bowing of the left tibia in congenital pseudoarthrosis.

- **Clinical features:** Short stature, fragility fracture, scoliosis, blue sclera **(Fig. 3.3)**. They also have hearing loss, wormian skull bones, increased cardiac anomalies (mitral prolapse, aortic regurgitation).

8. Congenital Pseudoarthrosis of Tibia (CPT)

CPT is congenital bowing of the tibia with anterolateral apex and pseudoarthrosis **(Fig. 3.4)**. It is associated with neurofibromatosis (NF-1).

9. Rickets

- It is a metabolic condition characterized by inadequate mineralization of the bone matrix in a growing skeleton.
- **Types:** *Hypocalcemic* rickets (due to calcium/vitamin D deficiency/Type 1 and 2 vitamin D resistant rickets) and *hypophosphatemic* rickets (renal phosphate wasting, poor phosphate intake).
- **Clinical features:** *Typical nutritional deficiency rickets (Calcium or Vitamin D) is characterized by* Craniotabes, frontal bossing, rachitic rosary, Harrison's sulcus, broadened wrist **(Fig. 3.5A)**, coxa vara, genu varum/valgum **(Fig. 3.5B)** and double malleolus sign. In *Type 2 vitamin D resistant rickets*, symptoms appear within 2 years of life. Other feature are alopecia and other ectodermal anomalies (multiple milia, oligodontia and ectodermal cyst). *Renal rickets or renal phosphate wasting (hypophostamic rickets)* is characterized by more deformities in lower limb, short stature, anemia and phosphate wasting in urine.

10. Osteomalacia

Osteomalacia is inadequate mineralization of bone matrix in an adult skeleton. It presents as generalized bone pain, fatigue, weakness, muscle tenderness and weakness, and rarely fractures of long bones. X-ray may show *Looser's zone in scapula, proximal femur and pelvis.*

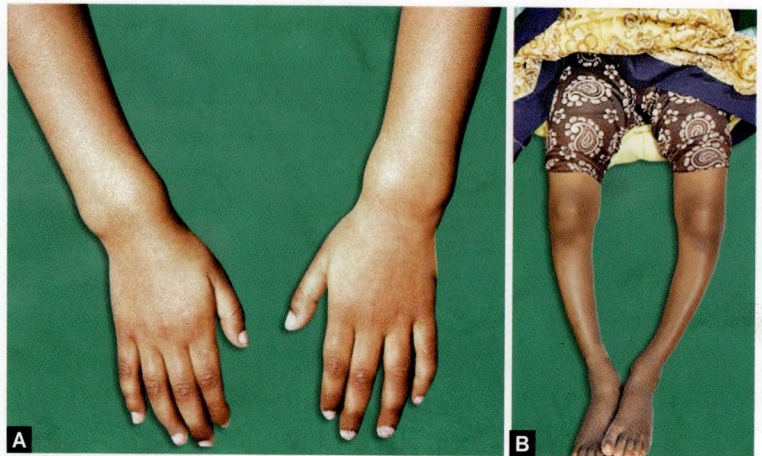

Figs. 3.5A and B: (A) Broadened wrist in rickets; (B) Bilateral genu varum in rickets.

11. Osteoporosis

Osteoporosis is decreased bone mass loss due to uncoupled osteoblast-osteoclast action resulting in microarchitectural defect in bone. Typically, it presents as generalized back pain and fragility fractures typically in cancellous bones (vertebra, hip, distal radius, proximal humerus, etc.) are one of the most important features. There may be exaggerated thoracic kyphosis (*Dowager's hump*).

12. Marfan's Syndrome

- It is an autosomal dominant disorder with defect in collagen and elastin formation.
- **Clinical features:** Most patients present with **tall stature** with scoliosis, unusually long limbs especially distal segments. They also have long narrow fingers (*arachnodactyly—spider fingers*), high-arched palate. Other features are ocular lens dislocation, aortic regurgitation, aneurysm and dissection.

13. Paget's Disease (Osteitis Deformans)

- Paget's is characterized by defective bone remodelling wherein there is initial increased bone resorption followed by bone deposition.
- **Clinical features:** Most commonly affected bones are pelvis and tibia. Other bones affected are femur, skull, spine and clavicle. Dull bone pain is most common symptom. Bowing

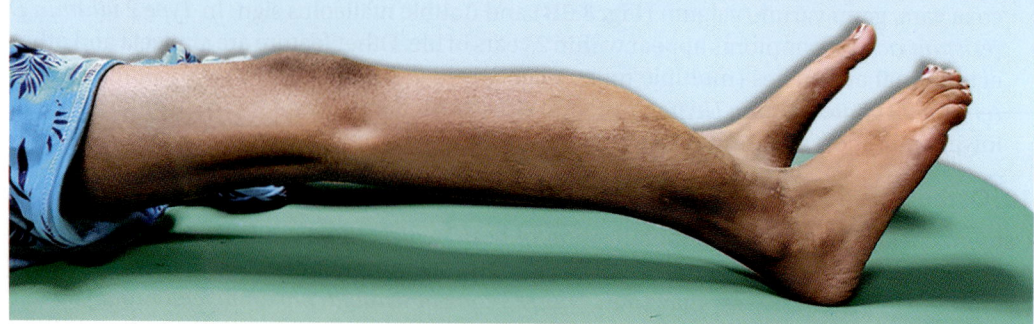

Fig. 3.6: Pagetic bowing of the tibia.

deformity is noted in long bones **(Fig. 3.6)**, kyphosis, and skull enlargement (increased hat size). Rarely, there can be secondary osteosarcomatous change in bone. Patients may have cardiac failure due to increased cardiac output.

CLINICAL EVALUATION OF PATHOLOGICAL JOINTS

Various common conditions, which affect single or multiple joints are:
1. **Degenerative osteoarthrosis:** Primary and secondary. Primary osteoarthrosis or osteoarthritis is age related and is due to wear and tear-related cartilage damage. Secondary osteoarthrosis is due to a specific underlying cause.
2. **Infective:** Tubercular arthritis, septic arthritis, gonococcal arthritis
3. **Inflammatory:** Rheumatoid arthritis (RA), SLE-associated arthritis, juvenile RA, ankylosing spondylitis (AS)
4. **Metabolic:** Gout, pseudogout, ochronosis
5. **Neuropathic arthropathy:** Charcot's joint
6. **Hematological:** Hemophilia
7. **Others:** Osteochondritis dessecans, synovial chondromatosis, Perthes' disease
   Almost all of the above conditions, especially if untreated, eventually affect the joint cartilage and cause arthritis. Arthritis can be classified and studied in many ways: primary and secondary, inflammatory and non-inflammatory **(Flowchart 3.1)**.

Note: Seropositive and seronegative implies RA factor positive and negative, respectively.

While evaluating a diseased or pathological joint, the consideration of age, gender, type of joint involvement, and occupation is essential.
1. **Age:** Typically, ankylosing and rheumatoid arthritis occur in younger men and women (between 20–50 years), whereas degenerative osteoarthritis is a disorder of patients more than 50–55 years. Gouty arthritis is common in younger patients, while pseudogout is common in the older patients. Gonococcal arthritis of a single joint is common in sexually active young adults.
2. **Gender:** While rheumatoid arthritis is more common in women, ankylosing spondylitis is more common in men.

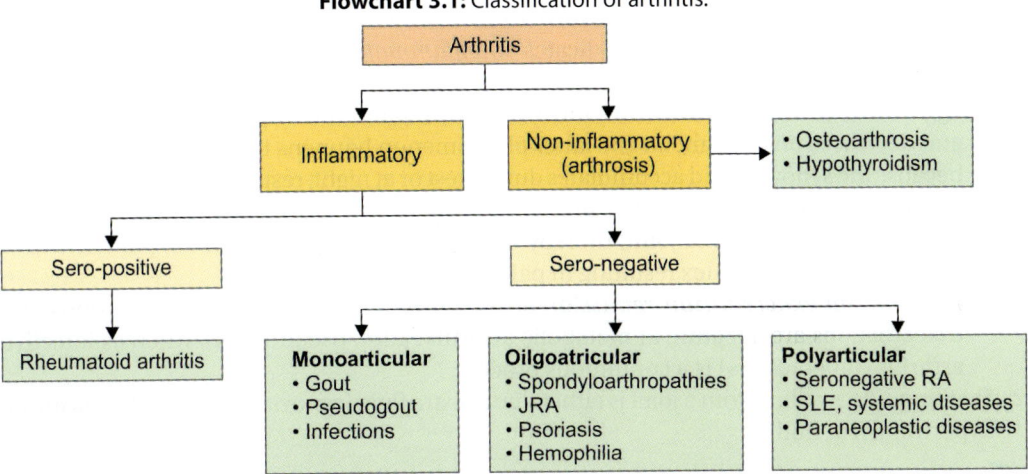

Flowchart 3.1: Classification of arthritis.

3. **Type of joint involvement**
   a. *Weight-bearing joint (Knee, hip, and ankle):* Primary degenerative osteoarthrosis
   b. *Axial joints: Sacroiliac and rest of the spine:* Seronegative arthropathy
   c. *Symmetric, small joints of wrist-hand and foot:* Rheumatoid arthritis (Metacarpophalangeal joint, proximal interphalangeal joint). However, note that monoarticular presentation is not uncommon.
   d. *Large joints:* Pseudogout; *Small joints:* Gout
4. **Occupation and activity:** People who stand and work are more prone to lower limb degenerative arthritis.

Chief Complaints and History of Presenting Illness

Patients with joint disorder complain of pain, swelling, deformity, stiffness, instability, and locking.
1. **Pain:** It is the most common complaint in a patient with arthritis. It is essential to note that *almost all joint conditions are painful except Charcot's arthropathy/neuropathic joint.* Charcot's arthropathy is painless destruction of the joint due to poor/absent protective sensory and proprioceptive signals to the spinal cord and brain. One must further probe into onset, duration, severity, character, progression, mechanical or rest pain, radiation, remission-exacerbation, aggravating and relieving factors.
   a. *Onset:* It could be acute or insidious.
      i. *Acute onset:* It is observed in acute septic arthritis, acute exacerbation of chronic inflammatory arthritis (RA), and metabolic arthritis (gout, pseudogout).
      ii. *Insidious onset:* It is noted in degenerative osteoarthrosis, inflammatory arthritis, tubercular arthritis.
   b. *Character of pain:* It could be *dull aching* (Degenerative osteoarthrosis), or *throbbing* (Septic arthritis). *Night cries are observed in tubercular arthritis.* In tubercular arthritis, the cartilage is destroyed due to the pathological process resulting in exposure of the subchondral bone. The joint is kept relatively immobilized in the daytime due to muscle spasms, minimizing the friction between the two joint surfaces. In contrast, muscles relax during sleep, allowing more friction between the joint surfaces resulting in night cries.
   c. *Mechanical or rest pain:* While mechanical pain is characteristic of degenerative osteoarthrosis and post-traumatic osteoarthrosis, rest pain is observed in infective, inflammatory, and metabolic arthritis. Also ask for **associated morning stiffness** lasting for more than one hour, which indicates *an inflammatory arthritis.*
   d. *Aggravating and relieving factors:* While the pain of degenerative osteoarthrosis aggravates on movement and reduces on rest, inflammatory pain increases with rest and decreases on movement. The latter phenomenon happens in inflammatory arthritis because the synovial fluid accumulates during rest or at night, resulting in capsuloligament stretching, causing pain. Once the patient mobilizes the joint, the excess synovial fluid disperses out of the joint, thereby decreasing the stretching of the pain-sensitive capsuloligament complex resulting in pain relief.
   e. *Intermittent exacerbation-remission or a continuous phenomenon:* Remissions and exacerbations are a feature of metabolic arthritis (gout, pseudogout), whereas infective arthritis (tuberculosis) is a continuous process.
2. **Swelling:** The swelling from a joint is either due to extra fluid (synovial/pus/blood) or synovial hypertrophy, or both.

3. **Deformity:** Most joint diseases gradually result in a deformed joint due to cartilage, capsule, and ligament damage. In the late stages of most arthritis, gross cartilage damage, subluxation, or dislocation of the joint contributes to the deformity.
4. **Loss of movement/stiffness:** Most joint disorders may affect the range of motion (ROM), which gradually decreases over several months to years after the onset of the disease. The loss of ROM happens due to arthritis, capsule-ligament contractures, osteophytes, muscle spasm, and deformity. In contrast, Charcot's arthropathy is characterized by excess movements (not loss of ROM) in different planes due to gross destruction of the joint surfaces and stretching of the capsuloligament complex. Sometimes, joint stiffness is felt in the mornings or after rest, which improves with activity. Morning stiffness is significant only if it lasts more than an hour. *Morning stiffness is the hallmark of inflammatory joint diseases, such as rheumatoid arthritis and ankylosing spondylitis.*
5. **Instability:** Instability of a joint is observed if there is damage to the stabilizing structures such as ligaments, capsule, articular surface, muscle-tendon complex, or neurological innervation.
6. **Locking:** It is one of the features of the joint disease wherein the joint intermittently gets stuck in a particular movement and cannot be further moved. Loose bodies (any joint), meniscal tears, and labral tears (shoulder, hip) are common causes of joint locking.

Past History

One must probe about the history of tuberculosis, current or in the past, as musculoskeletal tuberculosis is almost always secondary to primary elsewhere. History of trauma causing damage to the cartilage or meniscus may result in secondary post-traumatic osteoarthritis of the knee joint. Other relevant history of pre-existing co-morbidities, such as diabetes, hypertension, thyroid must be taken.

Family History

Family history is important in diseases such as hemophilia, RA and AS.

Personal History

Excess indulgence in alcohol and a non-vegetarian diet may result in gouty attacks. History of sexual activity without protection, especially in the case of multiple partners, may increase the possibility of gonococcal arthritis.

Drug History

Use of steroid intake due to some other medical (chronic asthma, skin disease) or surgical disorder may result in avascular necrosis of the hip. The use of pyrazinamide (one of the antitubercular drugs) can cause hyperuricemia and gout.

General and Systemic Examination

A thorough general and systemic examination is warranted as most of these joint disorders are systemic in origin or have a systemic association.

The general examination includes assessing vitals followed by pallor, icterus, clubbing, cyanosis, pedal edema, and lymph nodes.

Several examples of systemic involvement or associations are mentioned below.
1. **Rheumatoid arthritis:** Anemia, hepatosplenomegaly, lung fibrosis, rheumatoid nodules.
2. **Ankylosing spondylitis:** Iridocyclitis, cardiac conduction abnormality.

3. **Joint tuberculosis:** Pallor, look for any evidence of tuberculosis in lung, enlarged lymph nodes.
4. **Bouchard and Heberdon's node (in fingers) along with first carpometacarpal osteoarthrosis** is often present in moderate to severe cases of primary osteoarthritis of the knee.

Local Examination

1. **Gait:** It should be assessed in a standard fashion (*Refer to Chapter 14*).
2. **Attitude:** It should be described in a standard fashion.
3. **Inspection:** One must look at the swelling (localized or diffuse), deformity, skin, scar, sinus, muscle wasting and describe it in standard fashion.
    a. *Swelling* is the most common feature in almost all joint disorders. The joint swelling is easily visible in the superficial joints (elbow, wrist, knee, and ankle) **(Fig. 3.7)**, while it is not so evident in deeper joints (shoulder and hip).
    b. *Deformity:* Most chronic joint disorders may result in deformity due to the destruction of cartilage, combination of soft-tissue contracture and laxity followed by subluxation or dislocation.
       Some examples of common conditions and associated deformities are listed below.
         i. Osteoarthritis of the knee: *Genu varum*
         ii. Rheumatoid arthritis: *Genu valgum or windswept deformity (one knee in varum, other in valgum)*
         iii. Tuberculosis of the knee: *Triple deformity*, which is a combination of flexion, external rotation, and posterior subluxation of the knee.
         iv. Tuberculosis of the hip: Deformity of the hip varies in three stages of tuberculosis.
       It is important to note that degenerative arthritis results in asymmetric cartilage destruction according to the weight-bearing or loading pattern. In contrast, inflammatory, infective, and metabolic arthritis results in symmetric or more uniform joint destruction as the pathology is widespread in the joint irrespective of the weight-bearing or loading pattern.
    c. *The skin over the joint:* In an acute case of synovitis or infection, the skin may appear red, stretched, and shiny. However, chronic cases are accompanied by normal-looking skin.
    d. *Muscle wasting:* It is a feature of chronic arthritis indicating disuse atrophy.
    e. *Baker's cyst:* It must be looked for in all cases of chronic knee disorders **(Fig. 3.8)**.

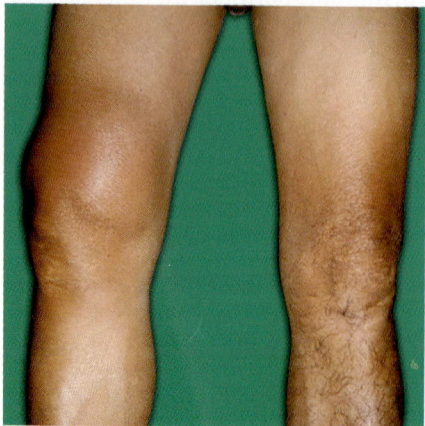

Fig. 3.7: Horse shoe shape swelling of the right knee joint.

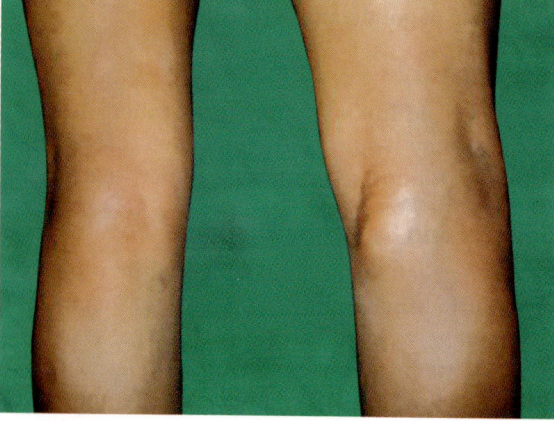

Fig. 3.8: Baker's cyst in the right popliteal fossa.

> Note that Baker's cyst is almost always a secondary finding due to an underlying primary pathology in the knee, such as inflammation/infection/degenerative condition.

    f. **Limb length:** One must compare the length of the two limbs. A joint disease can result in limb length discrepancy.
4. **Palpation:** One must feel for local temperature, tenderness (bone, soft tissue, and joint lines), synovial hypertrophy, and bony irregularity. Occasionally, loose bodies can be felt during palpation.
    a. *Local temperature:* It is raised in infective, inflammatory, and metabolic conditions.
    b. *Tenderness:* The tenderness should be assessed over bony and soft tissue landmarks in a standard fashion. The joint lines should be palpated, which are tender in arthritis.
    c. *Synovial hypertrophy:* The synovium is often hypertrophied (thickened) in infective and inflammatory disorders such as tuberculosis, rheumatoid arthritis.
    d. *Bony irregularity* over the bones forming the joint must be palpated. An irregular bone may indicate evidence of old malunited fracture, infection, etc.
5. **Movement:** It should be assessed in a standard fashion (*Refer to Chapter 1*).
   Note any deformity before initiating the movement assessment. Assess ROM on the normal side followed by index side. Active movements should be assessed first, followed by passive movement. Note whether movements are painful or painless. The crepitus can be felt during passive ROM, which either indicates a rough joint surface due to cartilage damage (arthritis) or a loose body in the joint. The crepitus of arthritis is usually fixed, i.e., it is elicited at the same sector of the ROM, whenever the joint is moved. In contrast, crepitus elicited in the presence of a loose body is variable, and is elicited whenever the loose body is caught between the articulating surfaces. Generally, there are some or more degrees of restriction of ROM in all arthritis, which increases with the severity of arthritis. In contrast, the late stages of Charcot's arthritis may reveal excess ROM (vide supra). The loss of ROM at a joint is known as stiffness, and ankylosis is a term used when joints have barely any demonstrable ROM (*Refer to Chapter 1*).

> Note that bony ankylosis is observed in a sequel of pyogenic arthritis, whereas fibrous ankylosis is observed in tubercular and rheumatoid arthritis.

6. **Measurement:** The length of the limb and muscle girth should be measured in a standard fashion (*Refer to Chapter 1*).
7. **Neurovascular examination:** Generally, the neurovascular examination is normal in joint disorders unless there is a compression over the neurovascular structure due to underlying pathology. However, it is relevant in Charcot's arthropathy.
8. **Special tests, if any:** It has been described in the respective chapters to follow.
9. **Lymph nodes:** Local lymph nodes must be palpated in infective tuberculosis or pyogenic arthritis) or inflammatory conditions (rheumatoid).
10. **Examination of one joint above and below:** It should be evaluated on standard lines.

Various Important Joint Diseases

This section will briefly describe various arthritis and joint diseases. However, many of these conditions are again discussed in specific regions.

1. Primary Degenerative Osteoarthrosis/Osteoarthritis (OA)

- It is a disease of the joints characterized by wear and tear of the articular cartilage followed by osteophyte formation.

- **Affects:** Men and women who are 50 years and above. Weight-bearing joints (knee, hip, and ankle) are more affected than upper limb joints.
- **Risk factors:** Obesity, occupation, habits (squatting, sitting cross-leg), smoking, and positive family history plays an essential role in the development of OA.
- **Presents with:** Mechanical pain in the affected joints with limited movements
- **Clinically:** Three major clinical features are joint line tenderness, crepitus, and limited ROM. Primary OA of a large joint is often associated with Heberden's and Bouchard nodes at DIP and PIP joints of fingers and OA of the 1st carpometacarpal joint.
  Typical OA knee: Genu varum and flexion deformity are common. Pain is felt while walking, stair climbing, squatting, and sitting cross leg and relieves with rest. Always look for Baker's cyst in the popliteal fossa!
- **Investigations:** Plain radiograph of joint—joint space reduction, osteophytes, deformity.
- **Treatment:** Medical management includes analgesics, chondroprotective agents, physiotherapy, braces, intra-articular injections of platelet-rich plasma or hyaluronic acid. *Surgical options* include arthroscopic debridement, arthrodesis, resection arthroplasty, realignment osteotomy, partial or total joint replacement.

2. Acute Septic Arthritis

- Although septic arthritis can affect any joint, the knee and hip are most commonly involved. It is common in children and the elderly. *Always look for the primary focus of infection elsewhere in the body.*
- **Bacteriology:** The most common causative organism is *Staph. aureus*.
- **Presents with:** Acute severe pain, swelling of the joint, and extreme difficulty in moving the joint (pseudoparalysis) along with high-grade fever. Neonates and infants may present with hypothermia, refusal to feed, excessive crying, and failure to thrive.

> **A note on gonococcal arthritis**
> - *Neisseria* gonococci causes gonococcal arthritis in otherwise healthy, sexually active young adults.
> - Associated with arthritis-dermatitis syndrome in approximately 60% of cases, whereas localized septic arthritis in almost 40% of cases.

3. Tuberculosis (TB) of a Joint

- It affects a person of any age. The lower limb and spine are more involved than the upper limb. TB of the shoulder is known as tuberculosis sicca, while TB spine is Pott's spine.

> Note that musculoskeletal TB is almost always secondary to a primary elsewhere (lung, GIT, genitourinary tract, and lymph nodes).

- **Presents with:** Chronic, insidious onset pain, swelling, deformity, and difficulty moving a joint. There may be *night cries, and other constitutional symptoms such as low-grade fever* (evening rise in temperature), night sweats, weight loss, and loss of appetite.
- **Clinically:** Swelling, deformity, muscle wasting, and painfully restricted movement. Cold abscess along with sinuses over the joint may be present. *Special clinical features of different joints (hip, knee, shoulder, and spine) are described in their respective chapters.*

Inflammatory Arthritis

4. Rheumatoid Arthritis (RA)

- Rheumatoid arthritis (RA) is a chronic, systemic, autoimmune, inflammatory disorder of unknown etiology that primarily involves synovial joints.
- **Risk factors:** Typically affects women > men (4:1) in the age group of 20–50 years. Family history is often positive (maternal side).
- **Genetics:** HLADR4+, DR1, DW5
- **Presents with:** Symmetrical polyarthritis (≥ four joints), especially involving small joints of hand and foot along with morning stiffness lasting more than an hour. Later, the disease process may spread to larger peripheral joints.
- **Pathologically:** There are three stages in rheumatoid arthritis: *Stage of synovitis, stage of arthritis, stage of the deformity and fibrous ankylosis.*
- **Clinically:** Typically, wrist, MCP, and PIP joints of the hand and various MTP and PIP joints of the foot are swollen and painful to move. Other joints such as elbow, knee, shoulder, hip, and ankle are often involved. Also, look for rheumatoid nodules over the extensor surface of the forearm. Typically, the spine is not involved except the upper cervical spine (C1-C2) area, where there can be atlantoaxial instability, basilar invagination, and subaxial subluxation.

> *An important note about monoarticular exacerbation in RA:* Any monoarticular exacerbation of pain and swelling in a patient with RA should be taken as septic arthritis unless proved otherwise.

- **The typical features in wrist and hand:** Boutonniere's and swan neck deformity, ulnar deviation of the fingers, Z-deformity of thumb, radial deviation of the wrist, MCP and DRUJ subluxation, trigger finger, and wrist arthritis.
- **The typical features in the foot:** Hallux valgus/varus, mallet and claw toes
- **Knee:** Genu valgus, Windswept deformity
- **Multisystem involvement in RA:** *Lungs* (Caplan's syndrome—pleural effusion, nodules, and bronchiolitis), *abdomen* (Felty's syndrome—splenomegaly with neutropenia), *vasculitis, mononeuritis multiplex, entrapment neuropathy* (carpal tunnel syndrome), and *keratoconjunctivitis sicca*
- **Investigations:** CBP, ESR (raised), CRP (elevated); RA factor, and anti-CCP are positive. Plain radiograph of the joint shows symmetric joint space reduction, periarticular osteopenia **(Figs. 3.9A and B)**, and deformity (late-stage).
- **Treatment:** *Medical management*—physiotherapy, bracing, NSAIDs, DMARDs (methotrexate, hydroxychloroquine, sulphasalazine, leflunomide), and steroids. Biological agents are added in resistant cases.
  Surgical options: Arthroscopic synovectomy, arthrodesis, resection arthroplasty, and total joint replacement.

5. Systemic Lupus Erythematosus (SLE) Related Arthropathy

- SLE is a chronic autoimmune disorder of unknown etiology that leads to the accumulation of autoimmune complexes in joints, skin, kidneys, lungs, heart, blood vessels, and nervous system. It affects women who are 15–45 years old.
- **Clinical features:** Symmetrical polyarthritis of small joints of hand and foot along with malar rashes. Arthritis *is migratory and non-erosive* (c.f. RA, wherein the arthritis is erosive). SLE

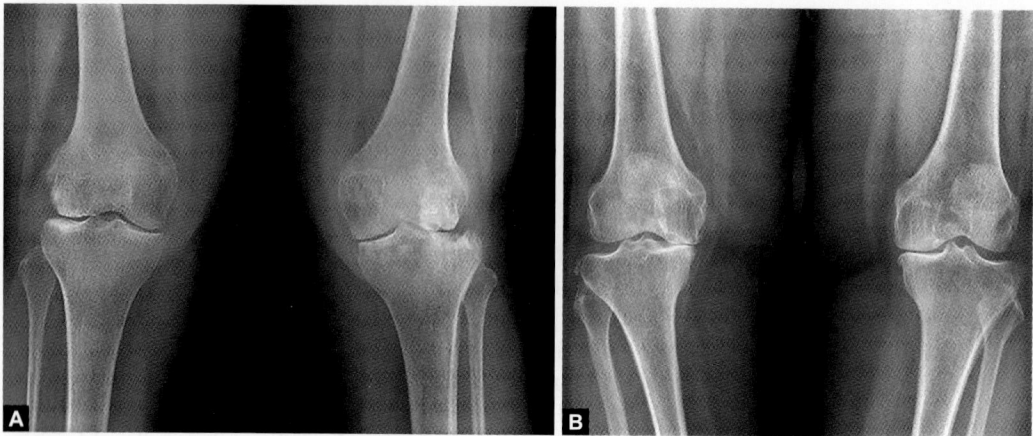

Figs. 3.9A and B: (A) X-ray of a patient with rheumatoid arthritis. Note symmetric reduction in joint space, periarticular osteopenia, bony erosion, valgus deformity, and lack of osteophytes; (B) X-ray of a patient with primary osteoarthritis. Note reduction in medial joint space only, osteophytes, and varus deformity.

deformities are similar to RA but predominantly due to ligament laxity, muscle contracture, and less joint destruction. Renal involvement is common.

6. Seronegative Spondyloarthropathies

The following features characterize these groups of arthritis:
- Male preponderance; age group of 20–40 years
- Usually HLA B27+
- **The pathological hallmark of spondyloarthropathy is "enthesitis."** Enthesitis is characterized by inflammation at the insertion of tendon/fascial/ligament (plantar fasciitis, tendo-Achilles tendinitis, etc.).
- **Important clinical features are:** Involves axial skeleton ± large peripheral joints (hip, shoulder, knee). Typicallly, these patients present with back pain with morning stiffness. The *cardinal feature is sacroiliitis.* Later, there is gradual involvement of lumbar, dorsal, and cervical spine. Peripheral joint involvement is usually oligoarticular and asymmetric. Extra-articular manifestations may be present.

Several important seronegative spondyloarthropathies are briefly discussed below.

A. **Ankylosing spondylitis (Marie–Strumpell disease/Bechterew's disease)**
   - Flagship disease of seronegative spondyloarthropathy
   - *Affects:* Typically affects men between 20–45 years. More common in men : women 2.5:1
   - ***Presents with:*** *Low back pain lasting >2–3 months, pain at rest, morning stiffness, relieves with activity, night pain with paraspinal muscle spasm.*
   - ***Clinically:*** SI Joint tests—tender SI joint, figure-of-four test positive; lumbar spine mobility— *Schober's test positive;* dorsal spine—*Roundback kyphotic deformity;* stiff cervico-dorsal spine—*occiput to wall distance increased; and chest expansion—decreased, < 2–3 cm.*

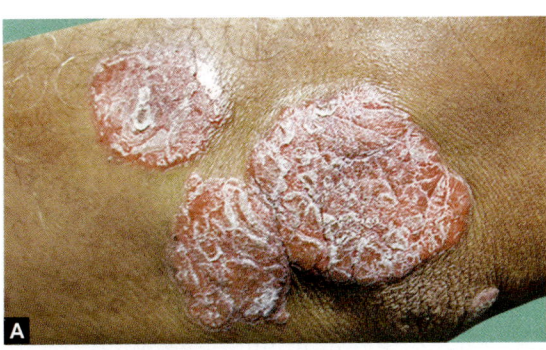 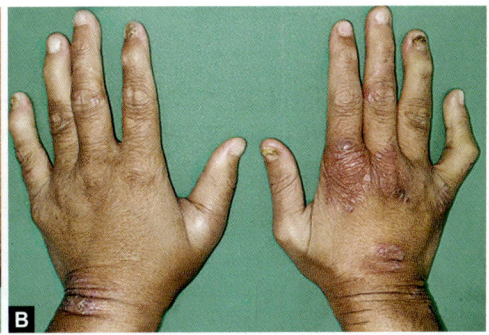

Figs. 3.10A and B: Typical scaly psoriatic lesions over the elbow. DIP involvement of the hand with nail changes.
Image Courtesy: Professor Prateek Gahalaut, SRMSIMS, Bareilly.

- **Extra-articular findings:** *Eyes:* Uveitis and iritis (40%); *Heart:* Cardiac conduction abnormality, aortic stenosis and regurgitation; *Lung:* Pulmonary fibrosis.

B. **Psoriatic arthropathy**
- It is a seronegative spondyloarthropathy characterized by the presence of *psoriasis*, small joint *erosive arthritis* (predominantly DIP joint and sometimes—PIP and MCP), *arthritis mutilans*, and *nail changes*.
- **Genetics:** 50% cases associated with HLA-B27.
- **Presents with:** *Low back pain* with *morning stiffness*. There are *Psoriatic lesions* over the body **(Fig. 3.10A)**. *Small joint of hand arthritis* is common. Commonly DIP is involved followed by PIP and MCP **(Fig. 3.10B)**. *Arthritis Mutilans (opera hand) is seen in severe cases wherein there are* telescoping phalanges due to destroyed IP joints. *Nail changes, such as* pitting, ridging, onychodystrophy, yellow discoloration of margins, subungual hyperkeratosis and onycholysis are also present.

C. **Reactive arthropathy (ReA) or Reiter's syndrome**
- Reactive arthropathy is a type of seronegative spondyloarthropathy, *which develops in response to a gastrointestinal or genitourinary infection* characterized by a classic triad of *non-purulent arthritis, non-gonococcal urethritis*, and *conjunctivitis*.
- **Etiology:** (a) *Bacteria with lipopolysaccharide component in the cell wall* (Chlamydia, Salmonella, Shigella, Campylobacter, Yersinia); (b) HLA-B27+; (c) *Molecular mimicry*.
- **Clinical features:** Males are more prone than females. It is characterized by urethritis, arthritis (asymmetric mono- or oligoarthritis), and conjunctivitis. They also complain of low back pain. *There may be Mucocutaneous lesions*, such as mucosal ulcers in the mouth, keratoderma blennorrhagicum and circinate balanitis.

D. **Enteropathic arthropathy**
- Enteropathic arthropathy is a seronegative spondyloarthropathy in association with inflammatory bowel disease such as ulcerative colitis/Crohn's disease.
- **Etiology:** Genetic predisposition, HLA-B27, Gut microbes
- **Presents with:** *Features of inflammatory bowel disease* (abdominal pain, diarrhea, altered bowel habit, and GI bleed), low back pain with associated morning stiffness, peripheral joint pain, uveitis, and skin lesion (erythema nodosum).

Crystal Arthropathy

7. Gout
- A crystal deposition disease is characterized by acute precipitation of uric acid (UA) crystal (monosodium urate) in the joint, followed by severe pain and swelling.

> *It is important to note that acute gout attacks result from fluctuation in serum uric acid levels rather than merely elevated uric acid levels in the serum.*

- **Typically affects** small joints of the foot, especially 1st MTP joint, ankle, finger, and wrist. (*Note: Pseudogout is observed in older individuals in larger joints*).
- **Risk factors:** *High cell turnover conditions* (malignancy, skin diseases like psoriasis), *poor excretion of UA from kidneys* (renal failure), dietary factors (high seafood intake, meat, alcohol, beer), and drugs (diuretics, aspirin, pyrazinamide).
- **Presents with:**
  a. *Acute gout:* Acute severe pain and swelling of the involved joint, which are extremely painful to move. 1st MTP joint of the foot is most commonly involved (Podagra).
  b. *Chronic gout:* It may present with painful, stiff, and deformed joints with recurrent exacerbation. Typically, Tophi (subcutaneous deposition of UA crystals) is observed over the great toe, ear, and olecranon.

8. Pseudogout
- It is a crystal deposition disease of *larger joints in older individuals* precipitated by deposition of calcium pyrophosphate dihydrate crystals.
- **Presents with:** Acute onset of pain and swelling in a large joint.
- **Clinically:** Swollen, painful, and erythematous joint with excruciating movements. Often, it gives a clinical impression of acute septic arthritis. However, other lab parameters suggestive of septic arthritis are normal.

Neuropathic Arthropathy

9. Charcot's Joint
- Charcot's arthropathy is chronic, progressive, painless destructive arthropathy of the joint due to loss of pain and/proprioceptive sensation.
- **Etiology:**
  - *Diabetes mellitus:* Presently, it is the most common cause of Charcot's arthropathy. Commonly, involves foot and ankle—mid-tarsals, tarsometatarsal, MTP, ankle; *Syringomyelia:* Most common cause in the upper limb (shoulder and elbow);
  - Others: *Hansen's disease, Meningomyelocele,* and *Tabes dorsalis.*
- **Clinical features:** *Painless, progressive massive destruction of the joint is the hallmark of Charcot's arthropathy.* The involved joint undergoes painless, gradually progressive deformity **(Fig. 3.11A)**. There may be trophic ulcers. The movements at the involved joint are exaggerated and painless.
- **Investigations:** Plain X-ray—gross destruction, dislocation of the joint **(Fig. 3.11B)**, joint space reduction, multiple, loose flakes of bone in the soft tissue space, dense-sclerosed bone, and occasional fractures.

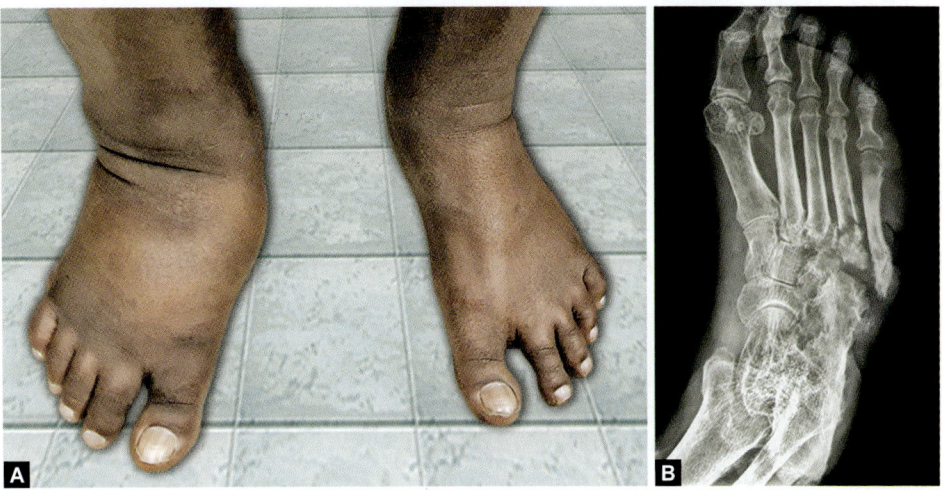

Figs. 3.11A and B: (A) Deformed right foot in Charcot's arthropathy; (B) X-ray of right foot showing destruction of tarsometatarsal joints, pathological fractures, debris and sclerosis.

Metabolic Arthropathy

10. Hemophilic Joint

- Hemophilic arthropathy is characterized by *repeated hemarthrosis and progressive joint degeneration.* It is an X-linked recessive disorder that manifests in males while females are carriers. Young men between 3–15 years are commonly affected. The knee joint is most commonly affected, followed by the elbow, ankle, and shoulder.
- **Genetics and type of hemophilia:**
    a. *Hemophilia A:* X-linked recessive, lack of factor VIII
    b. *Hemophilia B/Christmas disease:* X-linked recessive, lack of factor IX
    c. *Von Willibrand disease*: Autosomal dominant, rare, lack of factor VIII and platelet dysfunction, mostly mucosal bleed.
- **Clinically:** The clinical presentation depends upon the site of the bleeding (joint, muscles, nerves, and cysts). Patient may present with recurrent painful hemarthrosis, bleeding in muscles resulting in contractures, bleeding in nerves resulting in nerve palsy, and hemophilic cyst/pseudotumor formation.

CHAPTER 4

Clinical Evaluation of the Shoulder Joint

SURGICAL ANATOMY AND ITS CLINICAL SIGNIFICANCE

1. **Osteology:**
   - The shoulder joint [glenohumeral joint (GHJ)] is formed by the articulation of the humeral head and the glenoid cavity. However, functionally it is a combination of four joints, namely:
     1. Glenohumeral (GH) joint
     2. Acromioclavicular joint (ACJ)
     3. Sternoclavicular joint (SCJ)
     4. Scapulothoracic joint (STJ)

   > **Note:** A disease or affection at any of the four joints would affect the function of the entire shoulder girdle as there is an interplay between the movements of all the four joints. In addition, STJ is only a physiological and *not* an anatomical joint, as it does not have a synovial cavity.

2. **Functional anatomy of the glenohumeral joint:**
   - *Ligaments:* Three important GH ligaments stabilize the shoulder; superior, middle, and inferior (**Fig. 4.1A**). These three GH ligaments provide anteroinferior stability to the GHJ in different positions of the shoulder (GHJ). Among the three, IGHL is the main stabilizer. *Clinical significance:* During primary or recurrent anterior shoulder dislocation, the IGHL tends to stretch out (plastic deformation) along with a tear in the anteroinferior labrum (Bankart lesion).
   - *Labrum:* It is a circumferential fibrocartilaginous structure circumscribing the glenoid cavity (**Fig. 4.1A**). It deepens the glenoid cavity and creates a *chock-block effect* for stability. *Clinical significance:* A labral tear in shoulder dislocation disrupts the stability.
   - *Capsule:* The capsule of the shoulder is a major stabilizer of the joint. It extends from the *anatomical neck* of the humerus to the border or "rim" of the glenoid fossa. Excess laxity of the capsule could result in multidirectional instability of the shoulder.
   - *Rotator cuff and other surrounding muscles:* The rotator cuff comprises subscapularis, supraspinatus, infraspinatus, and teres minor muscles. The subscapularis is attached to the lesser tuberosity, whereas other three are attached to the greater tuberosity (**Figs. 4.1A and B; Table 4.1**). Apart from moving the shoulder in various directions, the rotator cuff muscles play an important role in dynamically stabilizing the shoulder joint.

   > **Important Note:** The overall function of the rotator cuff (subscapularis, supraspinatus, infraspinatus, and teres minor) is to "centralize the humeral head into the glenoid cavity through a mechanism called concavity compression." A centralized head enables the deltoid to efficiently elevate and abduct the arm, while the head remains centralized in the glenoid during the entire range of motion.

   - *Glenoid:* Glenoid is a pear-shaped part of the scapula that articulates with the head of the humerus. Any alteration in bony conformity of the joint surface, especially the glenoid would result in an unstable joint.

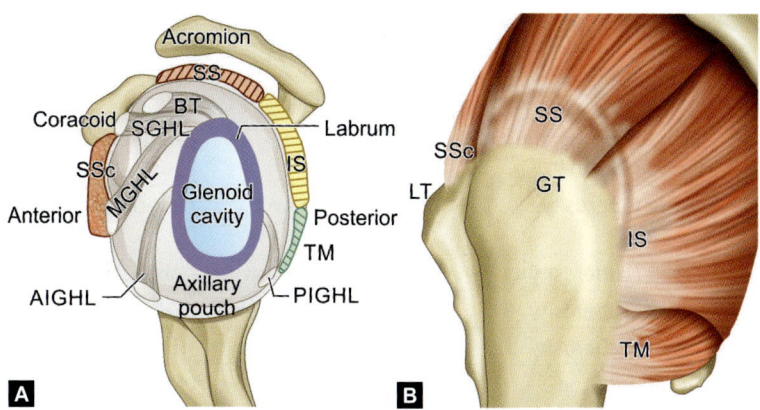

Figs. 4.1A and B: Anatomy of the shoulder joint. (A) Illustrative sagittal figure of the shoulder joint showing muscles and ligaments; (B) Rotator cuff insertion on the humeral tuberosity.

(MGHL: middle glenohumeral ligament; SGHL: superior glenohumeral ligament; SS: supraspinatus; BT: biceps tendon; PIGHL: posterior inferior glenohumeral ligament; TM: teres minor; AIGHL: Anterior inferior glenohumeral ligament; SSc: subscapularis; IS: infraspinatus. GT: greater tuberosity; LT: lesser tuberosity).

3. **Type of joints**
   - *Glenohumeral joint:* Synovial, ball and socket joint
   - *Acromioclavicular and sternoclavicular joint:* Synovial, plane joint
     ♦ Scapulothoracic joint: Not a true joint.
4. **Movements at the glenohumeral joint:** Flexion–extension, abduction–adduction, external, and internal rotation.
5. **Vascularity to the head of the humerus:** The vascular supply to the humeral head is via anterior and posterior circumflex humeral vessels. A comminuted fracture or dislocation of humeral head can jeopardise the circulation, resulting in avascular necrosis of humerus.
6. **Important facts about acromioclavicular joint stability:** The ACJ is stabilized by AC joint capsule and coracoclavicular (CC) ligaments (conoid and trapezoid).
7. **Important muscles around the shoulder (Table 4.1)**
   Before we proceed towards the clinical assessment of the shoulder, it is essential to know various pathological conditions affecting the shoulder and the relevance of age in those conditions as that helps establish a clinical diagnosis. **Boxes 4.1 and 4.2** summarize the common clinical conditions affecting the shoulder and clinical conditions in various age group, respectively.

HISTORY AND ITS EVALUATION

In patients with upper limb complaints, it is essential to ask their occupation and hand dominance as that might play a significant role in etiopathogenesis and management of the disease.

Chief Complaints and History of Present Illness

The patients with shoulder pathology often come up with specific complaints such as:
- Pain
- Difficulty in movement/overhead activities/reaching back
- Subluxation or dislocation

TABLE 4.1: Important muscles around the shoulder joint; their insertion, nerve supply, and action.

Muscle	Insertion	Nerve supply	Principal action at the shoulder joint
Deltoid	Over the upper one-third of the shaft humerus	Axillary nerve	Abductor, flexor, and extensor
Subscapularis	Lesser tuberosity	Upper and lower subscapularis nerve	Internal rotator
Supraspinatus	Greater tuberosity	Suprascapular nerve	Abductor
Infraspinatus	Greater tuberosity	Suprascapular nerve	External rotator
Teres minor	Greater tuberosity	Axillary nerve	External rotator
Latissimus dorsi	The floor of the intertubercular groove of the humerus	Thoracodorsal nerve	Extensor, adductor, and internal rotator
Trapezius	The posterior border of lateral one-third of the clavicle, acromion process, and spine of the scapula	Spinal accessory nerve	Rotation, retraction, elevation, and depression of the scapula
Serratus anterior	The costal aspect of medial margin of the scapula	Long thoracic nerve	Protracts and stabilizes scapula, assists in upward rotation
Pectoralis major	Lateral lip of the bicipital groove	Lateral and medial pectoral nerve	Clavicular head—flexion of humerus Sternocostal head—adduction of the humerus

BOX 4.1: Common conditions affecting the shoulder.

- **Idiopathic:** Primary frozen shoulder (adhesive capsulitis)
- **Degenerative:** *Most common category*
  - Rotator cuff tendinopathy/tendinitis
  - Calcific tendinitis
  - Rotator cuff tear
  - Acromioclavicular arthritis
  - Glenohumeral arthritis
  - Rotator cuff arthropathy
- **Traumatic:** Dislocation, fractures, associated brachial plexus injury, rotator cuff tear
- **Congenital:** Sprengel shoulder, Klippel–Feil syndrome
- **Infections:** Tuberculosis of shoulder (caries sicca), septic arthritis
- **Inflammatory:** Rheumatoid arthritis
- **Metabolic:** Gout, pseudogout, Milwaukee shoulder
- **Neurological:** Charcot's shoulder, brachial plexus palsy, other nerve injuries causing scapular winging
- **Neoplastic:** Benign/malignant tumors

- Cannot throw (overhead) the ball/an object with previous speed
- Catching, locking
- Swelling

> **BOX 4.2:** Common shoulder pathologies in various age groups.
> - **Infants and young ones:**
>   - Sprengel deformity, Klippel–Feil syndrome, and cleidocranial dysostosis
>   - Septic arthritis, osteomyelitis (can occur in older patients too!)
> - **15–35 years:**
>   - Shoulder instability, labral tears
>   - Superior labrum anterior posterior (SLAP) tear
> - **35–55 years:**
>   - Rotator cuff tendinopathy, partial rotator cuff tears
>   - Frozen shoulder
>   - Calcific tendinitis
>   - Acromioclavicular arthritis
> - **>55 years:**
>   - Rotator cuff tear
>   - Glenohumeral arthritis
>   - Rotator cuff arthropathy

Pain

It is the most common complaint, and is consistently observed in almost all shoulder pathologies.

- **Onset:** In most conditions, pain is insidious in onset. However, a few conditions can cause sudden pain such as:
  - **Calcific tendinitis:** It is one of the most common causes of sudden onset pain in the shoulder. The pain is often so severe that it may cause pseudoparalysis of the shoulder.
  - **Traumatic:** Patient gives a history of direct/indirect trauma to the shoulder.
  - Acute infection, acute exacerbation of inflammatory disorder such as rheumatoid arthritis.
- **Timing of pain or diurnal variation:** Although pain is induced during shoulder movements, most patients experience pain specifically at night, especially while attempting to sleep on the affected side. Many patients complain that they have not slept on the affected side for weeks or months.
- **Radiation:** The shoulder pain radiates to the tip of deltoid insertion, and sometimes up to the elbow or the mid-forearm. Rarely, it radiates toward the neck or scapula. *If the pain radiates towards the fingers, the origin of the pain is usually from the cervical spine (intervertebral disc prolapse).* Further, it is essential to note that both left shoulder pain and cardiac pain would radiate towards the left arm, and that must prompt the clinician to rule out an underlying cardiac disorder (history of cardiac disease, shortness of breath, palpitation).
- **Aggravating factor:** Pain in most shoulder conditions is felt at night, while lying on the index side, or during attempted movements. A constant pain may signify infection or a malignant tumor.
- **Relieving factor:** In most degenerative conditions, pain is less during the day-time or by taking analgesics.

Difficulty in Movements

The patients may find difficulty in moving their shoulder because of pain, stiffness, rotator cuff tear, loss of power (nerve paralysis), a dislocated subluxated/ dislocated joint, or a fracture. *(Refer to Chapter 1 for the inability or difficulty in moving a joint)*

Primary or Recurrent Dislocation/Subluxation of the Shoulder

Mostly, in such cases, the patient himself/herself reports history of repeated dislocation or subluxation. The dislocation could result after a traumatic/atraumatic episode. *Traumatic dislocations* are typically associated with structural lesions (labral tear, glenoid bony avulsion, Hill–Sachs lesion). In contrast, *atraumatic dislocations* are often due to muscle imbalance and capsular laxity.

Unable to Throw an Object Overhead

Sometimes, patients (especially overhead athletes) report a difficulty or inability to throw an object overhead (cricket ball from the boundary, Javelin bar) with previous velocity or difficulty in performing a powerful smash while playing badminton or tennis. These complaints are mostly seen in young patients (<40 years), especially those who play overhead sports. The possible causes for such a problem are:
- Superior labral anterior–posterior (SLAP) lesion
- Rotator cuff tears
- Weakness in rotators of the shoulder

Catching or Locking

It might be observed in instability, labral tears, or loose bodies, wherein the shoulder gets temporarily stuck in a particular position, and subsequently gets released during movement.

Swelling

Swelling is not common in degenerative shoulder pathologies. However, it might be observed in acute trauma, infection (septic arthritis, tuberculosis of shoulder), inflammatory disorders or extensive subacromial bursitis.

Occupational History

It is important as people in the different occupations are prone- to-specific shoulder pathologies. For example, workers with overhead activities are more susceptible to rotator cuff pathology; weight lifters often suffer from ACJ arthritis; and those who train hard on the bench press may suffer from labral tears.

Hand Dominance

It is important to know the dominant hand as it may influence decision making in treatment and rehabilitation. It also affects the kinematics of the shoulder.

Pain from Neighboring Areas Mimicking Shoulder Pain

Pathologies of a neighboring area such as neck, chest, and heart can also mimic shoulder pain. Rarely, diseased distant organs such as gallbladder, liver, and spleen can also add to the conundrum. Among all the neighboring areas, pain from the neck most frequently masquerades as shoulder pain, or it is present along with shoulder pain.

History of neck pain: While assessing the shoulder pain, the history should always include queries regarding complaints of neck pain, such as pain originating from the neck and radiating towards the shoulder and scapula. Note that cervical radiculopathy can be confused with any shoulder pathology. However, the site of shoulder and neck pain are pointed in a different location by the patient. A patient with neck pain keeps his hand over the nape of the neck or the medial border of the scapula, whereas the patient with shoulder pain keeps his hand over/

around the shoulder or at the deltoid tip. Further, shoulder pain usually does not radiate below the elbow. Nevertheless, one must note that shoulder and neck pathologies often co-exist, and diagnosis and treatment of both are essential for complete relief.

Cardiac origin pain: One must not forget that cardiac origin pain can radiate to the left shoulder giving rise to confusion in the diagnosis. However, cardiac pain is usually an exertional pain, which may be associated with dyspnea, sweating and palpitation. The patient may also have a history of pre-existing cardiac disease.

Chest pain: Occasionally, chest pain due to Tietze's disease or costochondritis can radiate towards the shoulder and arm, and the patient may perceive it as it is arising from the shoulder.

> Costochondritis is more frequent (than Tietze's disease), occurs in patients older than 40 years, is common in patients who perform repetitive and is characterized by tenderness over the costochondral junction of 2nd to 5th ribs. In contrast, Tietze's disease is rare, sudden in onset, present in patients younger than 40 years, and characterized by swelling and tenderness of the costochondral junction of the 2nd and 3rd rib.

Sub-diaphragmatic pathologies: Rarely, chronic liver disease, gallbladder, and splenic affections could result in referred pain over the shoulder.

Past History

Apart from all other comorbidities, the history of *"diabetes and thyroid dysfunction"* is most important in painful conditions of the shoulder. There is a strong association between frozen shoulder and these two diseases. Also, *epileptics* are more prone to primary/recurrent shoulder dislocations.

Personal, Treatment, Family, Menstrual, and Allergy History

It should be evaluated as per the standard protocol.

At the end of history assessment, many common clinical conditions can be reasonably diagnosed based upon a combination of age and other key complaints. **Table 4.2** summarizes the important snippets for the clinical diagnosis of common shoulder pathologies. However, all of them require confirmation with relevant tests.

EXAMINATION

General and Systemic Examination
As per the standard protocol.

Local Examination
After obtaining consent and ensuring privacy, one must provide a chaperone for the patients, especially vulnerable groups (children and elderly), and a female nurse while examining a female patient. The local examination must be performed after exposing the upper half of the body (adequately covered private parts in females).

Attitude

The shoulder is examined in sitting, standing, and sometimes supine position. The attitude of the index shoulder and upper limb should be described in a standard fashion. For example, the patient is sitting on a stool with right shoulder drooped, arm adducted and internally rotated, elbow flexed, forearm mid-prone, and wrist in neutral.

TABLE 4.2: Shoulder clinical diagnostic snippets.
- Think of **dislocations and labral pathologies in young patients** (15–30 years)
- Think of **rotator cuff tendinopathy and frozen shoulder** in middle age (35–55 years)
- Think of **rotator cuff tear in older age** (55 year onwards)
- Think of **glenohumeral osteoarthritis and cuff arthropathy** in elderly (>65–70 years) with complaints lasting for several years

Symptoms and sign	Most likely pathology/diagnosis
A 52-year-old clerk was referred to orthopaedics for 'evaluation of shoulder pain.' While talking to the patient, the clinician noticed that patient was keeping his hand over the neck, nape and over the scapula to describe his pain	*First rule out cervical causes of pain!* (Spondylitis/intervertebral disc prolapse) Cervical spine pathologies are quite common his in middle and older age individuals, and masquerade as shoulder pain
Most patients with recurrent dislocation tell the clinician that they have been dislocating their shoulders. The clinician has to confirm the diagnosis	*Recurrent dislocation shoulder* Beware of a self-dislocator—it is habitual dislocation!
A 46-year-old male with diabetes/hypothyroidism presents with increasing pain and stiffness in the right shoulder, unable to sleep on the affected side for eight weeks. There is a restriction in both active and passive movements	*Frozen shoulder* Note that many patients are first time diagnosed with DM/thyroid dysfunction in orthopedic OPD after they present with frozen shoulder
A 42-year-old carpenter complained of right shoulder pain during work and night while sleeping on the affected side for six months. Flexion–abduction ROM is terminally painful, while cuff strength is normal	*Rotator cuff tendinopathy*
A 49-year-old female presented with 'atraumatic' acute severe onset of pain in her right shoulder for two days making her shoulder almost paralyzed. She does not allow even the slightest movement	*Calcific tendinitis:* It is the most painful atraumatic condition in an acute setting. History is usually of few days to a week!
A 55-year-old male presents with the inability to actively elevate his shoulder following a fall (low-velocity injury) or a significant jerk while cutting a tree branch. However, his passive ROM is full	*Rotator cuff tear* Note: Rule out brachial plexus injury in high velocity injury
A 75-year-old male presents with increasing pain and stiffness in his left shoulder for two to three years. Both active and passive ROM are limited, and crepitus is felt	*Glenohumeral arthritis*

Inspection

General Findings

Swelling, scar, and sinus should be described in a standard fashion.

Specific Findings

a. **From front:** Look for contour and level of the shoulder, swelling, and Popeye sign.
   - **Shoulder contour:** The normal contour of the shoulder is maintained by the bulk of the deltoid muscle and underlying head of the humerus **(Fig. 4.2)**. A dislocated head of the humerus or the deltoid wasting (due to nerve palsy, multiple surgeries) will cause loss of shoulder contour **(Figs. 4.3 and 4.4A)**.

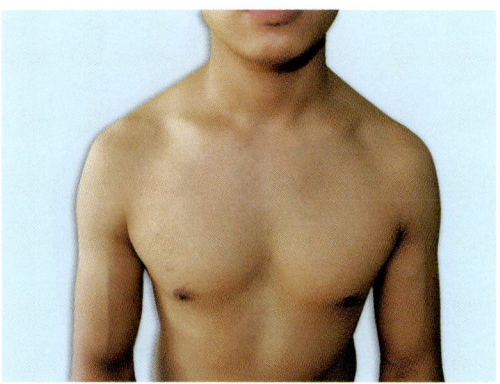

Fig. 4.2: Normal shoulder appearance with well-maintained contour noted from the front.

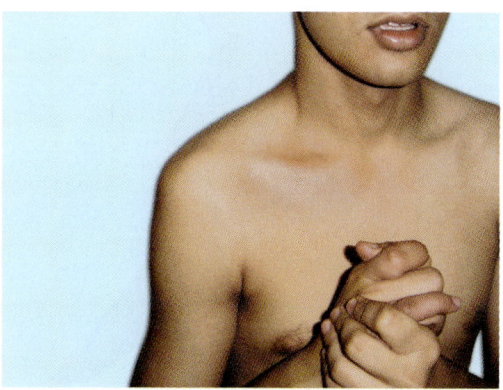

Fig. 4.3: Loss of right shoulder contour due to anterior dislocation of the shoulder.

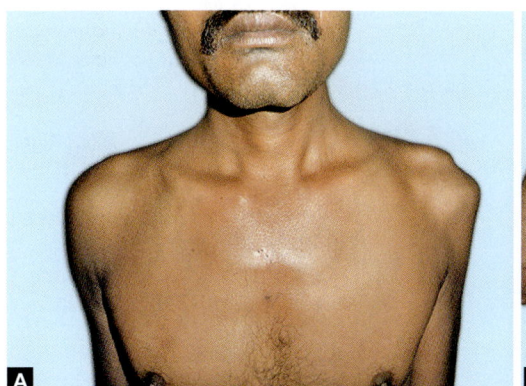
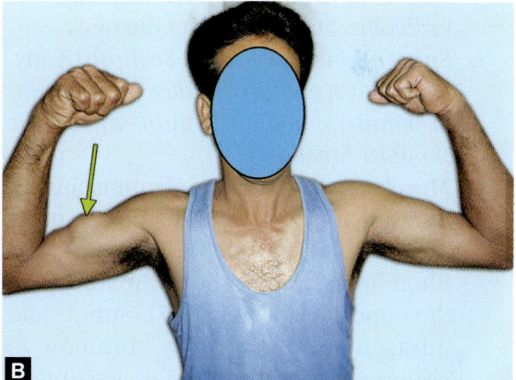

Figs. 4.4A and B: (A) Loss of left shoulder contour due to deltoid wasting; (B) Popeye sign over the right arm (green arrow).

- The ***level of the shoulder*** (drooped/elevated/same level) must be noted.
- The ***swelling or prominence*** of the SCJ, ACJ, and clavicle must be noted. Any bony deformity over the clavicle may indicate malunion or nonunion of clavicle. A prominent medial/lateral end of the clavicle could be due to a fracture, while a prominent ACJ/SCJ could be due to joint dislocation.
- ***Popeye sign:*** The mid- or lower-third of the arm may show a small bulge that increases in size when the elbow is flexed, indicative of rupture of long head of biceps **(Fig. 4.4B)**. It is often associated with rotator cuff tear, especially subscapularis tears.

b. **From the side:** Inspect shoulder and neck from the side, and look for any other obvious findings **(Fig. 4.5)**. For example, a surgical scar in the posterior triangle of the neck could indicate injury to the spinal accessory nerve resulting in trapezius palsy, which may explain shoulder abduction weakness.

c. **From the back (Fig. 4.6):** From behind, four important areas are inspected; *Neck,* rest of the *spine, muscle wasting* over and around the scapula, and *scapular alignment.*

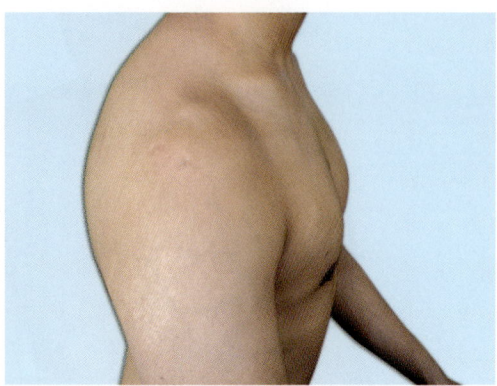

Fig. 4.5: Shoulder appearance from the side.

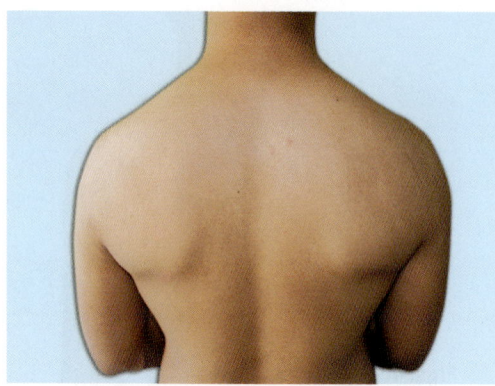

Fig. 4.6: Normal appearance of neck, shoulder, spine, and scapulae from the back.

- **Neck:** Hairline (low/normal), any tilt/torticollis, and webbing of the neck.
- **Spine and its curvature:** *Scoliosis*, if any. Note that *scoliosis can alter the scapular kinematics, which would affect the shoulder function.*
- **Muscle wasting:** Wasting of supraspinatus, infraspinatus, posterior deltoid, or other periscapular muscles (Trapezius and Rhomboids) should be compared from the opposite side (**Fig. 4.7**). Supra- and infraspinatus wasting is common in chronic cuff tear, whereas wasting of muscles, such as trapezius, deltoid, and other shoulder girdle muscles is observed in nerve palsies involving the cervical spine or brachial plexus.

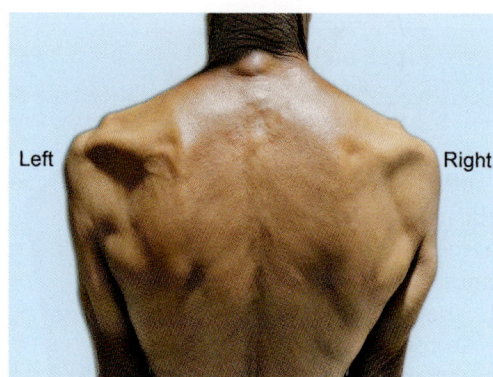

Fig. 4.7: Muscle wasting of supra- and infraspinatus of both sides (left more than right).

Winged scapula: In a 'winged' scapula, the medial (or in some cases, lateral) border of the scapula appears to be protruding from the back, like wings. Various neurological and musculoskeletal conditions can result in winging of scapula, which disturbs scapulohumeral rhythm; contributes to loss of power and limited motion (flexion and abduction) of the shoulder, and can be a source of shoulder pain.

- **Scapula:** Compare with the contralateral scapula and observe for level of superior and inferior angles, shape, and winging.
  - *Level of superior and inferior angle of the scapula:* Normally, the superior and inferior angles of the scapula lie at the level of the spinous process of the D2/D3 and D7/D8 vertebra, respectively. A high or low level of the scapular angles must be noted in winging, Klippel-Feil syndrome, and malunited scapula fracture (**Fig. 4.8A**).
  - *Shape of scapula:* Small or normal. It is small in Klippel-Feil syndrome, and Sprengel deformity (**Fig. 4.8B**).

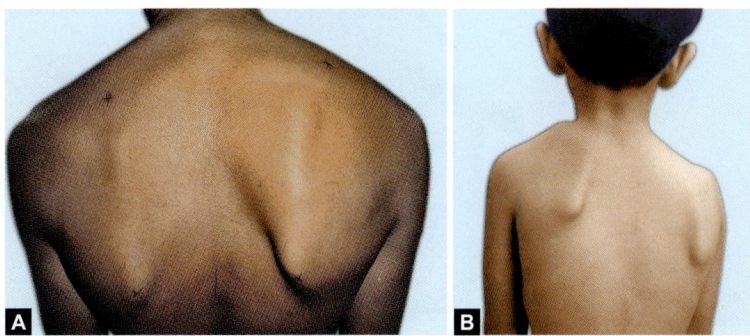

Figs. 4.8A and B: (A) Right scapular angles appear slightly higher than left; (B) Sprengel shoulder: Left scapula is higher and smaller in comparison to the right.

- *Winging of the scapula:* It is always pathological. One must note the type of winging, lateral or medial.
  Inferior and lateral winging: Observed in *trapezius palsy* due to loss of superomedial pull of the scapula by the trapezius.
  Superior and medial winging: Observed in *serratus anterior palsy* due to loss of anterior pull of the scapula by the serratus anterior.

Palpation

The palpation must assess local temperature, tenderness over various important bony and soft tissue landmarks, joint lines, and tissue laxity using Beighton score. Palpation of scar, swelling, sinus should be in standard fashion.

1. **The local rise in temperature:** Palpate by the dorsum of the hand over both the shoulders to compare for any rise in local temperature. It is raised in infections, inflammatory arthritis, tumors, and large subacromial bursitis.
2. **Tenderness:** Always palpate in a sequence to feel for tenderness over major soft tissue, bony landmarks, and joint lines. An appropriate sequence of palpation is mentioned below and shown in **Figures 4.9A to C**.

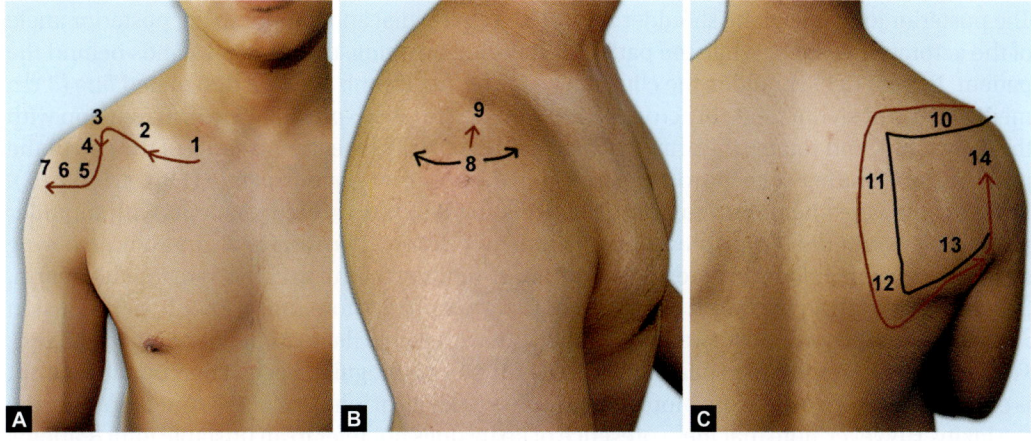

Figs. 4.9A to C: Palpation sequence for important bony landmarks of the shoulder. (A) Anterior aspect; (B) Lateral aspect; (C) Posterior aspect of the shoulder.

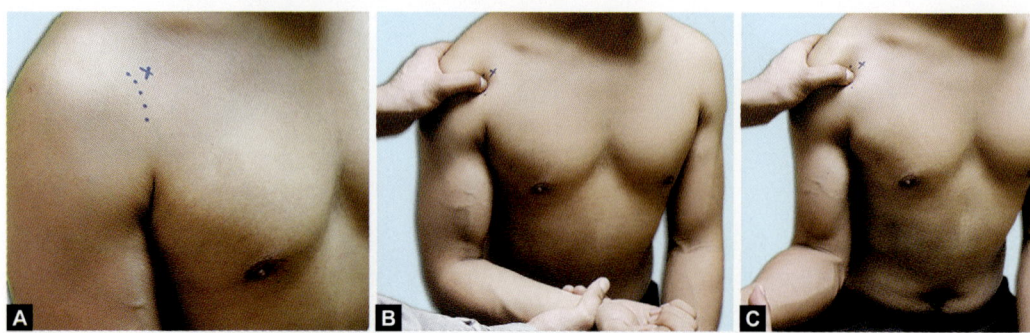

Figs. 4.10A to C: Palpation technique of the anterior joint line. (A) X mark over shoulder denotes coracoid process and dashed line represents anterior joint line; (B) With thumb over joint line, shoulder in internal rotation; (C) With thumb over joint line, shoulder in external rotation.

- *Sternoclavicular joint* (1), *Clavicle* (2), *Acromioclavicular joint* (3), *Coracoid process* (4), It is felt just below the lateral third of the clavicle. *Anterior joint line* (5), *Lesser tuberosity* (6), It is just lateral to the anterior joint line, *Bicipital groove* (7), Bicipital groove lies just lateral to the lesser tuberosity, wherein the bicipital tendon can be palpated; *Greater tuberosity* (8), It is lateral to the bicipital groove and occupies the entire lateral aspect of the top of the humerus. *Acromion* (9), *The spine of the scapula* (10), *Medial border of the scapula* (11), *Inferior angle of the scapula* (12), *Lateral border of the scapula* (13), and *Posterior joint line* (14). These various anatomical landmarks are tender in infections, fracture, and arthritis.

Method to Palpate Anterior Shoulder Joint Line

The joint line examination is done while patient is standing or sitting. The anterior GHJ line is just lateral to the coracoid process. For the right shoulder; the clinician keeps his left thumb just lateral to the tip of the coracoid process while the right hand holds the elbow and the proximal part of the forearm to rotate the arm internally and externally. The thumb can feel the gap of the anterior joint line between the rotating head and the anterior glenoid margin **(Figs. 4.10A to C)**.

Method to Palpate Posterior Shoulder Joint Line

The posterior joint line of the shoulder is located 3 cm medial and inferior to the posterior angle of the acromion process. While the patient is standing or sitting, the clinician stands behind the patient. For the right shoulder, the clinician keeps his left thumb over the designated line (3 cm medial to the posterior angle of acromion) and holds the elbow-proximal forearm junction with the right hand, and rotates the arm internally and externally. The thumb can feel the gap of the posterior joint line between the rotating head and the posterior glenoid margin **(Figs. 4.11A to C)**.

One must assess **ligament/soft tissue laxity** using **Beighton score** in patients with shoulder pathology, *especially if they present with recurrent dislocation.* This is a nine point scoring system assessing 1) elbow hyperextension >100, 2) bending thumb backwards to touch forearm, 3) bending little finger backward by 90° so that it stays parallel to forearm, 4) knee hyperextension >10°, and 5) ability to bend forward and touch foot with palms flat (without bending the knees). First four points are assessed bilaterally while fifth point is singular. Each action possible or not is equal to score of 0 or 1. Score more than 4 indicates laxity of joints. Higher is the score, more is the laxity. However, note that mere presence of laxity does not refer to an unstable joint. Patients who have instability can have higher laxity, but not all lax patients will be unstable.

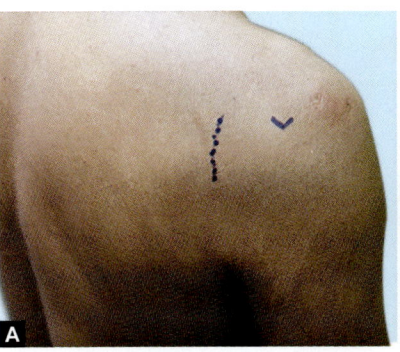 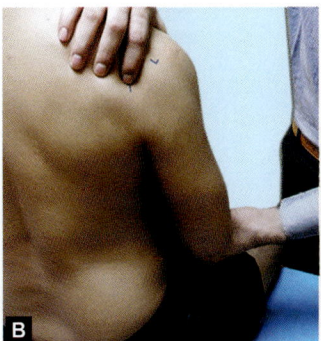 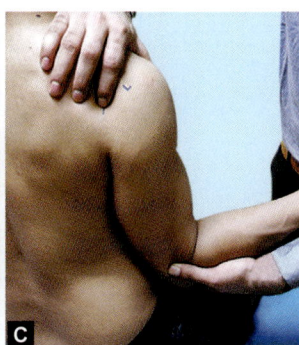

Figs. 4.11A to C: Palpation technique of the posterior joint line. (A) V mark denotes posterior acromion angle and dashed line represents posterior joint line; (B) With finger over joint line, shoulder in internal rotation; (C) With finger over joint line, shoulder in external rotation. (For clarity in picture, the clinician is standing in front of the patient and finger is kept over the joint line and not the thumb).

Movements

The shoulder (GHJ) is a ball and socket joint with movement possible in all three planes: *flexion–extension, abduction–adduction, and external–internal rotation* **(Figs. 4.12A to F)**. The normal range of movement (ROM) of the shoulder joint (GH) is mentioned in **Box 4.3**. One must follow undermentioned specific rules while assessing ROM of the shoulder.
  i. Always assess the normal side first for active ROM, followed by the index side.
  ii. Always assess the active followed by passive ROM. The assessment of active and passive ROM can give a clue to the possible diagnosis **(Box 4.4)**.
  iii. The crepitus can be assessed during passive ROM of the affected shoulder by keeping the hand over the shoulder.

However, before the passive ROM of the shoulder is performed, one must understand two important concepts:
1. During the shoulder movement at the GHJ, especially flexion and abduction, there is always concomitant movement at the scapulothoracic joint (STJ). Therefore, to assess the actual GHJ passive movements, the clinician must prevent the movement at the STJ by firmly keeping the hand over the scapula **(Figs. 4.13A and B)**. However, after 90° of flexion or abduction, the STJ movement cannot be prevented any further, and the scapula starts moving. Note that STJ movement interplays with GH movement in the ratio of 1:2 (30° of ST ROM to 60° of GH ROM). *Failure to obliterate STJ movement results in an erroneous assessment of actual GHJ ROM.*
2. Shoulder abduction is elicited in the plane of the scapula, whereas shoulder flexion-extension is elicited in the plane perpendicular to the scapula. The scapular plane lies 30° anterior to the coronal plane of the body as the scapula is tilted 30° forward over the rib cage. Hence, ideally, *flexion-extension is performed perpendicular to the scapular plane, which is 30° medial to the sagittal plane of the body, whereas abduction is performed in the plane of the scapula that is 30° anterior to the coronal plane of the body.*

Note: *Pseudopalsy* term frequently used in shoulder that implies that 'active forward elevation is less than 45-90°.' It is seen in rotator cuff tears or severe painful conditions.

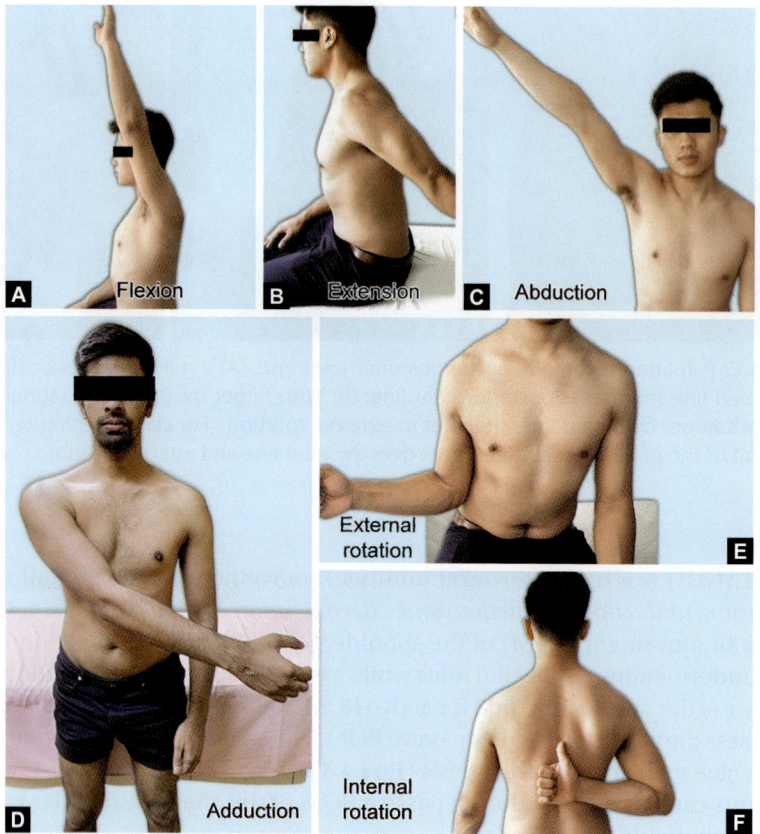

Figs. 4.12A to F: Demonstration of active ROM at the shoulder joint. (A and B) Flexion–extension; (C and D) Abduction and adduction; (E and F) External and internal ROM at the shoulder joint.

> **BOX 4.3:** Normal range of movement (ROM) at the shoulder joint.
>
> - **Flexion:** 0–180°
> - **Extension:** 0–60°
> - **Abduction:** 0–180°
> - **Adduction** *(across the body in front of the chest in coronal/frontal plane)*: 0–60°
> - **External rotation** *(with the arm adducted to the chest wall)*: 0–70°
> - **Internal rotation:** Patient is asked to place their thumb as high as possible over the spinous process of the vertebra. Usually, thumb reaches up to D6/D7 vertebra spinous process, and sometimes, up to spinous process of D3. *Note that internal rotation is clinically measured as 'where the tip of the thumb reaches with respect to a landmark' on spine (vertebra), PSIS, gluteal region, and greater trochanter.*

> **BOX 4.4:** Assessment of ROM can give a clue to the diagnosis.
>
> - **Restriction of only active ROM:** Rotator cuff tear, nerve injury (brachial plexus, axillary nerve)
> - **Gross restriction of both active and passive ROM:** Frozen shoulder, glenohumeral arthritis, and dislocated joint
> - **Terminal painful restriction of both active and passive ROM:** Rotator cuff tendinopathy, impingement syndrome, and subacromial bursitis
> - **Painful movements (active/passive) in the mid-abduction arc of 60–120°:** Painful arc syndrome

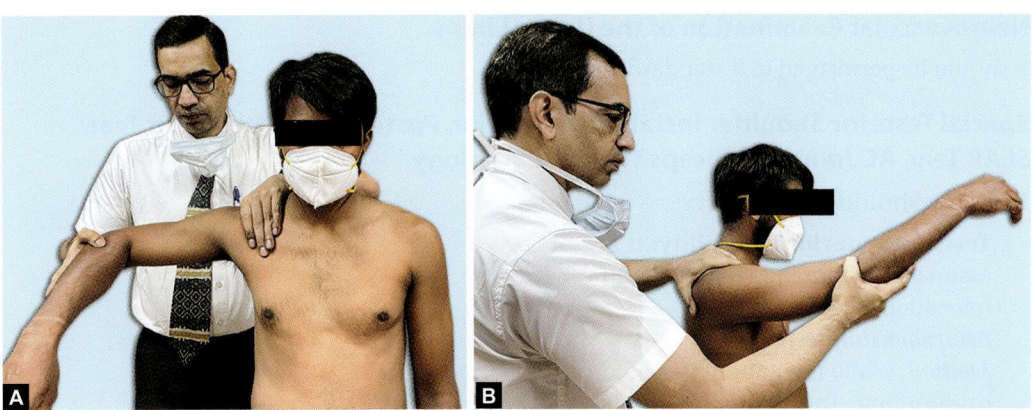

Figs. 4.13A and B: Assessment of passive ROM of the shoulder after stabilizing the scapula. (A) Abduction; (B) Flexion.

Measurements

The measurements of both upper limbs (limb length and circumference) are performed for comparison.
- **"The arm length"** is measured from the anterolateral angle of the acromion to the lateral epicondyle **(Fig. 4.14A)**.
- **"Forearm length"** is measured from the lateral epicondyle to the tip of the radial styloid process **(Fig. 4.14B)**.
- **"Measure the arm and forearm circumference for muscle bulk":** In an adult, arm and forearm circumferences should be measured 10 cm above and below the tip of the olecranon, respectively, on both sides for comparison. Alternately, it could be measured in the area of maximum girth of the arm and forearm.

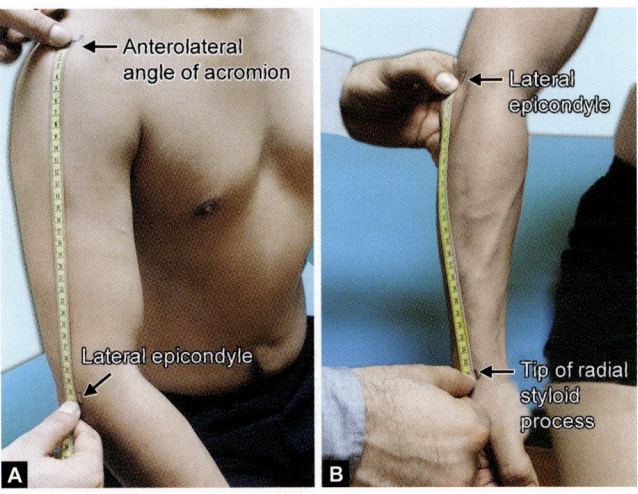

Figs. 4.14A and B: Upper limb length measurement. (A) Arm length measurement; (B) Forearm length measurement.

Neurovascular Examination of the Upper Limbs
It should be performed in a standard fashion.

Special Tests for Shoulder Instability (Anterior, Posterior), Rotator Cuff Tear, SLAP Tear, AC Joint and Biceps Tendon Pathology

Tests for Shoulder Instability

i. **Tests for anterior instability:** It is assessed by apprehension test and relocation-release test.

   Apprehension test:
   Method: While the patient is seated or standing, the clinician stands behind the patient's index shoulder. For the right side, the shoulder is gradually brought in 90° abduction and 90° external rotation by the clinician's right hand holding the elbow-forearm junction (which can further rotate the arm externally). The fingers of clinician's left hand are kept in front of the anterior joint line of the shoulder, while the thumb is kept over the posterior part of the humeral head. Then, the head is gently pushed anteriorly by the left thumb over the glenoid cavity, while other hand gently further externally rotates the arm **(Fig. 4.15)**. The fingers in front of the shoulder prevent excess anterior movement of the humeral head or a possible anterior dislocation.

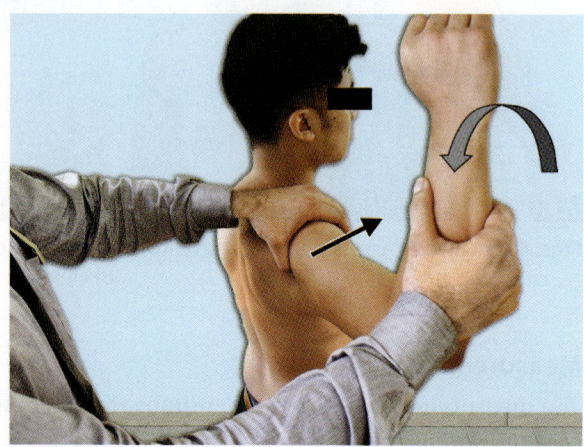

Fig. 4.15: Apprehension test (Black arrow indicates anterior thrust given to the humeral head by the thumb while curved arrow indicates external rotation of the arm).

   Interpretation: Apprehension, fear, or refusal to continue the maneuver by the patient is indicative of chronic anterior instability.

   Others tests for anterior instability are *relocation-release, Gagey's hyperabduction, and anterior drawer test*: Watch video for relocation-release test as it is one of the frequently performed test. The details of other tests are out of scope of this chapter for undergraduates.

ii. **Tests for posterior instability:** It is assessed by Jerk test.

   Jerk test
   Method: With the patient preferably sitting, the clinician stands in front or side of the patient. While stabilizing the scapula with one hand, the index arm is brought in 90° abduction, internal rotation, and *axially loaded toward the glenoid fossa* **(Fig. 4.16A)**. The arm is gradually adducted towards the horizontal plane, which may subluxate or dislocate the head posteriorly with a jerk in case of chronic posterior instability **(Fig. 4.16B)**. Again, taking the arm back to the plane of the scapula reduces the head with another jerk. This maneuver is repeated several times.

   Interpretation: In posteriorly unstable shoulder (due to capsulolabral tear and/or glenoid bone defect), the axially loaded posteriorly directed force subluxates or dislocates the head posteriorly, which reduces with a jerk when the arm is brought back in the scapular plane.

Tests for Impingement and Subacromial Bursitis

Impingement implies that the subacromial structures (rotator cuff and subacromial bursa) between greater and lesser tuberosity and acromial arch gets impinged/nipped during forward

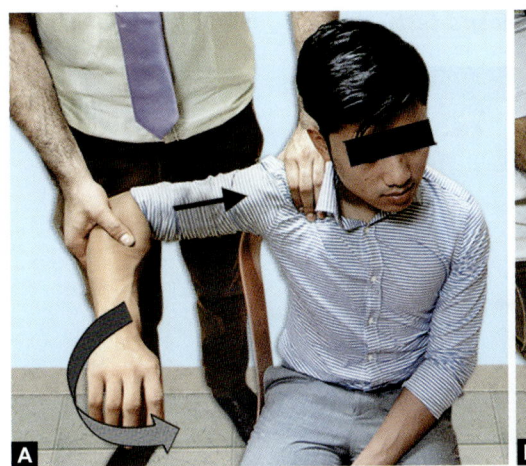
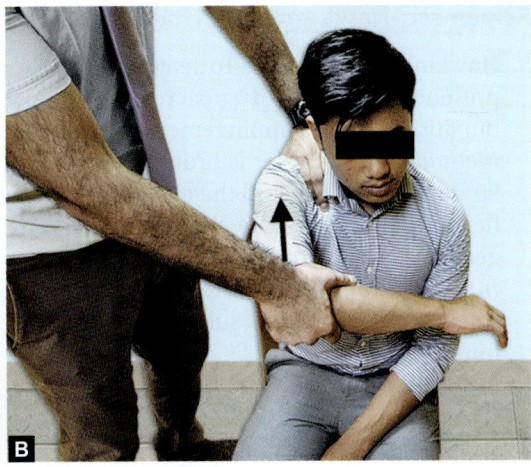

Figs. 4.16A and B: Jerk test. (A) An abducted, internally rotated (curved arrow) and axially loaded arm towards the glenoid (black arrow); (B) Internally rotated arm is gradually adducted in the frontal plane with maintained axial load, and with posteriorly directed force.

flexion or abduction. It occurs either due to narrowed subacromial space or thickened structures of the SA space.

Therefore, impingement indicates underlying pathology, such as rotator cuff tear/tendinopathy, subacromial bursitis, calcific tendinitis, mal- or non-united tuberosity fractures, or a frozen shoulder. Isolated impingement is uncommon, and one must assess the reason behind the underlying impingement.

1. **Neer's impingement sign:** To test impingement in the subacromial space.
   Method and interpretation: With the patient in supine/sitting/standing, a normal shoulder can be gradually forward flexed till 180° without pain **(Fig. 4.17)**. In the case of structural subacromial impingement, the patient would complain of pain usually after 140–150° of flexion.
2. **Neer's impingement test:** It is performed to differentiate between the pain arising from an impingement in the subacromial space or from the structures in the vicinity as the latter might mimic pain due to impingement from subacromial space.
   Method: First, inject 2–5 mL of 2% xylocaine into the index subacromial space. A few minutes later, perform Neer's sign.
   Interpretation: A negative Neer sign implies that the pain was due to the impingement of structures in the subacromial space. If Neer's sign is still positive, it implies that the source of the pain is not in the subacromial space. Reduction in pain/symptoms during post-injection Neer's sign implies that there is a source from subacromial space and elsewhere as well.

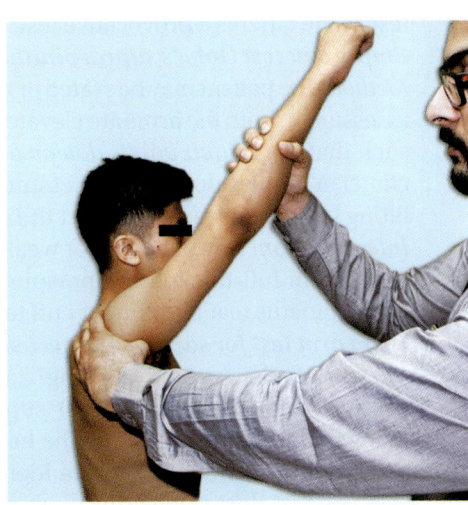

Fig. 4.17: Neer's sign.

==Remember:== *Neer's sign is performed before Neer's test.*

3. **Hawkins-Kennedy test:** To detect the presence or absence of "subacromial bursitis" as well as impingement.
   Method: The shoulder is brought to 90° forward flexion and the elbow is flexed to 90°. Then, the shoulder is gently internally rotated **(Fig. 4.18)**.
   Interpretation: Pain in the internal rotation is suggestive of subacromial bursitis.

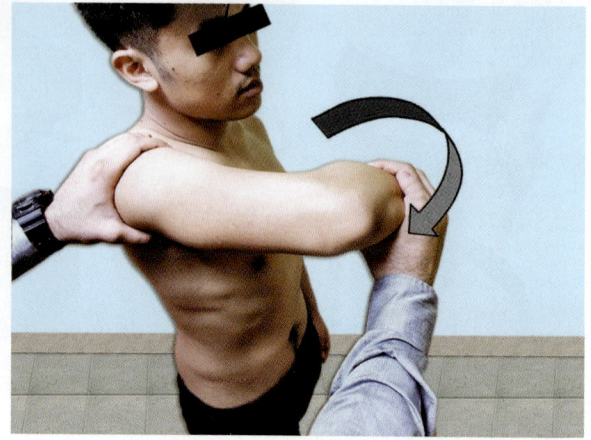

Fig. 4.18: Hawkin's sign. Gray curved arrow signifies internal rotation of the arm.

Tests for Rotator Cuff Tear

Typically, all the cuff tests are performed in standing or sitting. Further, the tests performed are comparative in terms of pain, strength or lag, presuming that the contralateral shoulder is normal.

i. **Supraspinatus tear:** The integrity of the supraspinatus tendon can be assessed with full can, empty can, and drop arm test.
   1. *Full can test*
      Method: While the patient is seated or standing, the clinician stands in front of the patient. For comparative assessment, both the arms are elevated 60–70° in the scapular plane and externally rotated such that the *thumb points upward* (like holding a full can of cola). Then, the clinician applies a downward pressure just above the wrist while the patient resists it by lifting his arm upward to abduct the shoulder **(Fig. 4.19A)**.
      Interpretation: Weakness in abduction strength with/without pain suggests the supraspinatus tear.
      Further, *if the full can test is painful and weak,* there is no need to repeat the empty can test as the latter is a provocative test.
   2. *Empty can test (Jobe's supraspinatus test)*
      Method: The patient may be seated or allowed to stand as per convenience. For comparative assessment, both the arms are elevated 60–70° in the scapular plane and internally rotated such that the *thumb points downward* (as if emptying an entire can of cola). Then, the clinician applies downward pressure just above the wrist while the patient resists it by lifting his arm upward to abduct the shoulder without shrugging it **(Fig. 4.19B)**.
      Interpretation: Any pain and/or weakness in this maneuver suggests supraspinatus tear. Apart from full-thickness supraspinatus tear, empty can test is also positive in partial supraspinatus tear and rotator cuff tendinopathy.
   3. *Drop arm test for supraspinatus tendon tear*
      Method: While a patient is sitting/standing, the clinician stands behind the patient and passively abducts the arm to 180° supporting arm at the elbow. Then, the patient is asked to lower the arm gradually till the hand touches the waist. This test is positive if there is pain while lowering the arm, sudden dropping of the arm, or weakness in maintaining arm position during lowering (with or without pain).

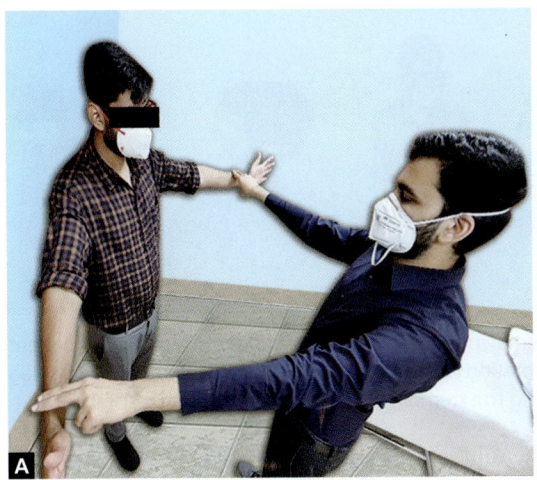
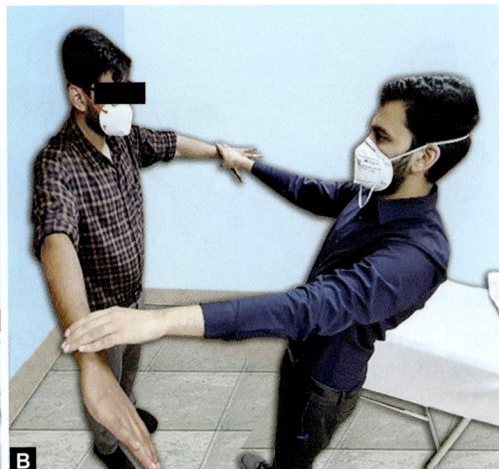

Figs. 4.19A and B: Tests for supraspinatus tendon. (A) Full can test with thumb-pointing upwards; (B) Empty can test with thumb-pointing downwards.

ii. **Infraspinatus tear:** Infraspinatus is an external rotator of the shoulder. Several tests are described for infraspinatus assessment, such as resisted external rotation test (RERT) and external rotation lag test at 20°.
   1. *Resisted external rotation test:* With the patient sitting or standing, the clinician keeps the patient's both arms in 0° abduction and neutral rotation at the shoulder while the elbow is held at 90° flexion. The patient is asked to externally rotate both arms against the resistance applied at the wrist and forearm by the clinician **(Fig. 4.20A)**. A poor resistance offered during RERT indicates infraspinatus tear.
   2. *External rotation lag test at 20°:* With the patient standing or seated, shoulder relaxed, the elbow is passively flexed to 90° and held with one hand of the clinician, and the affected shoulder is moved to 20° abduction in scapular plane by holding near the wrist with another hand **(Fig. 4.20B)**. The patient is then asked to maintain the external rotation position for a minimum of 10 seconds as the clinician releases the wrist. The sign is positive if the arm (indicated by wrist internal movement) falls back by >10° into internal rotation.
   3. *Patte's test:* With patient sitting or standing, abduct the shoulder to 90°, flex the elbow to 90°, and ask patient to externally rotate against resistance (of clinician). A weakness in rotating externally indicates infraspinatus tear.
iii. **Test for teres minor:** Since teres minor is also an external rotator of the shoulder, the tests for teres minor are almost similar to infraspinatus except for Hornblower's test. However, an increasing amount of lag or weakness while performing the tests pushes the interpretation of the test in favor of teres minor tear.
   1. *External rotation lag test at 90° (drop sign):* It is performed similarly as described above for infraspinatus **(Fig. 4.20C)**. However, it is performed in 90° abduction of arm. The sign is positive if the arm falls back by >10° into internal rotation. Larger the internal rotation drop, higher the chance of teres minor tear!
   2. *Hornblower's sign:* With the patient standing and both arms adducted to the chest, patient is asked to gradually bring both hands to the mouth keeping arm close to the chest. This maneuver involves external rotation (ER) at the shoulder. With the weak shoulder ER, any

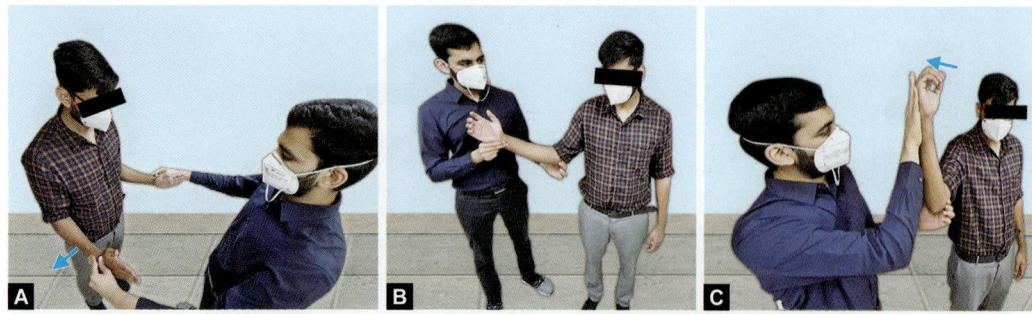

Figs. 4.20A to C: Tests for infraspinatus tendon. (A) External rotation resistance test (Blue arrow indicates patient resisting clinician's internal rotation force; (B) External rotation lag test at 20° abduction; (C) External rotation lag test at 90° abduction (Blue arrow indicates patient trying to externally rotate against clinician's resistance).

attempt to bring hand close to the mouth would require shoulder shrugging (which would elevate patient's elbow) and increased wrist extension **(Fig. 4.21)**. The elevated position of the elbow and extended wrist near mouth gives an appearance of 'blowing a horn'.

iv. **Subscapularis tear:** Subscapularis is an internal rotator, and all the tests described assess internal rotation strength. Two common tests are described below—Gerber's lift off and Belly press test.
  1. *Gerber's lift-off test:* With the patient seated or standing, the clinician asks the patient to bring his/her hand behind the back at the level of the mid-lumbar spine with shoulder extended and internally rotated, and keep the wrist-hand (in neutral of palmar flexion-extension) away from the back as much as possible against clinician's resistance.
     Interpretation: The test is concluded positive if the patient cannot keep his/her wrist-hand (in neutral) away from the mid-lumbar spine and cannot resist the clinician's push toward the back applied over the palm of the patient **(Fig. 4.22)**.

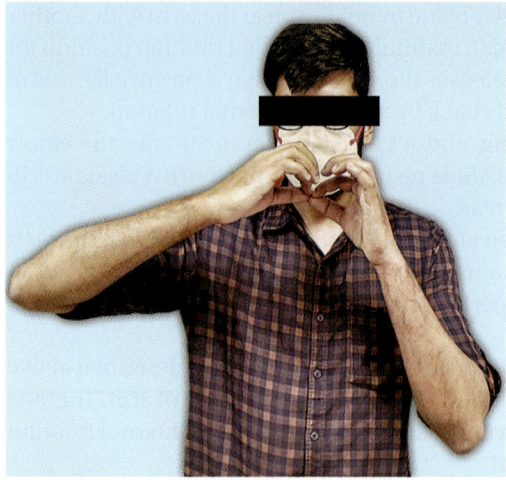

Fig. 4.21: Hornblower's test positive on right side (High elbow position of right side compared to contralateral normal side).

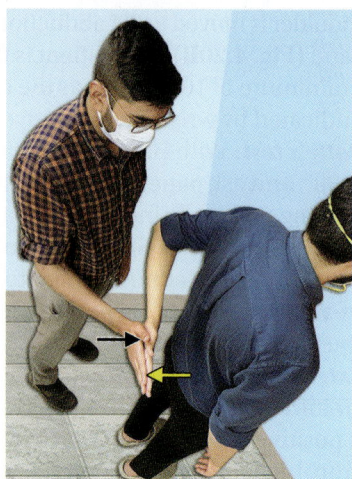

Fig. 4.22: Gerber's lift-off test (Black arrow denotes clinician's resistance while yellow arrow denotes patients effort to lift wrist-hand away from the back).

2. **Belly press (Napoleon) test:** The patient is asked to keep both his/her hands over the belly with the shoulder in maximal internal rotation so that the elbow comes in the line of the wrist-hand plane or ahead of the trunk in the coronal plane of the body. The test is considered positive if the elbow falls behind the wrist-hand plane or trunk. Further, to assess the strength, the clinician should push the elbow posteriorly and ask the patient to resist **(Fig. 4.23)**. In a patient with positive belly press test, the patient cannot resist the posterior elbow push by the clinician.

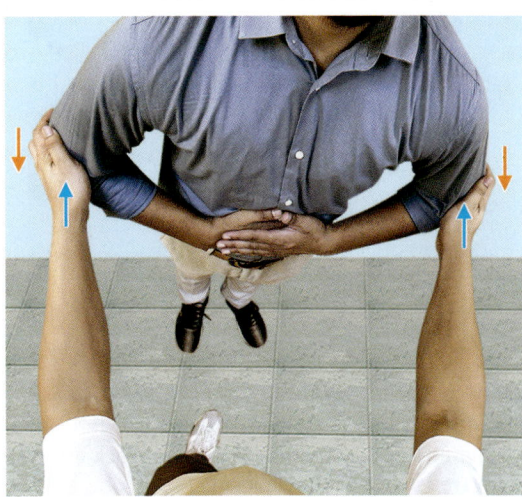

Fig. 4.23: Belly press test.

Tests for Superior Labrum Anterior Posterior (SLAP) Tear

The SLAP tear is characterized by a tear in the superior labrum at the root of the long head of the biceps, which often extends posteriorly and/or anteriorly. SLAP tear is usually observed in athletes or people who either play overhead sports (badminton, tennis, Javelin thrower, volleyball, etc.) or repeatedly perform overhead or throwing activities. Their chief complaint is an inability to throw or smash with 'previous velocity' with or without pain.

Commonly performed test to diagnose SLAP tear is O'Briens test.

O'Brien test

Method: While the patient is standing or supine, the shoulder is brought to 90° forward flexion, horizontally adducted by 10°, and then internally rotated completely so that the thumb points downward. Then the patient is asked to flex his arm upward (blue arrow), while the clinician gives downward resistance at the distal forearm. *It is important that patient should not shrug his shoulder while elevating the arm, which can be prevented by clinician firmly stabilizing the patient's shoulder* **(Fig. 4.24)**. Also, O'Brien is easier to perform in supine as the scapula is stabilized against the couch.

Interpretation: A positive test indicates weakness and/or pain during forward flexion.

Tests for Biceps Tendon Pathology: Bicipital Tendinitis

Speed's test:

Method: While the patient is standing, the shoulder is flexed 90° in the sagittal plane of the body with the forearm in full supination and elbow in extension. Then, the patient is asked to flex the shoulder further, while the clinician gives resistance against flexion over the distal forearm **(Fig. 4.25)** (*Note: The patient should not flex his elbow while elevating the arm*).

Interpretation: Any pain in the bicipital groove or anterior aspect of the arm along the course of the biceps tendon is considered a positive Speed's test.

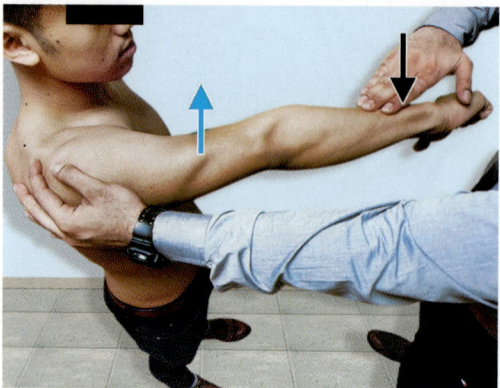 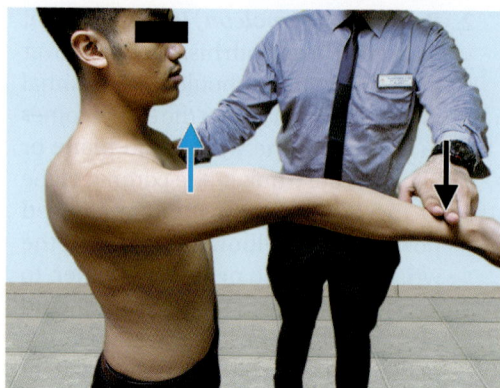

Fig. 4.24: O'Brien test. Blue arrow shows forward flexion attempt by the patient, while black arrow shows resistance by the clinician.

Fig. 4.25: Speed's test. Blue arrow shows forward flexion attempt by the patient, while black arrow shows resistance by the clinician.

Other test to assess biceps affection is *Yergason test*.

Tests for Acromioclavicular Joint Arthritis

1. **Acromioclavicular joint tenderness:** It is a quite sensitive and specific test for acromioclavicular joint (ACJ) arthritis.
   Method and interpretation: Gently palpate ACJ and feel for tenderness. The presence of tenderness over the ACJ indicates ACJ arthritis.
2. **Cross-chest adduction test (Scarf test):**
   Method: While the patient is standing or supine, the elbow is flexed and the shoulder is brought in 90° flexion. The shoulder is horizontally adducted across the chest by pushing the elbow, and the hand is made to cross the opposite shoulder **(Fig. 4.26)**.
   Interpretation: The patient with ACJ arthritis complains of pain over the ACJ area.

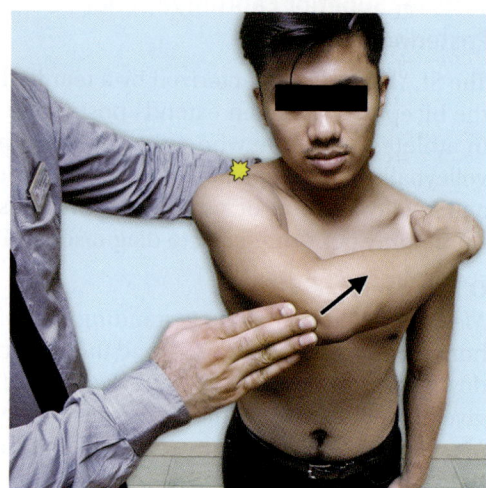

Fig. 4.26: Cross-chest adduction test: Black arrow indicates direction of push to the elbow. Yellow star indicates the site of pain at the AC joint during cross chest adduction.

Examination of the Joint Above and Below

Standard cervical spine and elbow joint examination must be performed in all cases of shoulder pathology. It is essential to examine the cervical spine in patients with shoulder pain as often the pain originating from cervical region can masquerade as pain originating from the shoulder.

Examination of the Lymph Nodes

Examination of lymph nodes of the neck and the axilla should be performed, especially when an infective or tumor pathology is suspected.

Shoulder Examination Proforma

1. **Attitude**
2. **Inspection**
    - *General findings:* All areas for overlying skin, swelling, scar, and sinus.
    - *Specifics findings of the inspection:*
        a. **From front:**
            - Shoulder contour, muscle wasting (deltoid), shoulder drooping, and swelling/prominence of SCJ/ACJ/other areas
        b. **From side:**
            - Shoulder from the lateral aspect
        c. **From back:**
            - Spine and its curvature, any deformity, neck, hairline level, and webbing
            - *Muscle wasting*: Supra- and infraspinatus, deltoid, and other periscapular muscles
            - *Scapula*: Level of scapula, size of scapula, the distance of medial border from the spine, winging
3. **Palpation:**
    - The local rise in temperature
    - *Tenderness*: Soft tissue and bony landmarks, joint line
    - Confirmation of palpatory characteristics of swelling, scar, and sinus
4. **Movements:** Active and passive
    - Flexion–extension, abduction–adduction, external and internal rotation
    - Crepitus, if any
5. **Measurements:** Limb length and arm-forearm circumference
6. **Neurovascular examination**
7. **Special tests:**
    - *Stability tests:* Apprehension test, relocation-release test, Jerk test
    - *Impingement tests:* Neer's sign and Hawkins test
    - *Rotator cuff integrity signs:* Supraspinatus (full can and empty can test), infraspinatus (resisted external rotation test, external rotation lag test at 20°, Patte's test), teres minor (Drop sign, Hornblower sign, external rotation lag test at 90°), subscapularis (Gerber's lift-off, Belly press test)
    - *SLAP tear test:* O'Brien test
    - *Biceps tendon pathology:* Speed's test
    - *ACJ pathology:* ACJ tenderness, cross-chest adduction test
8. **Joint above (cervical spine) and below (elbow)**
9. **Lymph node examination**

Common Conditions Affecting Shoulder and their Salient Features

1. **Recurrent anterior dislocation (traumatic):**
    - **Affects:** Young patients. It may be associated with ligament laxity.
    - **Presents with:** Mostly traumatic episodes (TUBS), occasionally atraumatic (AMBRII). Difference between the two is mentioned in the note box.
    - **Pathology:** Anteroinferior labral tear (Bankart lesion) along with the posterolateral head of humerus impaction injury (Hill–Sachs' lesion). Bony Bankart lesion is also quite common wherein the labrum is detached along with a glenoid bone fragment.
    - **Clinically:** Apprehension, relocation-release tests are positive.
    - **Diagnosis:** X-rays are usually normal. Sometimes, one can see a bony Bankart lesion or a deep Hill–Sachs' lesion; MRI is diagnostic for anterior labral tear and Hill–Sachs' lesion; CT scan is done in patients with recurrent dislocation to assess glenoid bone loss and Hill–Sachs' index.

➤ **Treatment:** Rehabilitation if it is a first episode/no bony bankart lesion. Recurrent episodes often require surgical stabilization.

TUBS: Traumatic, **U**nidirectional, **B**ankart lesion, often needs **S**urgical stabilization.
AMBRII: Atraumatic, **M**ultidirectional, **B**ilateral, **R**ehabilitation is the primary treatment. Surgery, if required—**I**nferior capsular shift and rotator **I**nterval closure is performed.

Note: Posterior dislocation is frequently seen in epileptic patients, electric shock, or ethanol intoxication and is often missed. Acute posterior dislocation patients have limited external rotation (c.f., patients with anterior dislocation who have limited internal rotation). X-ray shows the light bulb sign. *Treatment:* Closed reduction/Open reduction.

2. **Frozen shoulder/adhesive capsulitis/periarthritis shoulder:** Currently, frozen shoulder is more preferred term. Adhesive capsulitis is not preferred as there are no adhesions in the joint, while periarthritis is no longer advocated.
   ➤ **Definition:** Primary frozen shoulder is an idiopathic condition causing inflammation and fibrosis of the shoulder capsule and coracohumeral ligament, causing pain and global restriction in the movements without any other structural damage followed by gradual resolution in symptoms over a few months to years.
   Secondary frozen shoulder occurs following trauma, infection, inflammation, or post-surgery. It may not resolve on its own and may require surgical intervention.
   ➤ **Affects:** Middle age (40–55 years)
   ➤ **Risk factors:** Diabetes, thyroid dysfunction.
   ➤ **Presents with:** Pain and *progressive loss of ROM, both active and passive*; inability to perform overhead activities, difficulty in reaching behind head and back. Pain in the shoulder is severe, especially at night while lying on the affected side.
   ➤ **Pathology:** Inflammation followed by contracture of coracohumeral ligament (CHL), capsule, and synovium.
   Three clinicopathological stages affecting CHL, capsule, and synovium.
   ➤ **Freezing stage (0–6 months):** Severe pain, gradual loss of ROM
   ➤ **Frozen stage (6–12 months):** Pain decreases, profound loss of ROM
   ➤ **Thawing stage (12–18 months):** Further decrease in pain, ROM starts improving, gradually returning to normal or near normal.
   ➤ **Clinically:** Global (in all directions) loss of both active and passive ROM, painful ROM. Cuff strength is usually normal.
   ➤ **Diagnosis:** Mostly clinical. MRI/USG can be used to rule out underlying conditions as well as confirm frozen shoulder. MRI and USG can detect CHL and capsule contracture, rotator interval inflammation, and increased vascularity.
   ➤ **Treatment:** Largely conservative in the form of nonsteroidal anti-inflammatory drugs, physiotherapy, and intra-articular steroid injection. Treat the metabolic pathologies such as diabetes and thyroid dysfunction.
   If conservative treatment fails for >6–9 months, arthroscopic capsular release or manipulation under general anesthesia can be performed to regain the movements and alleviate the pain.
3. **Rotator cuff tendinopathy:**
   ➤ **Affects:** Middle-aged (35–55 years)
   ➤ **Presents with:** Mild-to-moderate pain experienced during activities and while lying on the affected side. Strength is usually maintained.

- **Pathology:** Tendinopathy of the rotator cuff, especially supraspinatus.
- **Clinically:** Terminally restricted ROM (both active and passive). Neer's and Hawkin's sign positive, empty can test often painful and may be slightly weak, while the full can test is strong.
  Cuff integrity test: Equivocal but mostly negative for any substantial weakness.
- **Diagnosis:** X-rays are normal. MRI/USG confirms the diagnosis. Diabetes and thyroid dysfunction should be evaluated.
- **Treatment:** Most cases resolve with conservative treatment—NSAIDs, physiotherapy, activity modification, and subacromial steroid injection. Resistant cases may require arthroscopic subacromial decompression (Subacromial bursa and acromial spur excision) with debridement of the frayed tendon.

4. **Rotator cuff tear:**
   - **Affects:** Older person >50–55 years. However, a traumatic tear can happen at a younger age too.
   - **Presents with:** Pain during shoulder movements and at night while lying on the affected side. There is difficulty elevating or moving the shoulder. Often, pseudopalsy is observed in acute posterosuperior (supra-and infraspinatus) cuff tears or massive cuff tears (tear in two or more tendons).
   - **Pathology:** Tear of one or more rotator cuff tendons from their attachment over the tuberosity. The tear could be traumatic or degenerative; the latter is more common than the former. Minor trauma such as a fall/jerk while lifting a heavy object is often superimposed over a degenerative tendon.
   - **Clinically:** *Loss of active movements but usually passive ROM is preserved* unless there is secondary stiffness. Wasting of cuff muscle is present in chronic tears. Tests for rotator cuff tears are positive depending upon which tendon is torn.
   - **Diagnosis:**
     - X-ray—mostly normal. In chronic cases, acromial spur and greater tuberosity sclerosis may be present. Massive cuff tears (with infraspinatus) reveal proximal migration of humeral head.
     - MRI—Most sensitive and specific investigation. It helps assessing the number of torn tendons, cuff retraction, fatty infiltration, and atrophy.
     - USG—dynamic, cheap, but operator dependent and less sensitive and specific than MRI.
   - **Treatment:** Conservative treatment can be offered as analgesics, and physiotherapy. If conservative treatment fails to improve pain and restore movements, Arthroscopic or open repair of cuff tear can be performed. In irreparable cuff tears, various surgical options are superior capsular reconstruction, tendon transfers, and reverse shoulder replacement.

5. **Rotator cuff arthropathy:**
   - **Affects:** 65–70+ years
   - **Presents with:** Pain, gross loss of strength and or inability to elevate the arm, reach the head or back.
   - **Pathology:** Massive tear of two or more rotator cuff tendons and arthritis of glenohumeral joint.
   - **Clinically:** Gross wasting of cuff muscles, cuff tests are positive, painful ROM, active ROM < passive ROM, and crepitus.
   - **Diagnosis:** X-ray shows the superior migration of the humeral head and arthritis of the GH joint (**Fig. 4.27**);

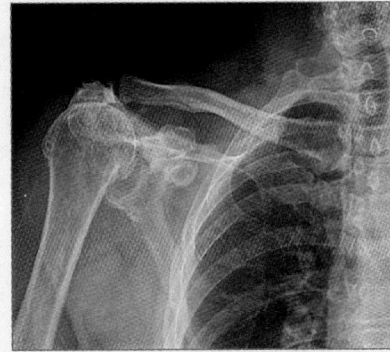

Fig. 4.27: Rotator cuff arthropathy with proximal migration of the humeral head.

MRI—to assess the cuff retraction, fatty infiltration, and atrophy; CT scan to assess the glenoid bony erosion and retroversion.
- *Treatment:* Conservative treatment—analgesics, physiotherapy, and subacromial steroid injection; definitive treatment is reverse shoulder arthroplasty with/without tendon transfers.

6. **Glenohumeral joint (GHJ) arthritis:**
   - *Affects:* Older patients, mostly > 60–65 years
   - *Presents with:* Pain and difficulty in movement. Note that the symptoms of GHJ arthritis are similar to frozen shoulder, but: (1) the duration is longer in GHJ arthritis; (2) symptoms continue to gradually worsen over months to years in GHJ arthritis, unlike frozen shoulder, which tends to recover partially or wholly in few months to years; and (3) patients with frozen shoulder are relatively younger than one with GHJ arthritis.
   - *Pathology:* Glenohumeral joint arthritis.
   - *Clinically:* Tenderness + over the joint line, crepitus is felt during ROM (*Note*: Crepitus is not a feature of the primary frozen shoulder). Both active and passive ROM are decreased.
   - *Diagnosis:* Plain X-ray shows decreased GHJ space, osteophytes (**Fig. 4.28**). CT scan is performed to assess glenoid erosion and inclination, while MRI is performed to assess rotator cuff status (integrity, atrophy, fatty infiltration)
   - *Treatment:* Conservative treatment NSAIDs, physiotherapy, intra-articular steroid, hyaluronic acid injection, and activity modification. If no relief, operative treatment is offered in the form of arthroscopic debridement of GH joint for early stages of GH arthritis; or shoulder replacement for advanced cases. Total shoulder replacement is performed, if the cuff is intact, not atrophied, while a reverse replacement is performed if there is a tear in the cuff or significant atrophy or fatty infiltration.

7. **Painful arc syndrome (PAS):**
   - It is not an isolated diagnosis per se but is a syndrome, as many pathological conditions can cause painful arc syndrome.
   - It is characterized by an arc of painful abduction (classically 60–120°) during shoulder abduction of 0–180°, wherein the initial and later part of abduction is painless (**Fig. 4.29**).

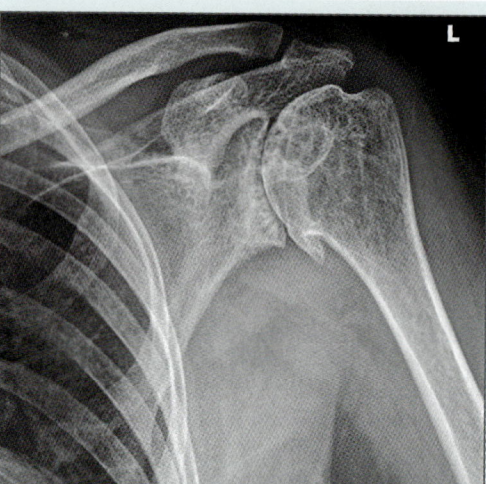

Fig. 4.28: Left glenohumeral osteoarthritis showing narrowed joint space and humeral osteophytes.

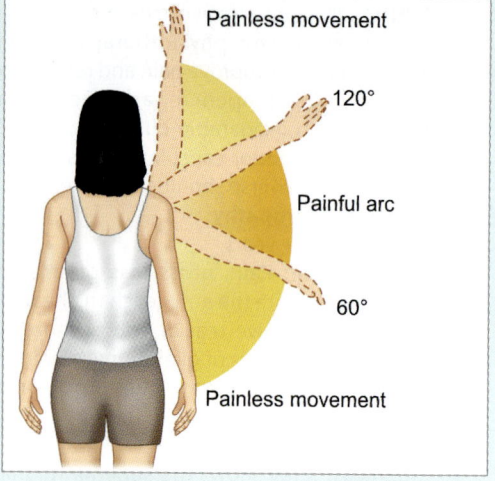

Fig. 4.29: Painful arc between 60 and 120° abduction of the shoulder.

- **Why does a painful arc happen?**
  Typically, the subacromial space is narrow between the abduction arc of 60–120°. However, if the subacromial structures (bursa and rotator cuff) are normal morphologically and subacromial space formed between tuberosities and acromial arch is normal, there is easy navigation of these structures in the subacromial space during the abduction arc of 60–120°. However, any pathology affecting these structures can cause painful negotiation in the abduction arc of 60–120°, resulting in PAS.
- The following conditions can cause PAS:
    - Subacromial bursitis (thick bursa)—rotator cuff tendinopathy (thick, frayed tendon)
    - Rotator cuff tears (floating, free margins of cuff)
    - Greater tuberosity avulsion malunion or nonunion (narrowed space)—acromial spur (narrowed subacromial space)
- *Treatment:* The treatment of PAS is treating the underlying condition.

8. **Calcific tendonitis:** It is one of the most acutely painful shoulder conditions, which is non-infective and atraumatic in origin.
    - *Affects:* Men and women in the 4th–6th decade
    - *Presents with:* Sudden onset, severe pain of the shoulder of a few days duration. Frequently, there can be pseudopalsy due to severe pain.
    - *Pathology:* Calcific deposits in the degenerated cuff. Supraspinatus is the most commonly affected tendon.
    - *Clinically:* Very painful and grossly restricted ROM in all planes. The patient does not allow the slightest movement.
    - *Diagnosis:* X-ray is always diagnostic (**Fig. 4.30**). There may be associated partial cuff tear, which can be detected on USG/MRI.
    - *Treatment:* Largely conservative in the form of NSAIDs, USG-guided barbotage, or subacromial steroid injection. Rarely, arthroscopic decompression of calcific spot may be required.

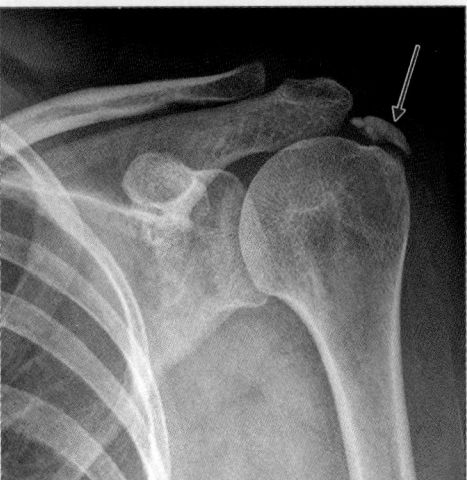

Fig. 4.30: Calcific tendinitis of left shoulder (Blue arrow).

CHAPTER 5

Clinical Evaluation of the Elbow Joint

RELEVANT SURGICAL ANATOMY AND ITS CLINICAL SIGNIFICANCE

1. **Osteology:**
   - The elbow joint is composed of the *humeroulnar* and *humeroradial articulation*. The *humeroulnar articulation* is formed by the spool-shaped trochlea and the proximal end of the ulna (trochlear notch), whereas the *humeroradial articulation* is formed by the hemispherical capitellum and the radial head **(Fig. 5.1A)**. The radial head also articulates with the ulna in the radial notch forming the proximal radioulnar joint.
     - The medial half of the trochlea is larger than the lateral and 6 mm below the medial edge, giving a slight valgus angulation (6–8°) to the elbow. This valgus angulation is known as carrying angle, which facilitates arm swing while walking without hitting the pelvis.
     - The **lateral condyle of the elbow** is formed by the *lateral epicondyle, capitellum, and lateral half of the trochlea* as these parts develop from the same growth plate. The anatomical configuration of lateral condyle is important in pediatric age group as fractures of lateral condyle are quite common.
   - The coronoid process of the proximal ulna is the *most important bony stabilizer of the elbow* **(Fig. 5.1B)**. A major fracture of coronoid process can render an elbow unstable.

Note: Condyle forms an articulation with another bone whereas epicondyle, which is the most prominent part on the condyle, provides sites for the muscle/ligament attachment.

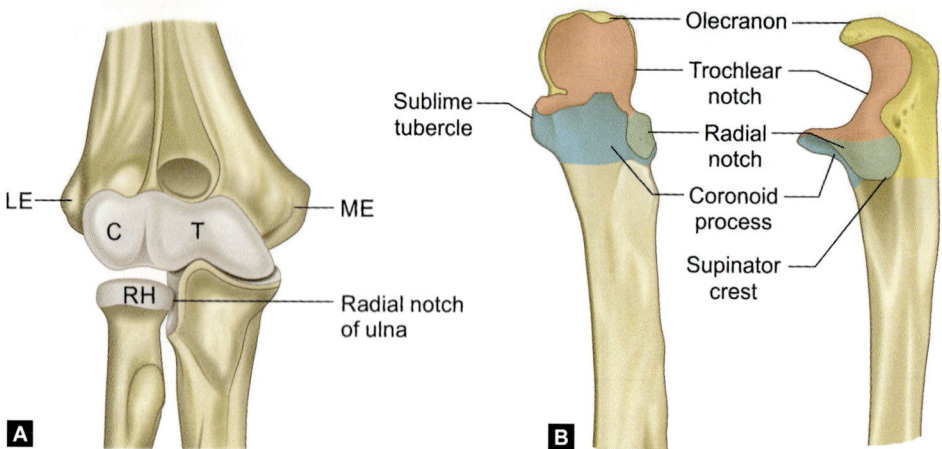

Figs. 5.1A and B: (A) Bony anatomy of the elbow and superior radioulnar joint; (B) Front and side view of the upper end of the ulna with coronoid process.
(LE: lateral epicondyle; ME: medial epicondyle; C: capitellum; T: trochlea; RH: radial head).

- The **superior radioulnar joint** is a pivot type synovial joint between the head of the radius and the radial notch of the ulna **(Fig. 5.1A)**. It is stabilized by the annular ligament. The elbow joint capsule and synovium encloses the superior radioulnar joint as well.
2. **Elbow stabilizing structures:** There are static (primary and secondary) and dynamic stabilizers of the elbow joint. *There are three primary static stabilizers:* Medial and lateral collateral ligament complex, and ulnohumeral articulation. *Secondary static constraints* include the radiocapitellar articulation and the joint capsule. *Dynamic stabilizers* comprise muscles crossing the elbow joint (biceps, brachialis, triceps, anconeus, and common flexor-extensor muscle mass). The lateral and medial ligament complex are briefly described below.
   A. *Lateral collateral ligament complex:* It has three components: radial collateral ligament (RCL), lateral ulnar collateral ligament (LUCL), and annular ligament **(Fig. 5.2A)**. Out of these three LCL components, *LUCL is most important in providing varus and external rotation stability during the entire arc of the flexion.* It is the most frequently injured ligament in the posterior dislocation of the elbow. The annular ligament originates from the radial notch of the ulna (or lesser sigmoid notch), wraps the radial head and inserts on the supinator crest of the ulna. It provides stability to the radial head during pronation and supination.
   B. *Medial or ulnar collateral ligament (MCL/UCL) complex:* MCL has three components: anterior, posterior, and transverse bands **(Fig. 5.2B)**. MCL is primarily responsible for valgus and posteromedial stability of the elbow, especially the *anterior band.*
3. **Type of joints:** The elbow is a synovial hinge joint (predominantly ulnohumeral), whereas the superior radioulnar joint is a pivot joint.
4. **Movements:**
   - *Elbow joint*: Flexion–extension
   - *Superior radioulnar joint*: Pronation–supination

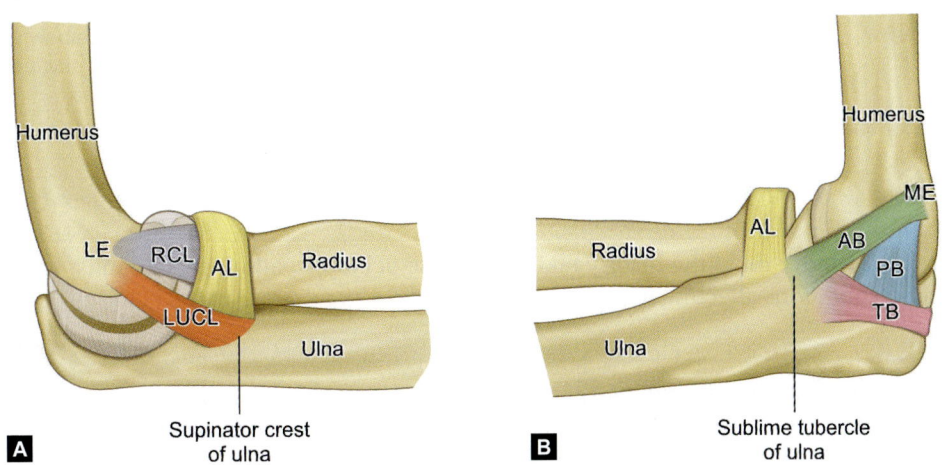

Figs. 5.2A and B: Ligaments of the elbow. (A) Lateral collateral ligament complex; (B) Medial collateral ligament complex.

(AL: annular ligament; LE: lateral epicondyle; LUCL: lateral ulnar collateral ligament; ME: medial epicondyle RCL: radial collateral ligament).

5. **Other important facts:**
   - ❑ ***Normal alignment*** for the elbow (carrying angle) in extension is 7–15° of the valgus, 4–8° for males and 8–14° for females. The function of carrying angle is to *keep the swinging upper extremity away from the side of the pelvis during walking.*
   - ❑ **3 bony points and their relations:** The three bony points of the elbow are the lateral epicondyle, the tip of the olecranon, and the medial epicondyle. The typical relation between them is that these three points form a scalene triangle in a 90° flexed elbow, whereas they lie in a straight line in an extended elbow. The idea of three bony point relation helps in differentiating between different pathologies of the elbow, such as supracondylar fracture, posterior dislocation elbow.
   - ❑ ***Anconeus triangle:*** It is located on the lateral side of the elbow and is formed by joining the lateral epicondyle, the radial head, and the tip of the olecranon. The center of the anconeus triangle represents the radiohumeral joint.
     Anatomical significance: Swelling in the anconeus triangle denotes intra-articular swelling, and the center of the triangle is a landmark for elbow joint aspiration.
6. **Important muscles around the elbow joint:** Common extensors originate from the lateral epicondyle, whereas common flexors originate from the medial epicondyle. Important muscles around the elbow, their insertion, nerve supply, and action are summarized in **Table 5.1**.

TABLE 5.1: Important muscles around elbow joint; their insertion, nerve supply, and action.

Muscle	Insertion	Nerve supply	Principal action
Brachialis	Tuberosity of the ulna	Musculocutaneous nerve	Primary flexor of the elbow
Biceps	Bicipital tuberosity of the radius	Musculocutaneous nerve	Flexor of the elbow, supinator of the forearm
Brachioradialis	Just above the radial styloid process	Radial nerve	Weak flexor of the elbow, supinator of the forearm
Triceps	Superior surface of the olecranon	Radial nerve	Extensor of the elbow
Anconeus	The posterior surface of the ulna	Radial nerve	Weak extensor of elbow prevents capsular pinching in the olecranon fossa
Pronator teres	Over upper one-third of shaft of radius	Median nerve	Pronator of the forearm
Supinator	Upper third of the radius	Posterior interosseous nerve	Supinator of the forearm

Before we move on to the history taking in a case of elbow pathology, one must know the common conditions affecting the elbow **(Box 5.1)**.

BOX 5.1: Common conditions affecting the elbow.

1. **Traumatic:** Malunited fractures leading to deformities such as cubitus varus/valgus, secondary osteoarthritis, post-traumatic stiffness, myositis ossificans, ligament injury leading to elbow instability, tardy ulnar nerve palsy, and pulled elbow
2. **Degenerative/overuse syndromes:** Tennis elbow, Golfer's elbow, olecranon bursitis
3. **Compressive neuropathies:** Cubital tunnel syndrome
4. **Infections:** Septic arthritis, tuberculosis
5. **Inflammatory:** Rheumatoid arthritis
6. **Metabolic:** Gout, pseudogout

HISTORY AND ITS EVALUATION

In patients with upper limb complaints, it is essential to *ascertain their occupation and hand dominance* as that might play a significant role in etiopathogenesis and management of the disease.

Chief Complaints and History of Present Illness

The patients with elbow pathology often come up with certain specific complaints:
- Pain
- Stiffness/difficulty in movement
- Swelling
- Deformity
- Tingling and numbness

Pain

The complaint of pain must be explored in detail in terms of location of pain, onset, duration, progression, diurnal variation, bilaterality, associated symptoms, and relation with repetitive trauma/overuse. An essential aspect of elbow pain assessment is the location of pain, which helps the clinician focus on the specific condition. **Table 5.2** mentions the common causes of pain around the elbow according to location.

TABLE 5.2: Common causes of elbow pain according to location.

Side of pain	Probable diagnosis
Medial elbow pain	• Golfer's elbow (medial epicondylitis) • Medial epicondyle fracture • Medial collateral ligament tear • Ulnar nerve neuritis
Lateral elbow pain	• Tennis elbow (lateral epicondylitis) • Lateral collateral ligament tear • Fracture of radial head, lateral epicondyle, lateral condyle, and capitellum
Anterior elbow pain	• Biceps tendinitis
Posterior elbow pain	• Triceps tendinitis, lecranon bursitis • Gouty/rheumatoid nodule
Global pain	• Osteoarthritis, rheumatoid arthritis, infection, tumor

- Pain can be *sudden or insidious in onset*, constant or intermittent in nature and generalized or localized in site.

Onset	Conditions
Sudden	Trauma, acute infection, metabolic condition (gout, pseudogout), or exacerbation of chronic inflammation (rheumatoid)
Insidious	Overuse syndromes, tendinopathy, arthritis, chronic infection, or a benign tumor
Constant	Infection, inflammation, or malignancy
Generalized	Intra-articular pathology, such as infection/inflammation/arthritis

Elaboration of trauma episode, if any:
- Trauma precedes several elbow pathologies such as deformities (cubitus varus, valgus, and flexion), pain-stiffness and instability. Young children presenting with cubitus varus/

valgus deformity are usually a result of inadequately treated or untreated fractures of the supracondylar humerus or lateral condyle humerus, respectively.
- The ***mechanism of injury*** is important to understand the fracture morphology. For example, fall on outstretched hand results most commonly in supracondylar fracture of the humerus.
- **Details of treatment:** Incomplete, inadequate (in form of native splinting), or no treatment could lead to malunion or nonunion of the fracture of the distal humerus. An unreduced radial head fracture can restrict pronation and supination of the forearm.
- **History of massage to the elbow:** Often present in case of myositis ossificans.
- **Progressive deformity of the elbow:** A typical malunion in cubitus varus is usually non-progressive unless associated with involvement of growth plate or avascular necrosis of the trochlea. Progressive cubitus valgus is observed in children with nonunion of the lateral condyle.

Stiffness/Difficulty in Movement

It could be due to pain, swelling (effusion), and other intra-articular (arthritis, adhesions, intra-articular fracture malunions) or extra-articular (contracture of capsule-muscle-tendon and other soft tissues, myositis ossificans) causes of stiffness.

Swelling

A joint swelling could be **traumatic** (fracture/dislocation/ligament tear), **infective** (septic or tubercular), **inflammatory** (rheumatoid, gout, pseudogout), or **tumourous** in nature. It can arise within the joint (effusion/synovial hypertrophy/both) or from an extra-articular source (bone, tendon, nerve, vessels).

Deformity

Mostly post-traumatic; occasionally infective, inflammatory, or metabolic. Various common deformities in elbow are—
- **Cubitus varus:** Decreased carrying angle and hence inward deflection of the forearm in relation to arm. The *most common cause of cubitus varus is a malunited supracondylar fracture of the humerus in children*. Other cause is avascular necrosis of the trochlea.
- **Cubitus valgus:** Increased carrying angle and hence outward deflection of the forearm in relation to arm. The *most common cause of cubitus valgus is nonunion of lateral condyle fracture of the humerus.*
- **Flexion deformity:** It is observed in post-traumatic stiffness, prolonged immobilization, inflammatory (e.g., rheumatoid arthritis), or infective conditions (e.g., tubercular arthritis).

Tingling and Numbness

The tingling and numbness in the forearm and hand can be due to nerve affection around the elbow, which may be seen in cubital tunnel syndrome (ulnar nerve compression behind the elbow). Sometimes, it could be arising from the proximal region, such as the cervical spine (intervertebral disc prolapse/spondylitis/cervical rib) or a brachial plexus. A detailed history and examination will help differentiate between local irritation of the nerve or proximal pathology.

Constitutional Symptoms

Ask about any constitutional symptoms such as fever, weight or appetite loss if there is a suspicion of infective, inflammatory or tumorous pathology.

Similar Symptoms on the Contralateral Elbow or Other Joints

Sometimes, there can be similar symptoms on the other side. Also, the pathology could be oligo- or poly-articular in the case of inflammatory (rheumatoid) or crystal arthropathies (gout, pseudogout).

After the detailed evaluation of all complaints, one must ask about the *effect of current disease over the activities of daily living.*

Past, Personal, Treatment, Family, Menstrual, and Allergy History

It should be evaluated in standard fashion. The details of occupation may give an idea about functional demand of elbow leading to pain.

At the end of history assessment, many common clinical conditions can be reasonably well diagnosed based upon a combination of age and key complaints. **Table 5.3** summarizes the important snippets for the clinical diagnosis of common elbow pathologies. However, all of them require confirmation with the specific examination.

TABLE 5.3: Elbow clinical diagnostic snippets.

Symptoms and signs	Most likely pathology/diagnosis
A 44-year-old carpenter presents with pain over the outer aspect of the elbow, which increases while working, or gripping objects. He points his fingers around the lateral epicondyle as the site of pain, and there is no swelling/stiffness/deformity	**Tennis elbow** However, one must always carefully check site of tenderness. Tenderness at lateral epicondyle is diagnostic of tennis elbow
A 38-year-old housewife complains of medial elbow pain, which increases with activity. She points her finger over the medial epicondyle as the site of pain	**Golfer's elbow** *Do not forget to examine the ulnar nerve!*
A 10-year-old girl presenting with cubitus varus deformity after a childhood injury	**Supracondylar fracture malunion** *In addition, suspect growth plate injury, if severe deformity, or if the three bony points are altered*
Young adult with a childhood elbow injury history now presents with numbness or pins and needle sensation of the little and ring finger along with cubitus valgus	**Tardy ulnar nerve palsy,** which is a complication of lateral condyle non-union with cubitus valgus
A young female presented with elbow stiffness following an elbow trauma, which was managed by above elbow cast for 4 weeks. Post-case removal, she was advised 'active' physiotherapy. However, she indulged in passive forcible movements and massage to the elbow to regain movements quickly	Suspect **myositis ossificans** (in view of massage and forcible passive movements)

EXAMINATION

General and Systemic Examination

It should be performed in standard fashion. The general and systemic examination is important in systemic diseases affecting the elbow joint, such as inflammatory arthritis, tuberculosis, etc.

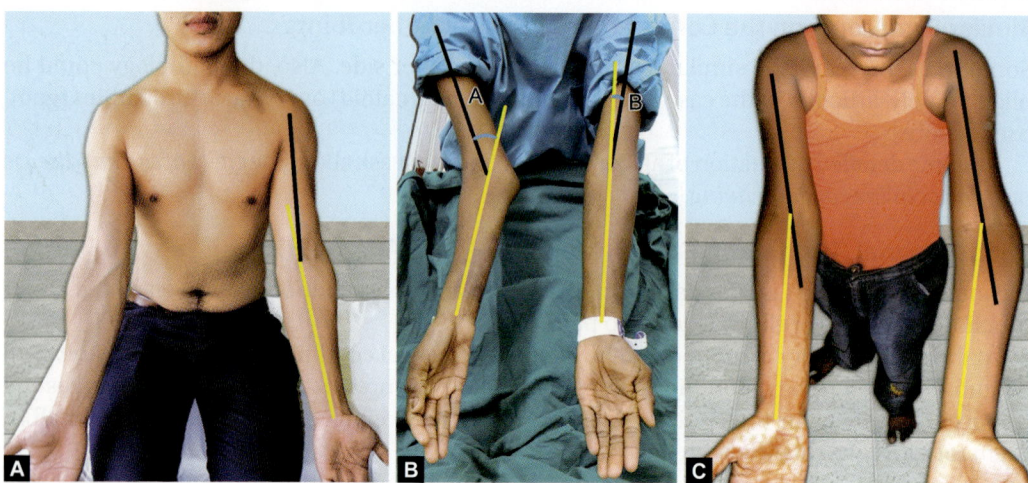

Figs. 5.3A to C: (A) Normal carrying angle in an extended elbow; (B) Cubitus valgus of right elbow. Angle A is more than B; (C) Right elbow with normal carrying angle, while left elbow shows cubitus varus with decreased/reversed carrying angle. In Figures A to C, black line represents arm axis while yellow angle represents forearm axis.

Local Examination

Attitude

The attitude can be described in the standard fashion.

Inspection

The index elbow must be inspected from all sides: front, medial, lateral and back.

General Findings

All around the elbow, swelling, scar, sinus, or ulcer should be described in a standard fashion.

Specific Findings

A. **Observe from the front:** Look for carrying angle, muscle wasting, swelling, and length of the limb.
1. **Carrying angle:** In a normally extended elbow, the forearm is in slight valgus with a normal carrying angle. The carrying angle is the angle formed between the longitudinal axis of the arm and forearm with the *elbow in neutral extension* and the *forearm in full supination* **(Fig. 5.3A)**. The normal carrying angle in the 4–8° in the males and 8–14° in females. *Look for any cubitus valgus or varus. Cubitus valgus* is a deformity wherein the extended forearm deviates away from the midline of the body **(Fig. 5.3B)**. The most common cause of cubitus valgus is nonunion of lateral condyle of the humerus. *Cubitus varus* is a deformity wherein the extended forearm deviates toward the midline of the body **(Fig. 5.3C)**. The most common cause of cubitus varus is malunited supracondylar fracture humerus.

> **Note:** Carrying angle is always checked in a completely extended elbow and supinated forearm. Hence, it should not be commented upon in cases with flexion deformity of the elbow or when the forearm cannot be completely supinated.

2. **Muscle wasting or hypertrophy:** Note wasting of arm and forearm muscles, if any. Wasting of muscle indicates chronic pathology.
3. **Swelling:** Look for any swelling in the cubital fossa or adjacent areas. Arm may show a *Popeye sign* or loss of *biceps bulk* due to rupture of the proximal biceps tendon, whereas distal biceps tendon rupture may cause '*reverse Popeye sign*'.
4. **Limb length discrepancy:** It should be noted in an extended elbow by observing the level of both elbow creases. If one elbow is in flexion deformity, the other elbow should also be placed in the same manner to note the discrepancy.

B. Observed from the side: Look for deformity in sagittal plane, anconeus triangle, and position of olecranon.

1. *Sagittal plane deformity:* A normal elbow can be completely extended with arm and forearm axis parallel to each other. A lack of complete extension indicates flexion deformity, while hyperextension indicates cubitus recurvatum (**Fig. 5.4**). Note that bilateral recurvatum is a normal finding in patients with ligament laxity. Most pathological conditions of the elbow result in flexion deformity.

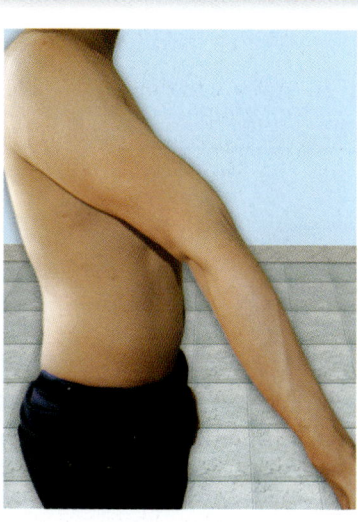

Fig. 5.4: Cubitus recurvatum (observed from side).

2. *Anconeus triangle:* Anconeus triangle is formed over the lateral aspect of a 90° flexed elbow by joining three bony landmarks: *lateral epicondyle, radial head*, and the *tip of the olecranon process* (**Figs. 5.5A and B**). The center of the anconeus triangle forms the center of the radiocapitellar joint. Any visible swelling in the anconeus triangle suggests intra-articular swelling (effusion/synovial hypertrophy/both).
3. *Position of olecranon*: In a normal elbow, the olecranon tip remains in line with the humeral shaft. In posterior dislocation, it moves posterior to the humeral shaft.

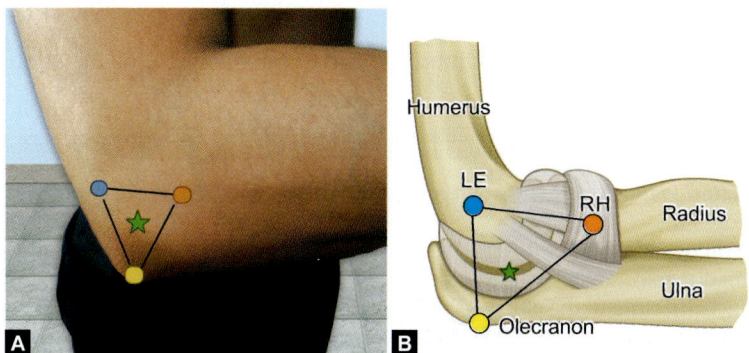

Figs. 5.5A and B: (A) Surface landmarks for anconeus triangle; (B) Illustrative figure of anconeus triangle. Blue, orange and yellow circles denote lateral epicondyle (LE), radial head (RH), and tip of the olecranon, respectively. Green star indicates center of the anconeus triangle, which overlies the radiocapitellar joint. Also, note that the tip of olecranon remains in line with the back of the humeral shaft.

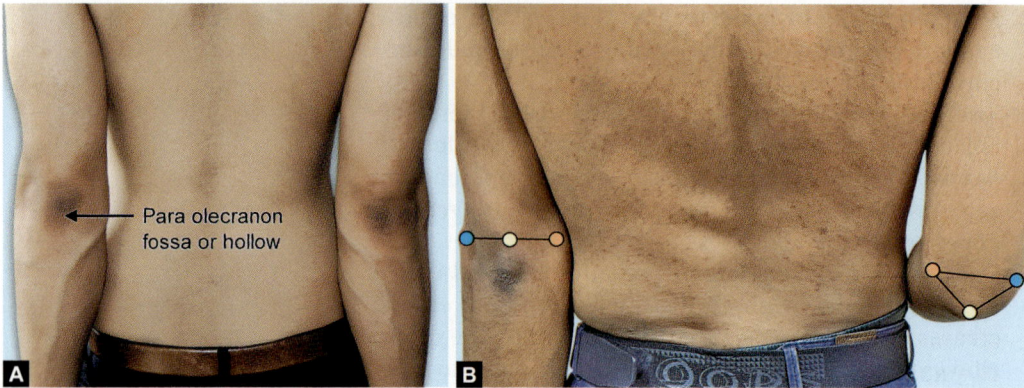

Figs. 5.6A and B: (A) Elbow from behind showing paraolecranon fossa; (B) Three bony point relationship—they are in straight line in an extended elbow (left elbow), while form a triangle in a 90° flexed elbow (right elbow). Blue circle: Lateral epicondyle; orange circle: Medial epicondyle; yellow circle: Tip of the olecranon.

C. Observed from behind: Both the elbows must be inspected posteriorly to see and compare olecranon position, paraolecranon swelling, and three bony point relation.
1. **Position of the olecranon:** It is altered in posterior dislocation of the elbow wherein the olecranon moves posteriorly.
2. **Para-olecranon fossa for swelling:** Normally, in an extended elbow, there is a hollow on either side of the olecranon called para-olecranon fossa **(Fig. 5.6A)**. It is obliterated in the presence of intra-articular swelling (effusion/synovial hypertrophy/both).
3. **Three bony points (lateral and medial epicondyle and tip of the olecranon) relationship:** It is important to note the relationship of these three bony points in an extended and 90° flexed elbow.
   ❑ *In extended elbow*: Three points should lie in a *straight line*
   ❑ *In 90° flexed elbow*: Three points must form a scalene *triangle* **(Fig. 5.6B)**
   Note that sometimes it is not possible to assess these bony points in 0 and 90° of elbow extension and flexion, respectively due to existing fixed deformities. However, one can still assess their relationship by keeping the contralateral (normal) elbow in the same position.
   The relationship of three bony points can be maintained or altered in various pathologies **(Box 5.2)**.

> **BOX 5.2:** Conditions around the elbow affecting the three bony point relationship.
>
> - **Conditions altering the three bony point relationship** (any condition where any of these three points are displaced):
>   ➢ Posterior dislocation of the elbow
>   ➢ Lateral/medial epicondyle fracture
>   ➢ Intercondylar fracture of the elbow
>   ➢ Olecranon fracture
>   ➢ Charcot's elbow
> - **Condition where the three bony point relationship is maintained:**
>   ➢ Malunited supracondylar fracture humerus.

4. ***Other swellings, scar, sinus over the back of the elbow and forearm:*** Localized swelling over the olecranon could be olecranon bursa (Student bursa/Popeye elbow). Sometimes, subcutaneous nodules can be observed over the extensor aspect of the forearm, which is seen in rheumatoid arthritis.

Palpation

Palpate around the elbow for local rise in temperature, bony and soft tissue landmarks, abnormal bony mass (myositis ossificans), ulnar nerve, and swelling, scar, sinus, ulcer, if any. *Ascertaining the relationship between important bony landmarks is one of the key aims of palpation.*

1. **Assess the rise in local temperature**, which may be increased in infective, inflammatory, and malignant tumors.
2. **Palpation of important bony landmarks:** One must palpate all the important bony landmarks such as supracondylar ridges, two epicondyles, olecranon process, the relationship between olecranon tip and epicondyles, radial head, proximal ulna, and the lower end of the humerus.

   These bony landmarks should be palpated for tenderness, their position and relationship with other bony prominences, presence of bony irregularity and thickness. The methodology to palpate several important bony landmarks is discussed below.

   i. **Palpation of the supracondylar ridges and two epicondyles—medial and lateral**
   Method: It is easy to feel the supracondylar ridges in a 90° flexed elbow. One must feel for the sharp lateral and medial supracondylar ridges over the lateral and medial aspect of the distal end of the humerus, respectively, by moving the index, middle, and ring fingers in an anterior-posterior direction. Once the ridge is felt, gradually descend over the ridge with the index finger alone. The first, most prominent point felt is the epicondyle, medial or lateral. Compared to the lateral supracondylar ridge, the medial supracondylar ridge is difficult to palpate as it is located in a deeper plane than the lateral one.

   ii. **Palpation of the tip of the olecranon process**
   Method: It is palpated by placing the index finger over the proximal part of the subcutaneous posterior ulnar border. The index finger should be gradually moved in the proximal direction. The most prominent point felt is the tip of the olecranon process. Just above the olecranon tip lies the olecranon fossa. Furthermore, the tip of olecranon is in line with posterior border of the humeral shaft. This relation helps assessing posterior dislocation elbow wherein the tip of olecranon moves posterior to the humeral shaft.

   iii. ***Ascertaining three bony points (two epicondyles and tip of olecranon) relationship***
   Method: The three bony points *"fall in a straight line in an extended elbow",* whereas the same forms a *"scalene triangle in 90° flexion"* **(Fig. 5.6B)**.

   > **Note:** It is not necessary to mention the type of triangle these three bony points form, but the triangles formed in the two elbows should be comparable with each other. The measurement of each side of the triangle should be compared to that of the normal side to ascertain the abnormality. **Box 5.2** discusses the conditions affecting the three bony point relationship.

   iv. **Palpation of the radial head**
   Method: Keep the elbow in 90° flexion to facilitate palpation of the radial head.
   The radial head is palpated about 1 cm below the lateral epicondyle along the shaft of the radius. Further confirmation of the radial head is done by pronating–supinating the forearm, during which the radial head can be felt rotating under the palpating thumb

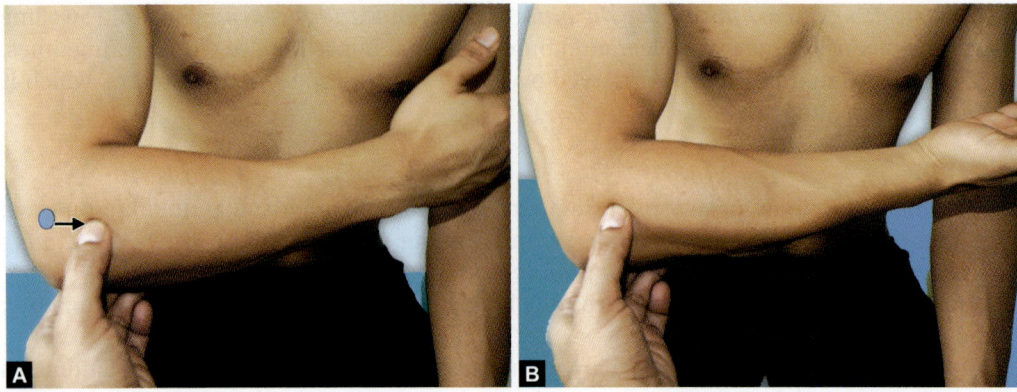

Figs. 5.7A and B: Radial head palpation is done with the elbow in 90° flexion, and the forearm is alternately pronated (A) and supinated (B). The blue circle indicates the lateral epicondyle position, and the black arrow indicates a point 1 cm distal to the lateral epicondyle (along the shaft of the radius) under which the radial head is palpated.

(Figs. 5.7A and B). Confirm the position of the radial head, freedom to rotate, bony tenderness and irregularity and compare with contralateral side.

An altered radial head position is felt in dislocated/subluxated radial head. There could be tenderness in a fractured radial head.

v. **Palpation of the anconeus triangle:** A swelling present in this triangle suggests an intra-articular pathology (synovial hypertrophy/effusion/both). Also, palpate for any tenderness in the triangle.

Apart from above-mentioned landmarks, also palpate shaft of radius, ulna and distal humerus.

3. **Palpation of various important soft tissue landmarks:** The flexor and extensor tendon attachment over the medial and lateral epicondyles, respectively; and triceps tendon over the olecranon, must be palpated.

Tenderness over important bony and soft tissue landmarks may suggest a specific pathology **(Box 5.3)**.

4. **Feel for any abnormal bony mass,** which indicates myositis ossification or a tumorous pathology.
5. **Ulnar nerve:** Palpate the ulnar nerve behind the medial epicondyle for any thickening, tenderness, or subluxability. *One of the common causes of thickened ulnar nerve is Hansen's disease.*
6. **Palpation of swelling, scar, sinus, ulcer, if any,** and its relevant description.

> **BOX 5.3:** Tenderness over important bony and soft tissue landmarks may suggest a specific pathology.
>
> - **Lateral epicondyle:** Tennis elbow
> - **Medial epicondyle:** Golfer's elbow
> - **Radial head:** Fracture
> - **Center of anconeus triangle:** Radiocapitellar joint affection
> - **Olecranon process:** Olecranon bursitis

Movements at the Elbow and Radioulnar Joint

Range of motion assessment is done on the standard lines: Assess existing deformity (if any), active and passive movement (painful, painless, and range of movement) and crepitus.

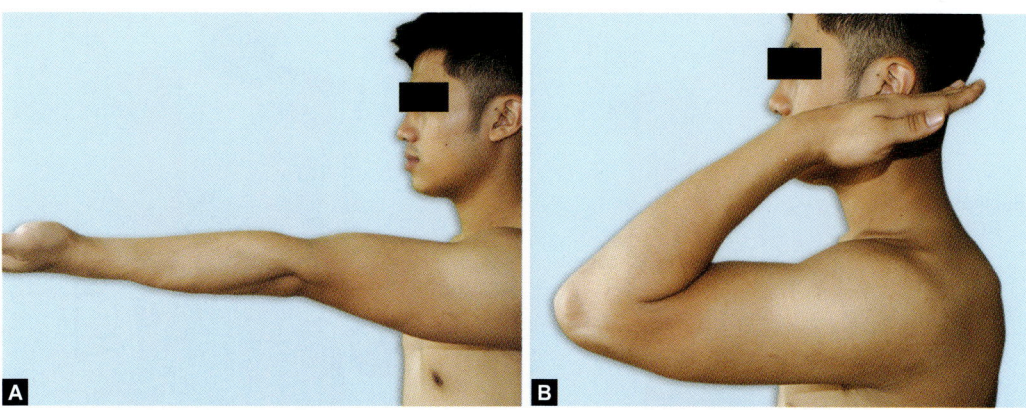

Figs. 5.8A and B: Elbow movements. (A) Extension; (B) Flexion.

- **ROM at the elbow joint:** The elbow joint permits flexion and extension **(Figs. 5.8A and B)**, while the radioulnar joint permits supination and pronation. The normal ROM at the elbow and radioulnar joint is mentioned in **Box 5.4**. However, conventionally while commenting elbow ROM, only flexion is mentioned unless there is hyperextension. For example, *while documenting elbow ROM, mention flexion 0–140°. Avoid documenting extension 140–0°. Only hyperextension is mentioned, if any.* Therefore, if an elbow has 10° of hyperextension and 140° of flexion, the ROM can be documented as -10°–0–140° *(Refer to Chapter 1 movement section for detailed description).*

> **Note:** Hinge joints (elbow, PIP, DIP, knee) ROM should be documented as the neutral position to maximum flexion movement arc. Extension ROM is mentioned only when the patient presents with hyperextension.

- **ROM at the radioulnar joint:** Pronation and supination of the forearm (radioulnar joint) should be checked by keeping both the arm and the elbow by the side of the chest with the elbow flexed to 90°. With a pen gripped in the patient's hand vertically and forearm in mid-prone, ask the patient to pronate and supinate the forearm. Note the arc of pronation-supination by the angle between the axis of pen and vertical midline axis **(Figs. 5.9A and B)**. *Any restriction of pronation–supination indicates the involvement of the radioulnar joint.* Box 5.5 mentions important conclusions about the elbow ROM.
- Crepitus is also elicited during the assessment of passive ROM of the elbow by keeping the hand over the elbow joint.

> **BOX 5.4:** Normal range of movements at the elbow and radioulnar (RU) joint.
>
> - **Flexion:** 0–145°. It may vary depending upon the bulk of the elbow and forearm.
>   *Note: Functional elbow flexion requirement is 30–130°.*
> - **Hyperextension, if any:** Normally 0° but occasionally it could be up to 10–20° (especially in a person with ligament laxity).
> - **Pronation at RU joint:** 0–70°
> - **Supination at RU joint:** 0–90°
>
> *Note: Functional pronation–supination requirement is 50–50° each.*
> Functional ROM is defined as the required ROM for individuals to maintain maximal independence, along with optimal conditions for ADL.

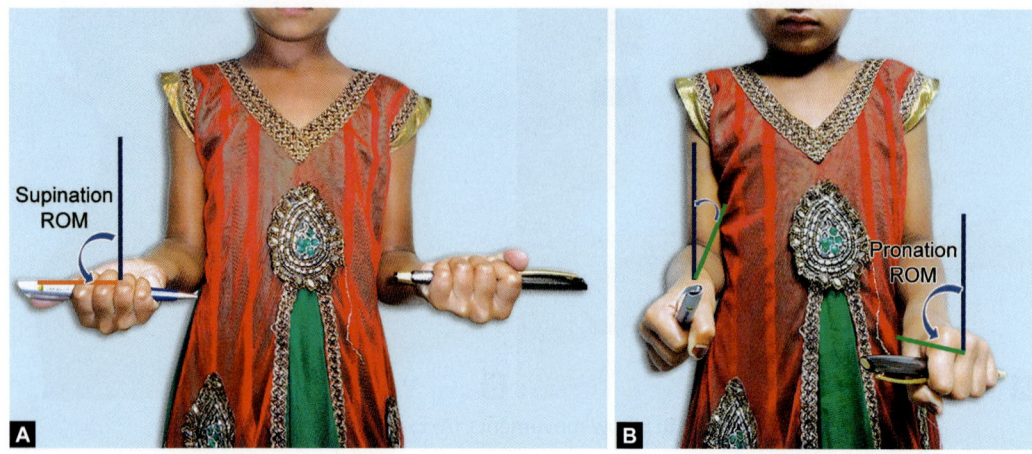

Figs. 5.9A and B: Supination-pronation at the radioulnar joint. (A) Supination is normal on both sides; (B) Restricted pronation on the right side. Black, orange and green lines represent midline vertical, supination, and pronation axis, respectively.

BOX 5.5: Important conclusions while assessing the range of motion around the elbow.

- **Restriction of flexion and extension in the elbow:** *Think about causes of a stiff elbow (joint)*—intra-articular pathology (intra-articular fracture malunion, arthritis, osteophytes, capsular contracture, adhesions) or extra-articular pathology (mechanical block like myositis ossificans, contracture of muscle-tendon, fascia, subcutaneous tissue, etc.)
- **Painful terminal extension:** Soft tissue or bony impingement in the olecranon fossa
- **Painless, exaggerated movement in all directions along with instability:** Charcot's arthropathy
- **Restricted pronation-supination:** Pathologies affecting radioulnar joint (radial head dislocation, radioulnar synostosis), myositis ossificans.

Measurement

One must measure limb length, carrying angle, the girth of arm and forearm, and sides of the triangle formed by the three standard bony points of the elbow and compare with contralateral side.

1. **Limb length discrepancy:**
   - *Arm length*: From the anterolateral angle of the acromion to the lateral epicondyle **(Fig. 5.10A)**.
   - *Forearm length*: From the lateral epicondyle to the tip of the radial styloid process **(Fig. 5.10B)**.
2. **Carrying angle:** It is the inner angle between the long axis of the arm and forearm. The normal carrying angle is 4–8° in males and 8–14° in females. *Prerequisite*: *The elbow should be fully extended, and the forearm should be fully supinated.* Note that the carrying angle cannot be accurately assessed if there is a flexion deformity at the elbow joint or if the forearm cannot be fully supinated.

   Method to measure: Keeping the elbow in 0° extension (not hyperextended) and forearm supinated, draw the long midline axis of the arm and forearm with a skin-marking pencil. The line joining the anterolateral angle of acromion and midpoint of the two epicondyle marks the arm axis. The line joining midpoint of the radial and ulnar styloid process and two epicondyle marks forearm axis. Extend the forearm axis line upward and arm axis line downward so that the two lines bisect each other over the anterior aspect of the cubital fossa. Now place the center of the goniometer at the anterior aspect of the cubital fossa over the bisected point, and align the two limbs of the goniometer along the arm and forearm axis. The inner angle between the intersection of two lines is the carrying angle **(Fig. 5.11)**.

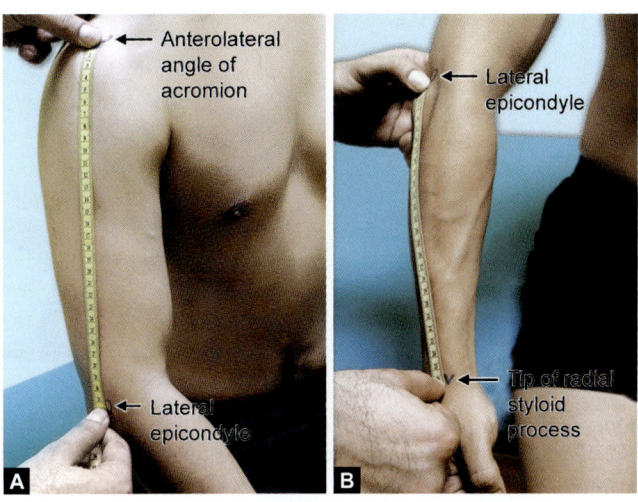

Figs. 5.10A and B: Upper limb length measurement.

3. **Wasting of arm and forearm muscles:** It should be measured at 10 cm above and below the tip of the olecranon for arm and forearm muscle wasting, respectively. Alternatively, it can be measured over maximal muscle mass of the arm and forearm.
4. **The three sides of the triangle** formed by standard three bony points (medial and lateral epicondyles and tip of the olecranon) must be measured and compared with the contralateral side.

Neurovascular Examination of the Upper Limb

A quick and relevant motor examination of the upper limb's five important nerves (axillary, musculocutaneous, median, ulnar, and radial) should be done. Quick motor-sensory assessment of upper limb nerves is mentioned in Table. In a patient with a definite nerve injury, a detailed neurological assessment is a must.

For vascular assessment, palpate brachial, radial and ulnar artery. The assessment of muscles around the elbow is briefly discussed at the end of the special tests.

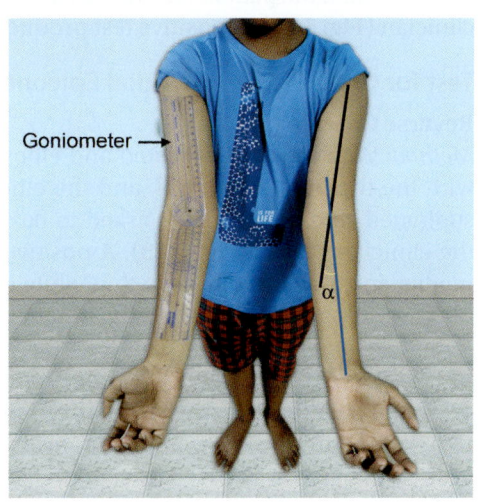

Fig. 5.11: Carrying angle measurement. Black and blue lines represent arm and forearm axis, respectively. Alpha angle represents carrying angle.

Special Tests for Tennis Elbow, Golfer's Elbow, and Elbow Instability

Tests for Tennis Elbow

Cozen's test:
Method: With the patient seated, elbow extended, forearm pronated, wrist radially deviated with hand fisted, the clinician stabilizes the elbow by holding it near the upper third of the

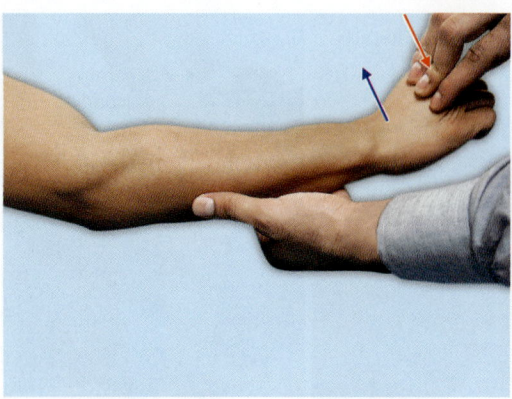 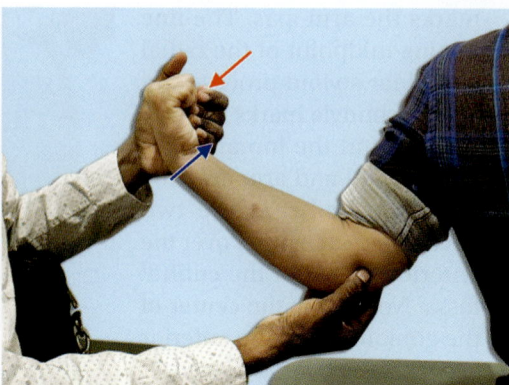

Fig. 5.12: Cozen's test. Blue arrow indicates dorsiflexion by the patient while red arrow indicates clinician's resistance.

Fig. 5.13: Reverse Cozen's test. Blue arrow indicates palmarflexion by the patient while red arrow indicates clinician's resistance.

forearm. Then the patient is asked to extend (dorsiflex) the wrist against resistance given by the clinician **(Fig. 5.12)**. A positive test produces pain over the lateral epicondyle.

Test for Golfer's Elbow (Medial Epicondylitis)

Reverse Cozen's test:
Method: With the patient seated and elbow in 90° flexion, the medial epicondyle is palpated with the thumb of one hand, and the elbow is stabilized by holding it. Then the forearm is supinated, and the patient is asked to flex (palmar flex) the wrist against resistance given by the clinician's hand **(Fig. 5.13)**. A positive reverse Cozen's test is indicated by pain over the medial epicondyle. Also, note that while evaluating Golfer's elbow, it is essential to rule out ulnar neuropathy by palpating the ulnar nerve.

Tests for Elbow Instability

1. **Medial collateral ligament stability:** The MCL can get torn in elbow dislocation or patients with repetitive overuse trauma in overhead throwers (baseball pitchers, Javelin throwers). MCL integrity is assessed by static valgus test.
   Static valgus stress test: While keeping patient's elbow in 30° flexion (unlocks the olecranon) and forearm fully supinated, the clinician holds the patient's elbow with his/her left hand and grasps the forearm with his/her right hand to apply valgus stress **(Fig. 5.14)**. Pain or an abnormal opening of the medial joint space of the elbow during the maneuver indicates a positive test. Compare with the opposite arm.
2. **Lateral collateral ligament stability:** The lateral collateral ligament can get torn because of singular acute trauma or a combination of fractures/dislocations, repeated injections over lateral side or inadvertent damage during elbow surgery. LCL integrity is assessed by static varus stress.
   Static varus stress test: Keeping the patient's elbow in 30° flexion (unlocks the olecranon) and forearm fully supinated, clinician holds the arm with the left hand and grasps the proximal forearm with his/her right hand and gives a varus stress. Observe for any abnormal opening

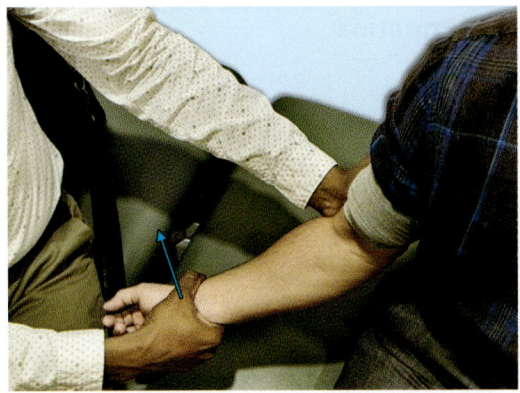 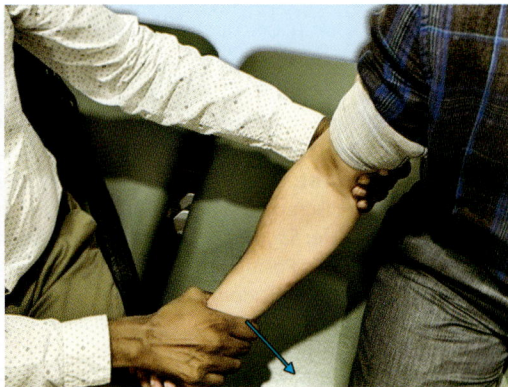

Fig. 5.14: Static valgus stress. Blue arrow indicates direction of valgus stress.

Fig. 5.15: Static varus stress test. Blue arrow indicates direction of varus stress.

of the joint space on the lateral side of the elbow or pain **(Fig. 5.15)**. Compare with the opposite side.

Examination of the Joint Above and Below

Standard assessment of shoulder joint, cervical spine, and wrist-hand area is essential in a patient with elbow pain for several reasons:
1. Pain due to cervical spine pathology (cervical spondylitis, IVDP) can radiate up to the elbow and mimic a local elbow pathology.
2. A patient who sustains an injury to the elbow following a fall on the outstretched hand may also have a concomitant injury to his wrist-hand (distal radius fracture, DRUJ disruption) or forearm (Essex-Lopresti lesion).

Regional Lymph Nodes of Cubital Fossa (Supratrochlear) and Axilla

In case of a suspected infected or a tumorous lesion around or below the elbow, one must examine the supratrochlear and axillary lymph nodes.

Elbow Examination Proforma

1. **Attitude**
2. **Inspection:**
   - *General findings:* All areas for skin overlying, swelling, scar, and sinus
   - *Specifics findings of inspection*
     a. **From front:** Carrying angle, cubitus varus/valgus, any other deformity, muscle wasting, limb length discrepancy, and cubital fossa
     b. **From side:** *Sagittal plane deformity*: Flexion/recurvatum deformity, anconeus triangle
     c. **From back:** Position of the olecranon, para-olecranon swelling, and three bony point relationship in extension–flexion
3. **Palpation:**
   - The local rise in temperature
   - *Tenderness*: Soft tissue and bony landmarks and anconeus triangle
   - Three bony point relationship, ulnar nerve, cubital fossa
   - Confirmation of palpatory characteristics of swelling, scar, and sinus
4. **Movements:** *Assess deformity, active and passive ROM, crepitus*
   - *Elbow joint*: Flexion–extension
   - *Radioulnar joint*: Pronation, supination
   - Crepitus, click; if any
5. **Measurements:** Limb length, arm-forearm circumference, carrying angle, three bony point relationship measurements
6. **Neurovascular examination, muscle strength around elbow**
7. **Special tests:**
   a. *Tennis elbow tests:* Cozen's test
   b. *Golfer's elbow test:* Reverse Cozen's test
   c. *Elbow instability test:*
      i. *MCL:* Valgus stress test
      ii. *LCL:* Varus stress test
8. **Joint above (shoulder, cervical spine) and below (wrist-hand)**
9. **Lymph node examination**

(MCL: medial collateral ligament; LCL: lateral collateral ligament)

Common Conditions Affecting Elbow and their Salient Features

1. **Congenital radioulnar synostosis:** Restricted pronation–supination since childhood
2. **Myositis ossificans**
   - ***Affects:*** Any age
   - ***Presents with:*** Painless loss of movements of the elbow, history of trauma/head injury. History of aggressive physiotherapy (passive mobilization), and massage may be present.
   - ***Pathology:*** Bony mass in the muscle (most commonly, brachialis)
   - ***Clinically:*** There are two clinical stages:
     - ♦ **Early myositis:** Presents as acute symptoms of increasing pain and swelling following a physiotherapy/massage. Locally, there is diffuse tenderness, swelling, and restricted movements.
     - ♦ **Late myositis:** Bony mass palpable on the anterior aspect of the elbow usually presents as a painless mechanical block during flexion.
   - ***Diagnosis:*** X-ray is diagnostic **(Fig. 5.16)**. Early cases reveal fluffy ossification (normal or cotton-wool appearance), whereas late cases show a bony mass around the elbow. CT is useful for planning as one can visualize bony mass in all the three dimensions.

- **Treatment:** Patients with early myositis require re-immobilization for a few days, anti-inflammatory drugs, ice pack, and wait and watch for bone mass to mature. Established myositis cases require mature bony mass excision and adhesiolysis. Watch for recurrence!
- **Differential diagnosis:** Parosteal osteosarcoma (in adults).

3. **Cubitus varus (Gunstock deformity) due to malunited supracondylar fracture of the humerus**
    - **Affects:** Children following a fall on the outstretched hand
    - **Presents with:** Painless deformity at the elbow following a history of fall on an outstretched hand, not treated/inadequately treated fracture. Usually, no functional deficit. Only, a cosmetic concern!
    - **Pathology:** Malunited supracondylar fracture of the humerus usually due to uncorrected medial rotation and horizontal tilt of distal fragment.
    - **Clinically:**
        - Cubitus varus/gunstock deformity (progressive/*nonprogressive*)
        - Decreased or reversed carrying angle
        - Typically, the three-bony-point relation is maintained. However, it may alter if there is any growth plate damage.
        - Irregular supracondylar ridges and supracondylar area of bone
        - Sometimes, flexion of the elbow is restricted; whereas extension of the elbow is exaggerated.
    - **Diagnosis:** Clinical diagnosis. X-rays are confirmatory.
    - **Treatment:** Conservative. Corrective osteotomy (Modified French), if major cosmetic concerns.

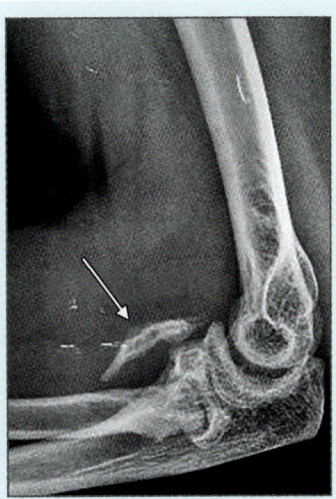

Fig. 5.16: Myositis ossificans of the elbow (arrow points over the bone mass).

Note: Cubitus varus can also occur after avascular necrosis of trochlea, growth plate damage.

4. **Cubitus valgus due to fracture non-union of lateral condyle of the humerus**
    - **Affects:** Affects children after a fall in childhood, may present in adulthood.
    - **Presents with:** Deformity of the elbow following a fall on the outstretched hand. Often from an untreated/inadequately treated lateral condyle fracture.
    - **Pathology:** Nonunion of the lateral condyle of the humerus occurs due to displacement of the lateral condyle fragment following pull and rotation by the common extensors.
    - **Clinically:**
        - Cubitus valgus deformity; progressive in children. It may be painful due to radiocapitellar/trochleohumeral articular incongruity.
        - Irregular supracondylar ridges on the lateral aspect.
        - Palpable step on the lateral distal humerus may be felt, three bony points relation is not maintained.
        - Elbow flexion and extension may be affected.
        - *Tardy ulnar nerve palsy* may be present at a later stage.
    - **Diagnosis:** X-ray shows nonunion lateral condyle, cubitus valgus. Look for joint incongruity.
    - **Treatment:** Anterior transposition of the ulnar nerve, corrective osteotomy for deformity, and internal fixation of the lateral condyle nonunion with/without bone grafting.

5. **Pulled elbow/Nursemaid's elbow**
    - Seen in children <5 years.
    - Occurs when children are pulled or lifted by their forearm; radial head subluxates inferiorly under the annular ligament.
    - The child cries incessantly and keeps his arm and forearm still.
    - **Managed by:** Pronation–supination along with flexion at the elbow reduces the subluxation with a "clunk."

6. **Tennis elbow (lateral epicondylitis)**
    - *Affects:* Middle-aged patients
    - *Presents with:* Painful elbow during activities, especially during pronation-supination
    - *Pathology:* Tendinosis of extensor tendons, especially extensor carpi radialis brevis (ECRB)
    - *Clinically:* Tender lateral epicondyle; Cozen's test is positive.
    - *Diagnosis:* Mostly clinical. Ultrasound and magnetic resonance imaging can confirm the tendinosis and partial tear of extensor tendons. Always rule out associated diabetes, thyroid dysfunction.
    - *Treatment:* Mostly conservative—tennis elbow splint, analgesic, physiotherapy, PRP or steroid injection, and activity modification. Rarely, open/arthroscopic debridement of the frayed-torn tendon.
7. **Golfer's elbow (medial epicondylitis)**
    - *Affects:* Middle-aged patients, less common than tennis elbow, more challenging to treat than tennis elbow.
    - *Presents with:* Painful elbow during activities, especially those which require flexion of the wrist. It may be seen in repetitive gripping, repetitive valgus stress.
    - *Pathology:* Tendinosis of the flexor-pronator mass.
    - *Clinically:* Tenderness presents over medial epicondyle.
        - Tenderness over and below the medial epicondyle. Some patients may have mild flexion contracture.
        - Reverse Cozen's test positive.
    - *Diagnosis:* Mostly clinical, USG, and MRI. Always rule out associated diabetes, thyroid dysfunction.
    - *Treatment:* Mostly conservative—brace, analgesic, physiotherapy, PRP or steroid injection, and activity modification. Rarely, open debridement of the frayed-torn tendon.
8. **Student's elbow/minor's elbow (olecranon bursitis)**
    - *Affects:* Young students whose elbow rubs against the table/chair while writing. It could also be inflamed in gout. Therefore, always rule out gout in young and adults patients.
    - *Presents with:* Painful swelling over the posterior aspect of the elbow (**Fig. 5.17**).
    - *Pathology:* Constant friction leading to bursitis of the olecranon bursa.
    - *Clinically:* Painful swelling over the olecranon. Rule out hyperuricemia!
    - *Diagnosis:* USG, MRI, serum gout levels.
    - *Treatment:* Activity modification, NSAIDs. Aspiration in some cases. Treat hyperuricemia, if any. Excision of the bursa in patients where it fails to subside with conservative treatment, and remains painful.

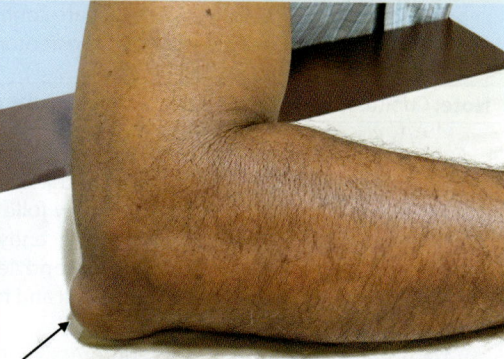

Fig. 5.17: Olecranon bursa (black arrow).

CHAPTER 6

Clinical Evaluation of the Wrist and Hand

SURGICAL ANATOMY OF THE WRIST JOINT AND ITS CLINICAL SIGNIFICANCE

1. **Osteology of wrist:**
   - A total of 27 bones form the wrist and hand.
   - Various bones that take part in the formation of the wrist are:
     i. The distal end of the radius and ulna
     ii. Eight carpal bones:
        - *Proximal row (radial to ulnar)*: Scaphoid, lunate, triquetral, and pisiform
        - *Distal row (radial to ulnar)*: Trapezium, trapezoid, capitate, and hamate
   - The wrist joint is not a single joint. It is formed by combinations of *radiocarpal, distal radioulnar*, and *intercarpal* joints.
     - **Radiocarpal joint:** It is the true wrist joint formed by distal radius, proximal row of the carpus, and articular disc overlying the ulna.
     - **Distal radioulnar joint (DRUJ):** It is formed between the ulnar head and sigmoid notch of the radius. It is most stable in supination and is stabilized by triangular fibrocartilage complex (TFCC).
2. **Ligaments of the wrist:** Various extrinsic (radius or ulna to carpal) and intrinsic (intercarpal) ligaments provide stability to the wrist. TFCC imparts stability to the DRUJ.
3. **Triangular fibrocartilage complex (TFCC):** TFCC is an ulnar sided structure that includes triangular fibrocartilage disc, radioulnar ligaments, ulnocarpal ligaments, ulnar collateral ligament, extensor carpi ulnar sheath, and meniscal homologue **(Fig. 6.1)**. The most important function of TFCC is to *stabilize the DRUJ*.
4. **Retinaculum around wrist:** There are two retinacula; flexor and extensor retinaculum.
   - The ***flexor retinaculum*** (FR) is located on the volar side of the wrist with its attachment on four carpals **(Fig. 6.2)**. *Nine tendons* (four flexor digitorum superficialis, four flexor digitorum profundus, and flexor pollicis longus) and *median nerve* pass underneath FR.

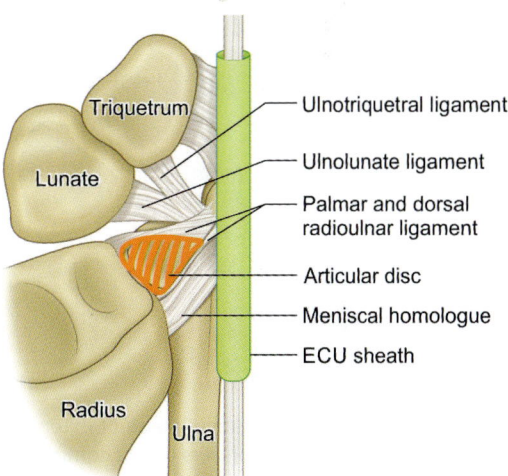

Fig. 6.1: Illustrative figure of triangular fibrocartilage complex along with its components.

Note that the median nerve passes under the FR, whereas the ulnar nerve passes outside the FR through "Guyon's canal" (located between the hook of hamate and pisiform).

- The ***extensor retinaculum*** is located on the dorsum of the wrist, which runs from distal radius to triquetrum and pisiform (and not ulna). There are six compartments under the ER through which various tendons of the extensor compartment, nerve, and artery traverse **(Figs. 6.3A and B, Table 6.1)**.

5. **Anatomical snuffbox:** The radial side of the wrist has an anatomical snuffbox which is bounded radially by abductor pollicis longus (APL) and extensor pollicis brevis (EPB), and ulnar side by extensor pollicis longus (EPL). The floor is formed by scaphoid and trapezium. It contains the cephalic vein, radial artery, and superficial branch of the radial nerve.
Clinical importance: The scaphoid is palpated in the anatomical snuff box. Post-traumatic tenderness and/swelling in the snuffbox could indicate fracture of the scaphoid. *It is also an area for autonomous zone for radial nerve sensory innervation.*

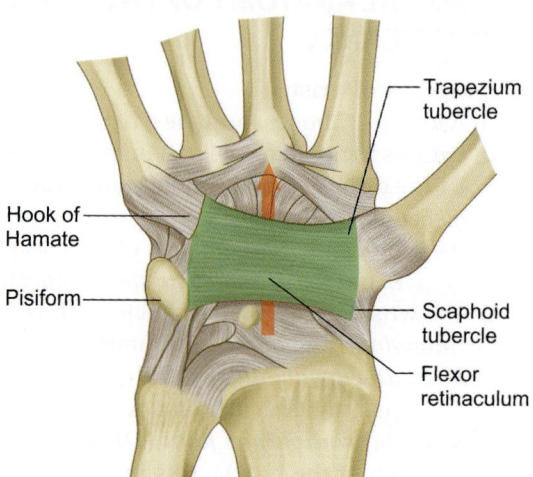

Fig. 6.2: Anatomy of flexor retinaculum (FR) attachment. Red arrow shows the space of the carpal tunnel underneath the FR.

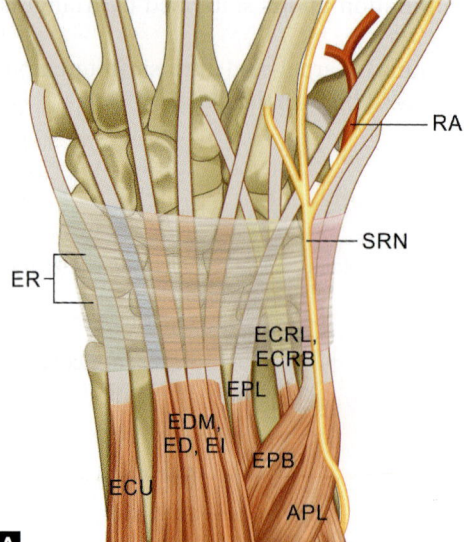

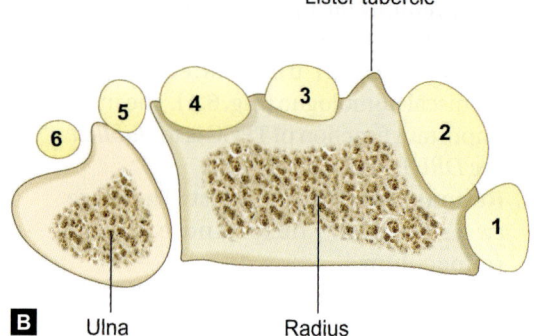

Figs. 6.3A and B: (A) Illustrative image of extensor retinaculum (ER) and structures passing underneath; (B) Schematic diagram of dorsal extensor compartments (1–6, from radial to ulnar side) under the extensor retinaculum.

(RA: radial artery; SRN: superficial radial nerve; APL: abductor pollicis longus; ECRL and ECRB: extensor capri radialis longus and brevis; EPL and EPB: extensor pollicis longus and brevis; ED: extensor digitorum; EI: extensor indicis; EDM: extensor digiti minimi; ECU: extensor carpi ulnaris).

TABLE 6.1: Contents of six compartments of extensor retinaculum (from radial to ulnar side).

1st	2nd	3rd	4th	5th	6th
APL and EPB	ECRL and ECRB	EPL	ED, EI, PIN, and PIA	EDM	ECU

(APL: abductor pollicis longus; EPB: extensor pollicis brevis; ECRL and ECRB: extensor carpi radialis longus and brevis; EPL: extensor pollicis longus; ED: extensor digitorum; EI: extensor indices; EDM: extensor digiti minimi; ECU: extensor carpi ulnaris; PIN: posterior interosseous nerve; PIA: posterior interosseous artery)

6. **Types of joint and its movements:**
   Radiocarpal: Ellipsoid joint allowing dorsi- and palmar flexion, radial and ulnar deviation.
   DRUJ: Diarthrodial trochoid synovial joint allowing pronation and supination.
   Intercarpal: Gliding joint allowing slight flexion-extension and abduction-adduction.
7. **Important muscles around wrist joint:** Important muscles around the wrist are mentioned in **Table 6.2**.

TABLE 6.2: Important muscles around wrist joint their insertion, nerve supply, and action.

Muscle	Insertion	Nerve supply	Action
FCR	Palmar aspect of second MC base	Median	Palmar flexion and radial deviation
FCU	Pisiform, the hook of hamate and fifth MC	Ulnar	Palmar flexion and ulnar deviation
ECRL	Dorsal aspect of second MC base	Radial	Dorsiflexion and radial deviation
ECRB	Dorsal aspect of third MC base	PIN	Dorsiflexion and radial deviation
ECU	Dorsoulnar aspect of the fifth MC	PIN	Dorsiflexion and ulnar deviation

(FCR: flexor carpi radialis; ECRL: extensor carpi radialis longus; ECRB: extensor carpi radialis brevis; FCU: flexor carpi ulnaris; ECU: extensor carpi ulnaris; MC: metacarpal; PIN: posterior interosseous nerve)

8. **Three nerves** (median, ulnar, and superficial radial) enter the wrist-hand complex and supply various muscles and carry sensation from the skin of the hand. Note that the posterior interosseous nerve, which lies in the 4th compartment of the ER, ends after supplying dorsal wrist capsule and has no cutaneous innervation.
9. The **arterial circulation** of the wrist-hand is through the superficial and deep palmar arches formed by radial and ulnar artery. Due to excellent anastomosis between vessels through arches, gangrene is hardly observed even if one of the vessels is blocked.

SURGICAL ANATOMY OF THE HAND AND ITS CLINICAL SIGNIFICANCE

The Hand Comprises Metacarpals and Phalanges (Fingers)

1. **Osteology:** Five metacarpals in hand; each finger has three phalanges: proximal, middle, and distal, whereas the thumb has two phalanges: proximal and distal phalanx. All fingers have two joints, proximal and distal interphalangeal. Thumb has only one joint, interphalangeal joint. Metacarpals distally form joint with phalanges (metacarpophalangeal-MCP) and proximally form joint with carpal (carpometacarpal).
2. **Muscles, aponeurosis and ligaments:**
   a. *Extrinsic and intrinsic muscles of the hand:* Extrinsic muscles originate from the forearm and insert over bones of the wrist and hand, whereas intrinsic muscle has both its origin and insertion over bones of the wrist and hand.

b. ***Palmar aponeurosis:*** It covers the volar aspect of the hand. Arising from the distal edge of the flexor retinaculum, it divides into one superficial and four deep slips, one for each finger. Superficial slip is attached to dermis, while the deep slips insert into deep transverse metacarpal ligament. The palmar aponeurosis protects deeper structures (nerves, artery, tendons). Its contracture results in 'Dupuytren's contracture.'
   c. ***Ligaments of the hand:*** Many ligaments in hand, such as MCP collateral ligaments, volar plate, and deep transverse ligament provide support to the various joints of the hand.
3. **Major joints and movements:** All joints are synovial type.
   a. ***1st carpometacarpal (CMC) [thumb]:*** Saddle joint; Adduction-abduction, flexion-extension, opposition-reposition and circumduction.
   b. ***Metacarpophalangeal joints:*** Condyloid joint; Flexion, extension, abduction, and adduction.
   c. ***Interphalangeal joint:*** Hinge joint; Flexion, extension.
4. **Three basic functions of the hand**: *Pinch, grasp, and hook*
5. **Important muscles of the hand:** They are mentioned in **Table 6.3**.

Before we proceed towards the clinical assessment of the wrist-hand, it is essential to know various pathological conditions affecting the wrist-hand as that helps establish a clinical diagnosis. **Box 6.1** summarizes the common clinical conditions affecting the wrist and hand.

HISTORY AND ITS EVALUATION

Chief Complaints and History of Present Illness

In patients with upper limb complaints, it is essential to ask their occupation and hand dominance as that might play a significant role in etiopathogenesis and management of the disease.

The patients with wrist and hand conditions present to outpatient with several common complaints such as:
- Pain
- Swelling
- Difficulty in movement
- Deformity
- Weakness in the grip
- Tingling and numbness

Note: Two questions remain the key to initiate the evaluation of the history of present illness. One, when were you apparently all right, and two, how did it start?

Pain

It is the most common complaint. Apart from probing into onset, duration, progression, nature, aggravating and relieving factors, associated sensory symptoms, the location of pain in the wrist and hand provides vital clues regarding the diagnosis. **Table 6.4** mentions the common conditions affecting the wrist-hand in radial-dorsal-ulnar-volar fashion.
   a. The ***onset of pain*** could be sudden or insidious in different conditions, as mentioned below.
      ❑ *Sudden onset, moderate-to-severe intensity pain is a characteristic of* trauma (fractures, ligament injury), acute infection (pyogenic tenosynovitis, felon, paronychia), and acute inflammation (inflammatory tenosynovitis, joint synovitis).
      ❑ *Insidious onset, usually dull aching pain is observed in*—arthritis, chronic infection (Tuberculosis), chronic tendinopathy, chronic ligament injuries, and tumors. Insidious onset, moderate-to-severe, burning type could be present in complex regional pain syndrome (CRPS).

TABLE 6.3: Important intrinsic and extrinsic muscles of the hand, their nerve supply, and action.

Area	Important muscles	Action	Nerve supply
Thenar eminence	APB, opponens pollicis, and FPB	Abduction, opposition of thumb, and flexion of thumb at MCP joint, respectively	Recurrent branch of the median nerve. The superficial and deep head of FPB are supplied by median and ulnar nerve, respectively
Palm (radial side)	Adductor pollicis	Adduction of thumb	Deep branch of ulnar nerve
Hypothenar eminence	Opponens digiti minimi, flexor digiti minimi, and abductor digiti minimi	Opposition, flexion at MCP joint, and abduction of little finger, respectively	
	Dorsal interossei	*Finger abduction away from middle finger,* flexion at MCP and extension at IP joint along with lumbricals	
Central	Palmar interossei	*Finger adductors toward middle finger,* flexion at MCP and extension at IP joint along with lumbricals	Deep branch of ulnar nerve
	Ulnar "two" lumbricals	"With the help of interossei"—flexion at MCP and extension at IP joint	
	Radial "two" lumbricals	"With the help of interossei"—flexion at MCP and extension at IP joint	1st and 2nd common palmar digital nerve branches of the median nerve
Other important extrinsic muscles of the volar aspect			
	FPL	Flexion of thumb at IP joint	Median nerve
	FDS	Flexion of all fingers at PIP joint	
	FDP lateral two tendons	Flexion of the index and middle finger at DIP joint	
FDP medial two tendons		Flexion of the ring and little finger at DIP joint	Ulnar nerve
Other important extrinsic muscles of the dorsal aspect			
	EPL	Extension of thumb at IP joint	Posterior interosseous nerve
	ED	Extension of finger (2nd–5th) at MCP joint	
	EI	Extension of index finger at MCP joint	

(APB: abductor pollicis brevis; FPB: flexor pollicis brevis; FPL: flexor pollicis longus; FDS and FDP: flexor digitorum superficialis and profundus; MCP: metacarpophalangeal; IP: interphalangeal; PIP: proximal interphalangeal; DIP: distal interphalangeal; EI: extensor indicis; ED: extensor digitorum; EPL: extensor pollicis longus)

> **BOX 6.1:** Common conditions affecting the wrist and hand.
> - **Congenital:** Syndactyly, hypoplastic thumb
> - **Traumatic:** Fractures of metacarpal and phalanx—malunion, nonunion; Mallet and Jersey finger
> - **Infections:** Tenosynovitis, tuberculosis of phalanx (spina ventosa), paronychia, felon
> - **Neoplasm:** Phalangeal enchondroma, giant cell tumor of tendon sheath
> - **Degenerative:** 1st CMC joint osteoarthritis, Bouchard and Heberden nodes
> - **Inflammatory:** Rheumatoid arthritis, psoriatic arthritis, tenosynovitis
> - **Neurological:** Carpal tunnel syndrome, Guyon's canal syndrome, Wartenburg syndrome
> - **Metabolic:** Gout, pseudogout
> - **Others:** Dupuytren's contracture, glomus tumor (nailbed), ganglion of the tendon sheath

b. **Nature of pain and diurnal variation:** The pain is often throbbing and severe at night in felon, paronychia, acute tenosynovitis, and malignant tumor. *A patient with carpal tunnel syndrome may wake up at night with pain and tingling in hand, which gets relieved by moving or shaking the wrist several times.*

c. **Aggravating and relieving factors:** Pain arising from conditions such as tendinopathy, chronic ligament injuries and primary osteoarthritis is usually mechanical in nature, which increases on activity and decreases at rest. In contrast, pain arising out of inflammation (rheumatoid), infection, and malignant tumor would be felt even at rest.

d. **Associated sensory symptoms:** Pain associated with a burning sensation or altered sensation could be of neurological origin such as carpal tunnel syndrome or complex regional pain syndrome.

Swelling

One must probe a swelling regarding onset, duration, location, whether intermittent or permanent, relieving and aggravating factors, association with fever, stiffness, and discoloration. The swelling could be localized or diffuse.

TABLE 6.4: Common causes of wrist pain according to the location around the wrist.

Structures/area affected	Tendon	Bone	Joint	Ligament	Nerve	Others
Radial side	De Quervain's tenosynovitis	Scaphoid fracture, radius fracture	CMC arthritis		Wartenburg syndrome/Cheiralgia paraesthetica (superficial radial nerve)	Madelung deformity
Dorsal aspect	Extensor tenosynovitis	Lunate fracture/Dislocation, Kienbock's disease	Radiocarpal arthritis			Ganglion cyst
Ulnar side	FCU and ECU tendinitis	Ulnar styloid fracture	DRUJ arthritis	TFCC injury	Ulnar nerve compression in Guyon's canal	
Volar aspect	Flexor tendon tenosynovitis	Hamate fracture			Carpal tunnel syndrome	Ganglion cyst

(CMC: carpometacarpal; DRUJ: distal radioulnar joint; FCU: flexor carpi ulnaris; ECU: extensor carpi ulnaris; TFCC: triangular fibrocartilage complex).

- **Localized swelling:** It is observed in Ganglion, Heberden nodes, Bouchard nodes, and small tumors. The ganglion is one of the most common localized swellings of the wrist. It is usually present on the dorsum of the wrist. Bouchard and Heberden nodes are observed in primary osteoarthrosis, which are localized to proximal interphalangeal joints (PIP) and distal interphalangeal joints (DIP), respectively. The most common hand tumor is enchondroma of the phalanx.
- **Diffuse swelling:** It is observed in several conditions, such as traumatic (fractures, soft tissue injury), infection (cellulitis, pyogenic, CRPS).

Difficulty in Movements

Any difficulty in movement at the wrist and hand joints could be due to pain, swelling, stiffness, deformity, and loss of power. One must probe into what has caused the above-mentioned symptoms.

Deformity

Typical deformities in malunited Colles' fracture, rheumatoid hand, mallet finger, Dupuytren's contracture, and Madelung's contracture often provide a direct clue to the diagnosis.

Weakness in the Grip

A 'give away' feeling could be a symptom of wrist instability, which could result after a injury to DRUJ or TFCC.

Tingling, Numbness

These sensory symptoms in hand result from neurological affections, which could be local or proximal. Common *local causes* of neurological symptoms are carpal tunnel syndrome and Guyon's canal syndrome, whereas common *proximal causes* are cervical spine affections (cervical spondylitis/intervertebral disc prolapse), thoracic outlet syndrome, and proximal compressive neuropathies (cubital tunnel syndrome). A detailed history and localizing signs help differentiate between various causes of such symptoms. CRPS is another common condition that can cause an altered sensation, along with swelling and skin color change (mottled, pinkish).

Complaints in the Proximal Joints (Neck, Shoulder, and Elbow)

Patient must be asked about any complaints in the proximal joints as a proximal pathology could result in distal manifestation in the wrist-hand. For example, C5-6 intervertebral disc prolapse, thoracic outlet syndrome, or cubital tunnel syndrome could present as pain and tingling in hand, and that can be mistaken as carpal tunnel/ulnar tunnel syndrome.

Disruption in Activities of Daily Living

One must assess how the current problem of the wrist and hand has affected the *activities of daily living*. *Hand dominance* is also quite important during treatment, rehabilitation and disability assessment.

Past, Personal, Treatment, Drug, Allergies, and Other Relevant History

One must thoroughly probe past, personal, treatment, drugs, and allergy history to assess its impact or association with the current complaint(s).

Co-morbidities such as *diabetes mellitus and thyroid dysfunction* can predispose to various pathologies such as tendinopathies (De Quervain's), Dupuytren's contracture, tenosynovitis and carpal tunnel syndrome. History of smoking, alcohol intake, and anti-epileptic drug intake are associated with Dupuytren's contracture. Occupational history may give clues regarding the current hand problem. For example, repetitive typing on a computer, chain saw workers, or pneumatic tool drillers are more prone to carpal tunnel syndrome. Avocations (minor habit/hobby) such as too much typing on an electronic gadget could result in De Quervain's disease (blackberry thumb).

Table 6.5 summarizes the important snippets for the clinical diagnosis of common wrist-hand pathologies. However, all of them require confirmation with the specific examination.

TABLE 6.5: Wrist-hand clinical diagnostic snippets.

Symptoms	Most likely pathology/diagnosis/cause
Traumatic conditions	
A 27-year-old banker presents with pain over the wrist for three days following a fall on an outstretched hand. There is no noticeable swelling, tenderness is present over the anatomical snuffbox, and extreme dorsi- and palmar flexion is painful	*Scaphoid fracture*
A 17-year-old cricketer presents with pain, deformity and difficulty in moving DIP joint following a hit from a ball at the tip of finger	• **Mallet finger**, if the patient has a flexion deformity at the DIP joint and cannot actively bring it to the neutral position • Think of **Jersey finger**, if there is bluish discoloration of the pulp and volar DIP joint, and cannot actively flex the DIP joint
Non-traumatic conditions	
A 44-year-old lady presents with insidious onset radial side wrist pain, which aggravates with thumb movement. There is the tenderness over the radial styloid with a positive Finkelstein test	*De Quervain's tenosynovitis* Note: Always check the region of the 1st CMC joint, especially in older patients, as it is one of the most common sites of primary arthritis in hand
A 55-year-old lady presents with insidious onset of painful movement of the thumb (brushing, pinching) associated with mild swelling and tenderness at the base for six months	*1st CMC joint arthritis*
A 54-year-old diabetic patient presents with pain in the ring finger for 6 weeks, more in morning hours, with preserved active and passive movements. There is tenderness over the distal palmar crease with locking/triggering of the finger	*Trigger finger*
A 38-year-old lady presents with insidious onset of pain, tingling/paraesthesia in hand since six months which gets aggravated at night and while doing activity requiring steady and repetitive force. Pain and tingling are relieved when she shakes her hand a few times, only to return after falling asleep again	*Carpal tunnel syndrome* Always rule out hypothyroid, diabetes, and other etiologies, if carpal tunnel is suspected!
An 18-year-old girl presents with an insidious swelling over the dorsum of the wrist for three months. The size of the swelling keeps varying. Mostly, it is painless, while sometimes it is painful!	*Wrist ganglion* Note: Wrist ganglions (dorsal and volar side) are the most common swelling observed in young women!

Contd...

Contd...

Symptoms	Most likely pathology/ diagnosis/ cause
A 52-year-old man who has diabetes and is on anti-epileptic drugs presents with deformity in the ring, and little finger with the inability to straighten the finger. There are painless cord-like bands running longitudinally in the palm	*Dupuytren's contracture*
A 34-year-old woman presented with painful swelling in the PIP and MCP joints of the hand along with associated morning stiffness lasting more than an hour	*Inflammatory arthritis (Rheumatoid arthritis)*

EXAMINATION

General and Systemic Examination

It should be performed in a standard fashion. It is important to note that many systemic pathologies such as rheumatoid, psoriasis, and SLE can also affect the hand.

Local Examination

Attitude

Usually, the wrist-hand examination is performed in a sitting position. The attitude of the wrist and hand can be described in a standard fashion. Normally, **with supinated forearm** with the dorsum of the hand lying on the table, the fingers reveal a *normal flexion cascade* at rest which is the posture/alignment of fingers with some flexion at all the joints of the digits, beginning with less flexion at the index finger and progressing to more flexion at the little finger **(Fig. 6.4A)**. Any abnormal cascade must be noted **(Fig. 6.4B)**. Furthermore, with the forearm fully pronated and wrist-hand lying flat on a table, the wrist-hand as a whole is centered over the forearm where an imaginary line through the *middle finger is in alignment with the shaft of the radius* **(Fig. 6.4C)**.

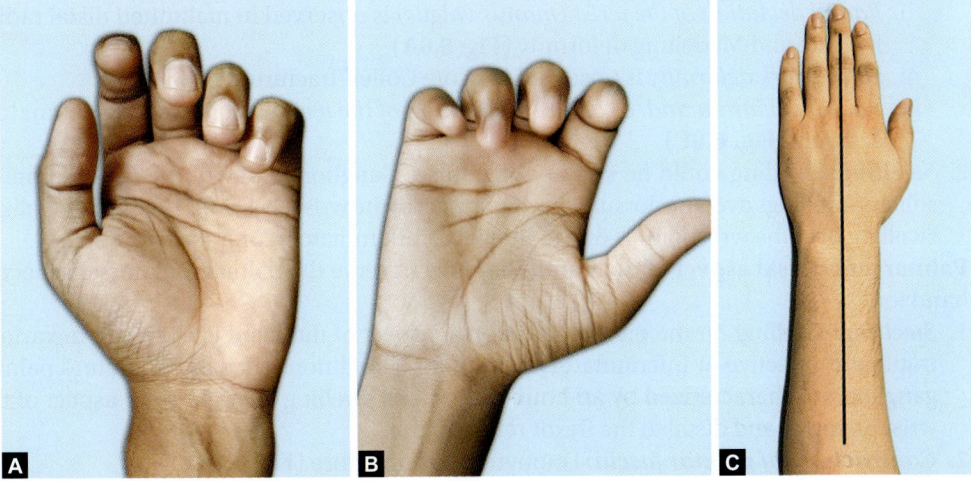

Figs. 6.4A to C: (A) Normal cascade with progressive finger flexion from index to little finger; (B) Loss of normal finger cascade [ring finger is flexed more, and little finger is deviated radially]; (C) Hand-Wrist-forearm alignment as visualized from dorsum (axis of middle finger, 3rd metacarpal, and radius are in the same line).

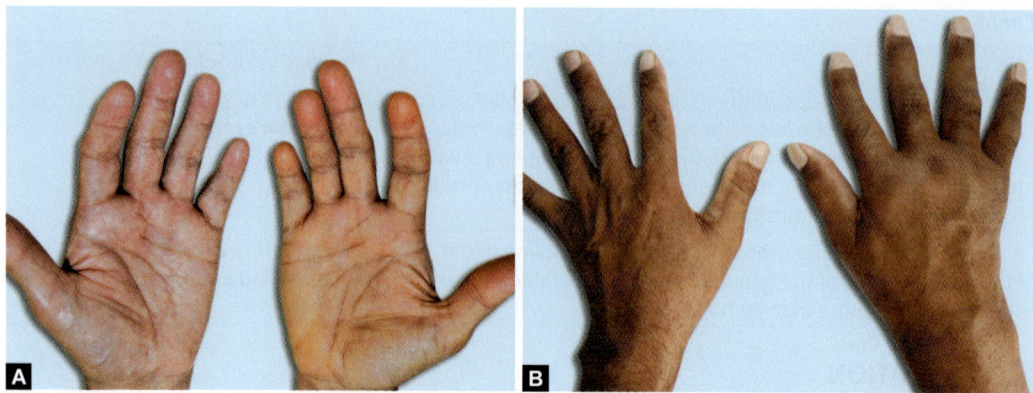

Figs. 6.5A and B: (A) Skin changes (shiny, reddish/bluish/mottled) observed over left hand in CRPS; (B) Hair loss along with spindle-shaped fingers of the right hand.
(CRPS: complex regional pain syndrome).

Inspection

Inspect the wrist and hand from the volar and dorsal aspects.

General Findings

Look for scars, ulcer, and sinus. Observe *skin changes*, such as mottled red-blue spots with trophic changes over the nails in CRPS **(Figs. 6.5A and B)**.

Specific Findings

Look for specific findings at wrist, palm (volar and dorsal), and fingers.
a. **Wrist:** Look for deformities and swelling.
   1. *Deformity:* Certain deformities in the wrist are a typical presentation of conditions such as:
      i. *Radial deviation of the wrist (manus valgus)* is observed in malunited distal radius fracture and Madelung deformity **(Fig. 6.6A)**.
      ii. *Dinner fork deformity* is observed in acute Colles' fracture **(Fig. 6.6B)**.
      iii. *Radial deviation and/or volar subluxation of the wrist* is observed in rheumatoid arthritis **(Fig. 6.6C)**
   2. *Swelling:* Swelling could be solitary or diffuse. Ganglion is one of the most common solitary swellings over the dorsum or volar aspect of the wrist **(Fig. 6.6D)**, while generalized swelling over the wrist joint is due to infective, inflammatory, or traumatic etiology.
b. **Palmar and dorsal aspect of the hand:** Carefully observe the palmar and dorsal aspect of hand for:
   1. *Swelling:* Swelling on the palmar and dorsal aspect of the hand is observed in various traumatic, infective or inflammatory conditions. Conditions such as compound palmar ganglion are characterized by an hour-glass shape swelling over the volar aspect of the wrist proximal and distal to the flexor retinaculum.
   2. *Contractures of palmar fascia:* Dupuytren's contracture **(Fig. 6.7A)**
   3. *Muscle wasting:* Interossei, thenar, and hypothenar eminence wasting is observed in upper limb nerve palsies **(Fig. 6.7B)**. *Note: 1st webspace is the best place to observe interosseous muscle wasting.*

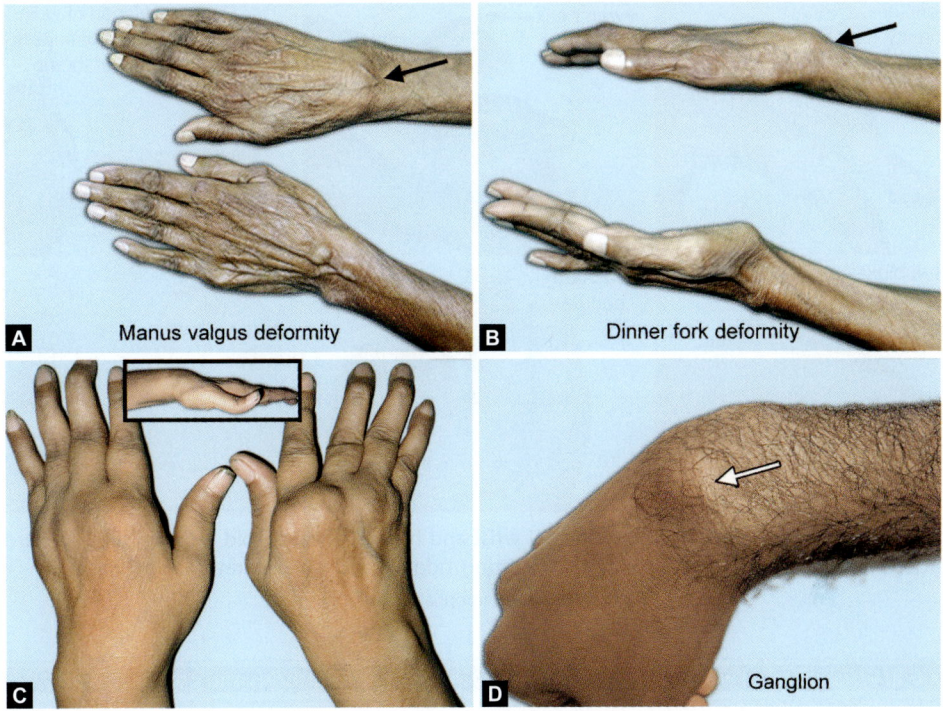

Figs. 6.6A to D: (A) Manus valgus deformity (right wrist); (B) Dinner fork deformity (right wrist); (C) Typical deformity of rheumatoid wrist—radial deviation of wrist, and volar subluxation of wrist (inset); (D) Ganglion over dorsum of the wrist.

c. **Fingers:** Observe for any deformity, swelling, nail and pulp changes.
   1. *Deformity:* Observe for any deformities in the fingers (claw hand, mallet or Jersey finger, deformities of RA or psoriasis, or osteoarthrosis). Several common hand deformities of RA are shown in **Figures 6.8A to D**, and **Box 6.2** mentions common deformities of wrist-hand in rheumatoid and psoriasis.

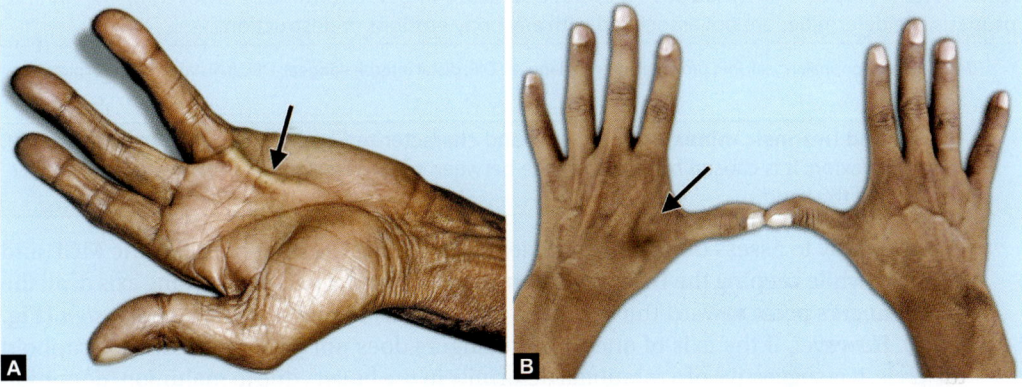

Figs. 6.7A and B: (A) Dupuytren's contracture (black arrow shows contracted palmar fascia); (B) Wasting of the interosseous muscle of the left hand (black arrow in left 1st interosseous space).

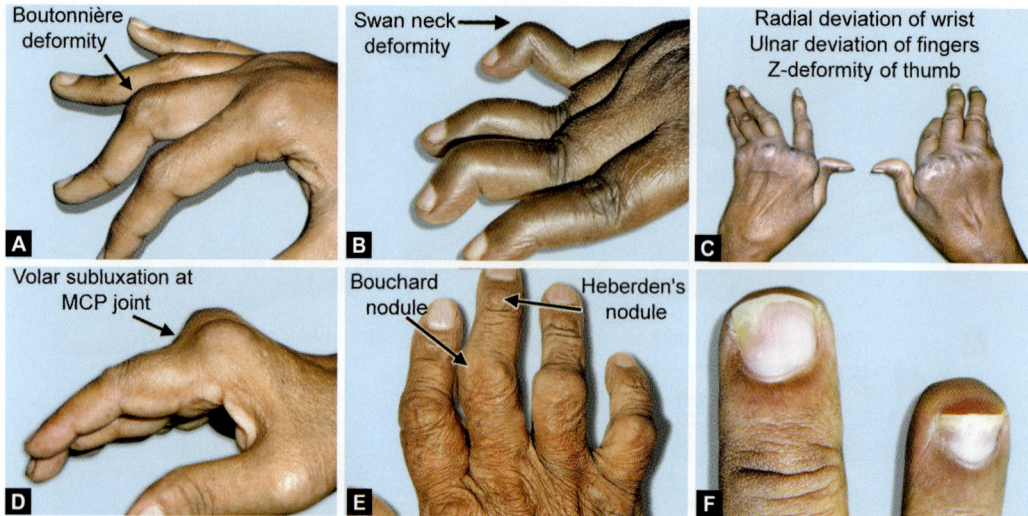

Figs. 6.8A to F: (A to D) Various deformities of wrist and hand in rheumatoid arthritis; (E) Bouchard and Heberden's nodule in primary osteoarthritis; (F) Pitting, ridging, and nail separation in psoriasis.
(MCP: metacarpophalangeal).

> **BOX 6.2:** Various typical wrist and hand deformities in rheumatoid arthritis and psoriasis.
>
> - **Rheumatoid arthritis:** MCP and PIP swelling, Boutonnière and swan-neck deformity, ulnar drifting of fingers, Z-deformity of thumb, volar subluxation at MCP joint, dorsal DRUJ subluxation, and radial deviation and volar subluxation of the wrist.
>   ➤ *Boutonnière deformity:* Flexion at PIP and hyperextension at DIP joint
>   ➤ *Swan-neck deformity:* Hyperextension at PIP and flexion at DIP
> - **Psoriasis:** Note that unlike RA where MCP and PIP joint is involved, psoriasis commonly affects PIP and DIP joints. *Sausage-shaped digit* (swelling at PIP), *arthritis mutilans* and *nail changes* (pitting, ridging, and onycholysis) are characteristic of psoriatic hand. Arthritis mutilans (opera glass hand) is a rare destructive arthritis of the hand with severe deformities characterized by telescoping fingers (like opera glass) due to resorption of bone and dissolution of joints of the fingers.
>
> **Note:** Systemic lupus erythematosus (SLE) can also cause finger deformities. However, unlike RA and psoriasis, the deformities are not associated with any bony erosions or destruction.

(MCP: metacarpophalangeal; PIP: proximal interphalangeal; DIP: distal interphalangeal; DRUJ: distal radioulnar joint)

> **Claw hand (intrinsic minus hand):** Claw hand characterized by MCP hyperextension with PIP and DIP flexion. It is caused by an imbalance between paralyzed intrinsic and overactive extrinsic muscles of the hand.

A simple way to assess deformity in fingers is by asking the patient to flex the MCP and PIP joint while keeping the DIP joint extended. In a normal person, the long axis of all the flexed fingers point toward the scaphoid tubercle, also known as the *cascade sign* **(Fig. 6.9A)**. However, if the axis of one or more fingers does not point towards the scaphoid tubercle, it is suggestive of a rotational deformity in the fingers due to malunion/nonunion in phalanges or metacarpal or a persistent dislocation in joints **(Fig. 6.9B)**.

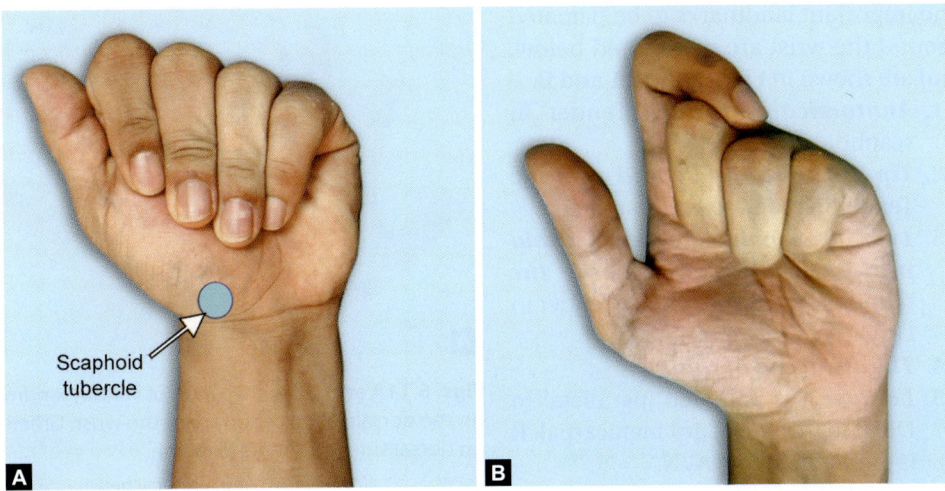

Figs. 6.9A and B: (A) Typical cascade of fingers flexed at the MCP and PIP joint pointing toward the scaphoid tubercle; (B) Loss of normal cascade due to malrotation of index finger following a malunited 2nd metacarpal fracture.

2. **Swelling:** Observe for any swelling over the finger joints (MCP, IP). Look for characteristic swellings such as Bouchard and Heberden nodes at PIP and DIP joint, respectively, which are often observed in primary osteoarthritis **(Fig. 6.8E)**.
3. **Nail and pulp changes:** Several common nail changes and associated conditions are mentioned below:
   - *Pitting, ridging, crumbling, and separation of the nail:* Psoriasis **(Fig. 6.8F)**
   - *Bluish-black discoloration:* Raynaud's phenomena
   - *Infections around nailbed:* Paronychia
   - *Subungual hematoma*
   - *Infection of the finger pulp:* Felon.

Palpation

During palpation of wrist and hand, one must feel the *local rise in temperature, tenderness over soft tissue and bony landmarks, joint line, bony irregularities, swellings, synovial hypertrophy, and radial-ulnar styloid process relationship.*

a. **The local rise in temperature:** Rise in local temperature is felt in inflammatory, infective, or tumor conditions. In contrast, the hand may feel cold in ischemic conditions such as Raynaud's disease and thoracic outlet syndrome with a vascular compromise. Warm or cold feeling with altered sweating pattern in hand is common in CRPS, while anhydrosis (dry feeling) is a feature of nerve injury.
b. **Tenderness around wrist:** Start palpating the wrist sequentially clockwise or anti-clockwise so that no injuries are missed. Conventionally, the wrist examination usually begins with the palpation on the dorsoradial side from the anatomical snuffbox **(Fig. 6.10)** proceeding circumferentially towards the ulna.

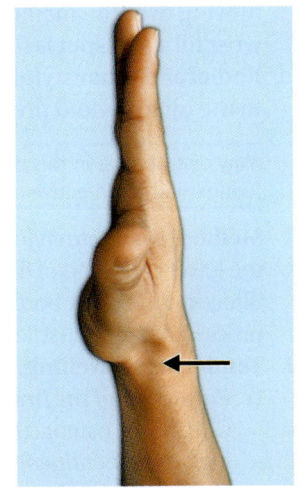

Fig. 6.10: Anatomical snuffbox (arrow).

The important landmarks to be palpated around the wrist are mentioned below, and are shown in **Figures 6.11A and B**.
1. *Anatomical snuffbox:* Tender in scaphoid fracture
2. *Tip of the radial styloid process:* Tender in radial styloid fracture
3. *1 cm "proximal to the radial styloid process for tenderness over the tendons of APL and EPB":* Tender in De Quervain's tenosynovitis
4. *The distal end of radius*
5. *Lunate:* It is palpated just distal to DRUJ in the line of 3rd metacarpal. It is tender in lunate AVN.
6. *Distal end of ulna:* Tender in fractures
7. *Ulnar styloid process:* Tender in fracture
8. *Distal radioulnar joint:* Tender in DRUJ arthritis
9. *Fovea:* It is a soft spot just inferior to the tip of the ulnar styloid process, which is tender in TFCC injuries
10. *Wrist joint line:* Tender in wrist arthritis, synovitis
11. *Median nerve*
12. *Ulnar nerve*

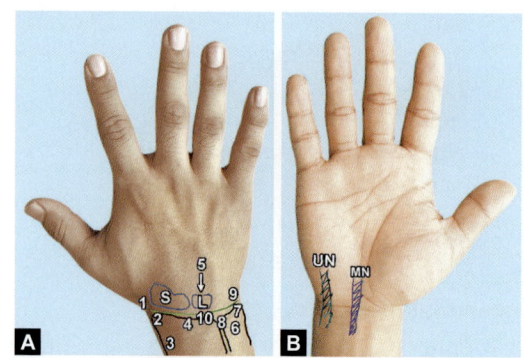

Figs. 6.11A and B: (A) Palpation of various landmarks on the dorsal; (B) Volar surface of the wrist. Green line on dorsal side represents joint line.
(MN: median nerve; UN: ulnar nerve).

c. **Wrist joint line tenderness:** It is easy to palpate the dorsal joint line of the wrist compared to the volar side as the former is more superficial, whereas the latter is situated deep within the thick volar soft tissues, flexor tendons and median nerve.
Method of palpating dorsal joint line: The patient's right hand is grasped with the clinician's right hand holding the first and second metacarpal. Then, the clinician uses his left hand's thumb and palpates the second and third metacarpal shaft and further palpates proximally moving over the metacarpals while the right hand alternately dorsiflexes-palmarflexes the wrist till a soft spot is felt, and that is wrist joint line **(Fig. 6.11A)**.
d. **Radial and ulnar styloid process relationship:** The radial styloid process tip is 8–14 mm distal to the ulnar styloid process.

Any disturbance in this relationship is an indicator of deformed distal radius or ulna (post-traumatic, congenital, or infective cause).

Method to palpate styloid process: The radial styloid process lies in the anatomical snuffbox over the lower-most end of the distal radius, and the ulnar styloid process is the distal-most end of the ulna over the ulnar border, where it is seen as a dorsal prominence. On palpation of both styloid processes, radial must lie distal to the ulnar. This must be compared with the normal side **(Fig. 6.12)**.
f. **Tenderness, swelling, and bony irregularity in all other areas and joints of the hand:**
- ❑ **Palpation of the first carpometacarpal (CMC) joint** is important as it is tender in the first CMC joint osteoarthritis (primary or secondary). *Palpate all other metacarpals, thenar, hypothenar eminence, MCP and IP joints.*
- ❑ **Dorsal and palmar tendon palpation:** Feel for any tenderness and nodules along the tendons traversing the hand on the dorsum and palmar aspect of the hand. The *nodules of the trigger finger* are typically on the flexor tendon over the volar aspect of the MCP joint and

can be felt moving if the patient is asked to flex and extend the fingers.
- **Pulp of all fingers:** Pulp space infections (felon)
- **Nailbeds:** Tender in glomus tumor, paronychia.

Movements at the Wrist, Metacarpophalangeal, and Interphalangeal Joints

The range of movements (ROM) should be assessed at the wrist, MCP and IP joints of the thumb and fingers. At all the joints, check for any fixed deformity, active followed by passive movement (painless/painful), crepitus, and hand function.

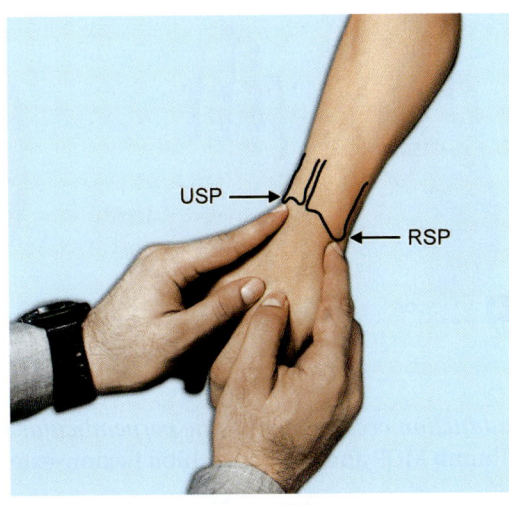

Fig. 6.12: Relationship between two styloid processes. (USP: ulnar styloid process; RSP: radial styloid process).

Range of movements at the wrist joint: Wrist exhibits five movements: radial deviation, ulnar deviation, palmar flexion, dorsiflexion, and circumduction **(Figs. 6.13A to D)**. The wrist movements involve movement both at the radiocarpal and midcarpal joint.

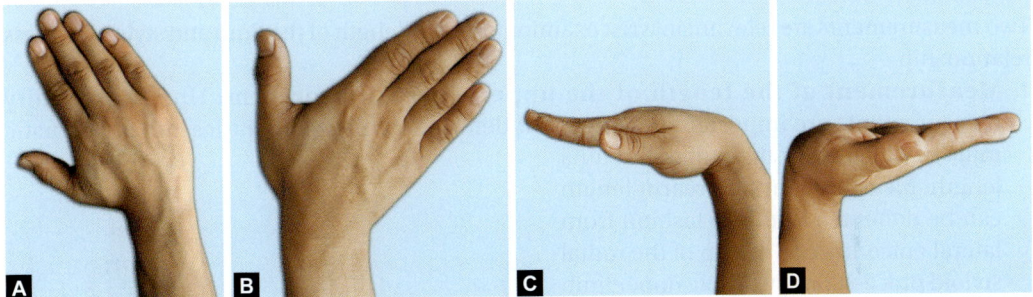

Figs. 6.13A to D: Wrist ROM. (A) Radial deviation; (B) Ulnar deviation; (C) Palmar flexion; (D) Dorsiflexion.

Method to elicit passive ROM at the wrist joint: To elicit passive ROM of the wrist, hold distal part of the forearm with one hand and 2nd to 5th metacarpals with another hand to elicit various ROM. **Box 6.3** mentions normal wrist ROM.

Note: Compared to ulnar deviation, radial deviation at the wrist joint is less as the longer and more distally projecting radial styloid process (compared to ulnar styloid) abuts against the scaphoid during the radial deviation. The palmar flexion is more than dorsiflexion due to the volar tilt of articular surface of the radius.

Range of movements at the thumb: Movements of the thumb occur at the first CMC joint, MCP, and IP joints of the thumb. Principal thumb motions at the CMC joint are flexion–extension, adduction–abduction, opposition, and circumduction. *Note that flexion-extension of thumb CMC joint occur 'in the plane of the palm' (coronal plane), while abduction–*

BOX 6.3: Normal ROM at the wrist joint.
- *Dorsiflexion:* 0–70°
- *Palmar flexion:* 0–80°
- *Radial deviation:* 0–20°
- *Ulnar deviation:* 0–35°

(ROM: range of movements)

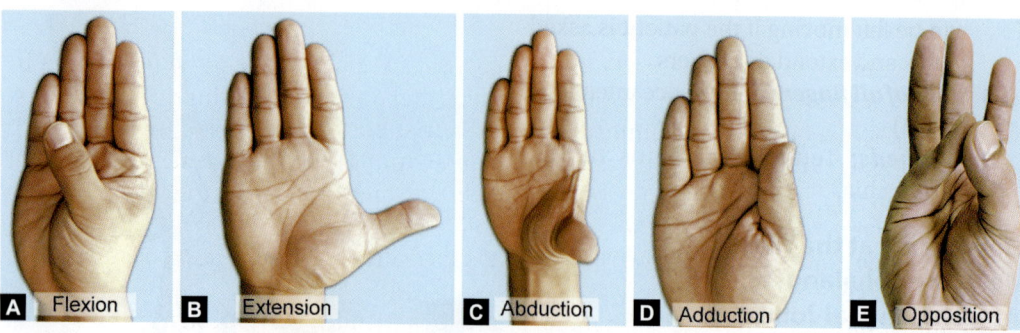

Figs. 6.14A to E: Thumb movements.

adduction occur in the 'plane perpendicular to the palm' (sagittal plane) **(Figs. 6.14A to E)**. Thumb MCP and IP joints exhibit flexion-extension.

Range of movements at MCP and IP joint of fingers: MCP joint allows flexion– extension–adduction–abduction, and IP joint allows flexion–extension.

Assessment of hand function: It is also important to assess various functions of wrist and hand by assessing the *pinch, grasp and hook strength and release of all the fingers after a grip.*

Measurements

Two measurements are relevant in wrist examination: The length of the limb and styloid process relationship.

1. **Measurement of the length of the upper extremity/forearm:** Upper extremity measurements are important in congenital deformities/physeal injuries/other traumatic injuries which affect the radius and ulna length. Measurement of forearm length can be done in a standard fashion from lateral epicondyle to the tip of the radial styloid process. Rarely, whole upper limb measurement might be required.

2. **The distance between the two styloid processes (Fig. 6.15):**
   Method: Draw a line over the midline axis of the forearm extending from the mid-forearm to the wrist joint (black line). Then, drop perpendiculars from two styloid processes (blue and yellow lines). The distance between the two perpendiculars represents the distance between the two styloid processes (white arrow).

3. **Measurement of arm and forearm muscle girth:** It is relevant in muscle wasting of the arm and forearm.

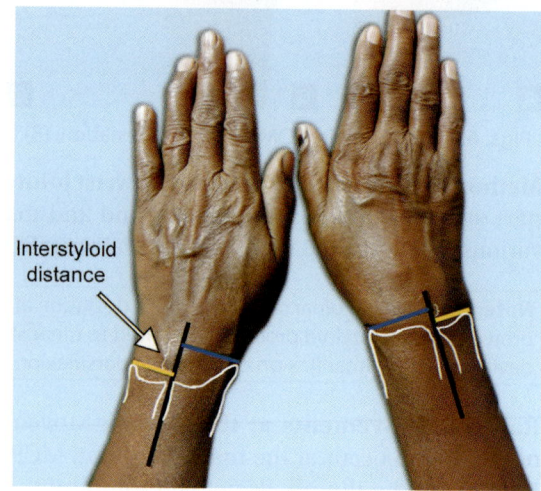

Fig. 6.15: Measurement of the interstyloid distance between two styloid processes. The interstyloid distance is decreased on right side.

Neurovascular Examination of Upper Limbs

It should be done in a standard fashion. The sensory assessment should be performed by assessing the sensations over autonomic zones of radial, median and ulnar nerve over 1st dorsal webspace, volar side of the index finger, and ulnar border of the hand, respectively. A quick motor assessment of three nerves could be done by observing any muscle wasting over the forearm, thenar, hypothenar eminences, and over the interosseous muscles. Further, quick motor assessment of three nerves should involve:

1. **Ulnar nerve:** Abduct fingers against resistance, especially little finger, Froment's sign
2. **Median nerve:**
   a. *Anterior interosseous branch:* Flexion of thumb IP and index DIP (OK sign)
   b. *Recurrent motor branch:* Palmar abduction of the thumb (pen test)
3. **Radial nerve:** Extension at the wrist, MCP and thumb IP joints. Note that radial or posterior interosseous nerve per se is not affected in local pathology of the wrist-hand complex.
   A detailed neurological examination is warranted in case of doubt.
   Vascular assessment involves assessing radial and ulnar pulse, Allen's test, and capillary refill test.

Special Tests

Various special tests are performed to assess pathological conditions involving the wrist and hand, such as carpal tunnel syndrome (CTS), De Quervain's tenosynovitis, first CMC osteoarthritis, patency of radial and ulnar artery, DRUJ instability, and TFCC injury.

Tests for Carpal Tunnel Syndrome

1. **Phalen's sign:** The patient is asked to completely palmar flex both his wrists by opposing the dorsum of both hands against each other **(Fig. 6.16A)**. Development of tingling and/or numbness within 60 seconds in the median nerve distribution area is indicative of CTS.
2. **Reverse Phalen's sign:** The patient is asked to completely dorsiflex both his wrists by opposing the palm of both hands against each other **(Fig. 6.16B)**. Development of tingling and/or numbness within 60 seconds in the median nerve distribution area is indicative of CTS.
3. **Durkan's median nerve compression test:** It is the *most sensitive test for CTS*. The median nerve under the FR is compressed by the clinician's thumb *for 30 seconds* **(Fig. 6.16C)**. Any tingling and numbness within 30 seconds in the median nerve distribution area is considered as positive Durkan's test.

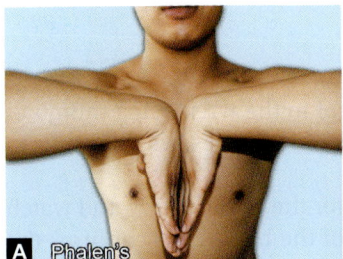 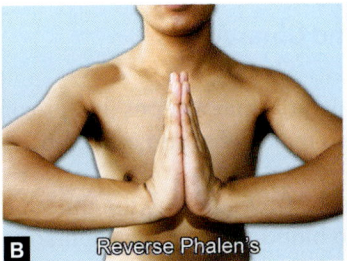 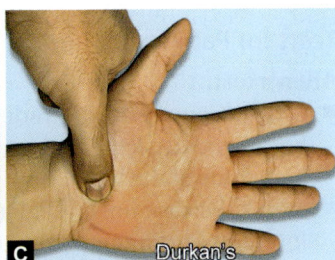

Figs. 6.16A to C: Signs of carpal tunnel syndrome.

Note: Both in Phalen's and reverse Phalen's sign, the patient is asked to hold wrist in a specific position for 60 seconds, while pressure over the flexor retinaculum is applied for 30 seconds in Durkan's test.

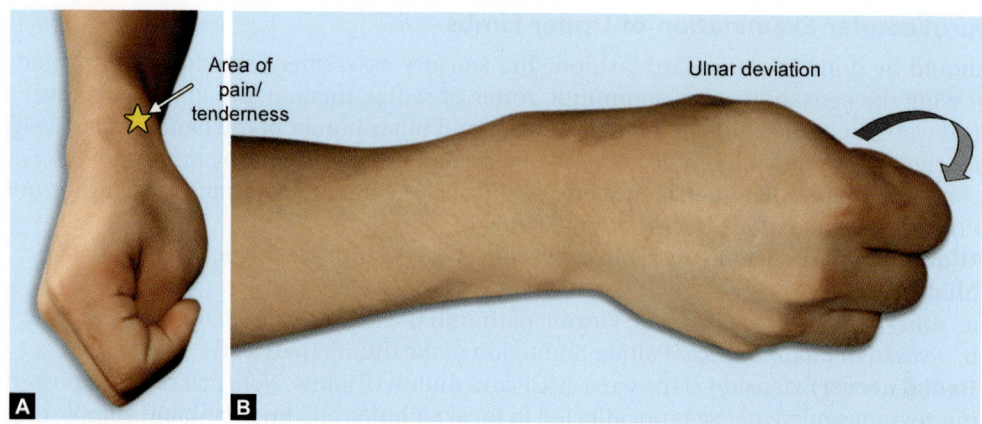

Figs. 6.17A and B: (A) Tenderness and occasional swelling along the radial border of the wrist in De Quervain's tenosynovitis (Yellow star); (B) Eichhoff test (gray curve arrow indicated ulnar deviation of the wrist).

Tests for De Quervain's Tenosynovitis (Texting Thumb/Blackberry Thumb)

In De Quervain's disease, there is tenosynovitis of abductor pollicis longus and extensor pollicis brevis tendons (tendons of 1st extensor compartment), resulting in pain and tenderness along the radial border of the wrist and occasional swelling **(Fig. 6.17A)**. Two commonly performed tests are Finkelstein and Eichhoff test.

Finkelstein test: The thumb is just drawn into ulnar deviation without closing the fist/drawing wrist into ulnar deviation.

Eichhoff test: The thumb is flexed, drawn into ulnar deviation, held inside the fist **(Fig. 6.17A)**, and the patient either actively ulnar deviates the wrist **(Fig. 6.17B)** or it is passively deviated by the clinician. A positive sign indicated by sharp pain along the radial border of the wrist.

Tests for First Carpometacarpal Joint Arthritis

Grind test: The patient's thumb is held between the clinician's thumb and index finger, and the wrist is held and stabilized by the other hand of the clinician. Then, axial stress is given along with the rotatory movement of the thumb of the patient while keeping the wrist stabilized. Pain during such maneuver is indicative of first CMC arthritis.

Tests for Patency of Radial and Ulnar Artery

Allen's test:
- Step 1: Compress both radial and ulnar arteries just proximal to the wrist using thumb of both hands. Ask the patient to make a fist and open-close it several times, which results in blanching of the hand.
- Step 2: Release only radial artery by removing the thumb over the radial artery and watch for hand turning pink due to blood refilling the capillaries of the hand. This confirms the patency of the radial artery.
- Now *repeat step 1* and release only the ulnar artery and watch for the hand turning pink. This confirms the patency of the ulnar artery.

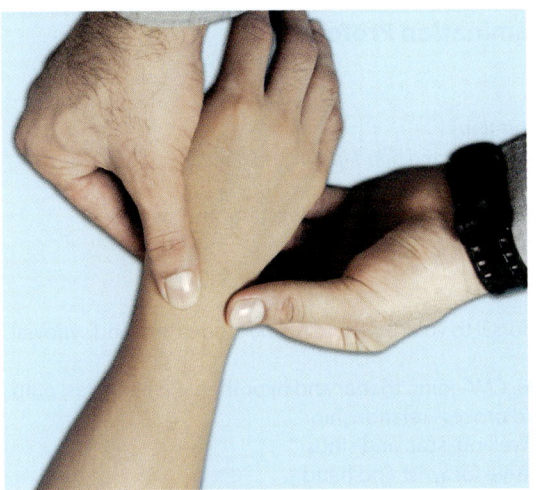

Fig. 6.18: Piano key sign.

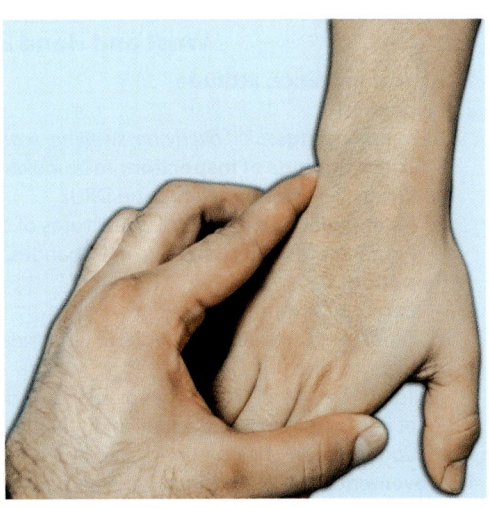

Fig. 6.19: Tests for TFCC injury–Foveal tenderness.

Tests for Dislocation/Subluxation of DRUJ

Piano key test assesses ballottement of the ulna and compare with opposite side.
- **Method:** Keeping the patient's forearm in pronation, the clinician stabilizes the distal end of the radius of the patient by holding it between the thumb and index finger of one of his/her hand, while the distal end of the ulna is held between the thumb and index finger of other hand. Now, the ulna is subjected to dorsal and volar ballottement forcibly and is compared with the contralateral side **(Fig. 6.18)**. Significant side-to-side differences should be noted; approximately 3 mm of dorsal and 5 mm of volar translation in neutral rotation is normal. The test should be performed in midprone and supination too.
- **Interpretation:** An abnormal volar-dorsal movement indicates unstable DRUJ.

> **Note:** During piano key sign, there can be elicitation of crepitus arising out of DRUJ indicating DRUJ arthritis or TFCC articular disc injury.

Tests for TFCC Injury

Fovea sign: While keeping the forearm in pronation, palpate for foveal tenderness, which is a soft spot lying between the ulnar styloid process and FCU. Foveal tenderness is indicative of TFCC injury **(Fig. 6.19)**.

Examination of the Joint Above

A quick assessment of elbow, shoulder and cervical spine is a must to rule out radiating pain from a proximal source or an additional proximal pathology.

Lymph Node Examination

It is essential to examine the epitrochlear (around the elbow) and axillary lymph nodes in patients with infection, inflammation or tumorous lesions of wrist-hand.

Wrist and Hand Examination Proforma

1. **Hand dominance, attitude**
2. **Inspection**
   General findings: *Skin overlying, swelling, scar, and sinus*
   Specifics findings of inspection: *To be looked over wrist and hand (palm and fingers)*
   a. **Wrist:** Deformity, swelling, and DRUJ
   b. **Palm (volar and dorsal):** Contractures of the palmar fascia, muscle wasting, and swelling
   c. **Fingers:** Deformity, swelling, nail changes, and cascade sign
3. **Palpation:**
   - Local rise in temperature
   - Tenderness around wrist (radial to ulnar side, dorsal to volar), wrist joint line tenderness, and synovial hypertrophy
   - Tenderness of all other areas of hand (tendons, CMC joint, thenar and hypothenar eminences, pulp of fingers and nailbed), radial and ulnar styloid process relationship
   - Confirmation of palpatory characteristics of swelling, scar, and sinus
4. **Movements and hand function:** Active and passive for wrist and hand
   - **Wrist:** Dorsiflexion, palmar flexion, abduction and adduction
   - **Thumb CMC joint:** Flexion, extension, abduction, adduction, opposition
   - **Thumb MCP and IP joint:** Flexion and extension
   - **MCP joints of fingers:** Flexion, extension, abduction, adduction
   - **IP joint of fingers:** Flexion and extension
   - Crepitus, click; if any
   - **Hand function:** Pinch, grasp, hook, and finger release
5. **Measurements:** Limb length, arm–forearm circumference, and the distance between radial and ulnar styloid process
6. **Neurovascular examination**
7. **Special tests:**
   - **Carpal Tunnel tests:** Phalen's and reverse Phalen's test, Durkan's test
   - **De Quervain's disease:** Finkelstein, Eichhoff test
   - **First CMC arthritis:** Grind test
   - **Radial and ulnar artery patency:** Allen's test
   - **DRUJ subluxation/dislocation:** Piano key test
   - **TFCC injury:** Fovea sign
8. **Joint above**—Elbow, shoulder, cervical spine
9. **Lymph node examination**—epitrochlear, axillary

(DRUJ: distal radioulnar joint; TFCC: triangular fibrocartilage complex; CMC: carpometacarpal; MCP: meta- carpophalangeal; IP: interphalangeal)

Common Conditions Affecting Wrist-hand and their Salient Features

Degenerative
1. **Ganglion:**
    - **Affects:** Young age, more common in females
    - **Presents with:** Usually, small pea size swelling on the dorsum of the wrist, in the vicinity of the wrist joint **(Fig. 6.20)**. Sometimes, swelling is on the volar aspect. Often, size varies with time. Intermittently painful.
    - **Pathologically:** Not a true cyst. Many theories; synovial herniation/ mucous cyst formation/degeneration of connective tissue, and cyst formation. Often, it communicates with the wrist joint.
    - **Clinically:** Firm or hard on palpation. Dorsal or volar swelling, which becomes prominent on dorsiflexion/palmar flexion of the wrist, respectively. It may/may not be tender.
    - **Diagnosis:** Magnetic resonance imaging (MRI)/ultrasound (USG) can establish the diagnosis.
    - **Treatment:** Conservative—observation. Aspiration and intracystic steroid injection. However, the chance of recurrence is high.
    - *Surgical excision*, if frequently painful, or recurrence after aspiration.

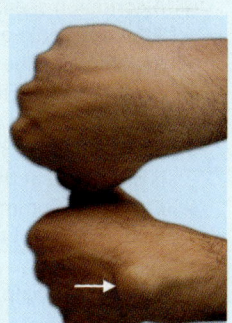

Fig. 6.20: Ganglion over the dorsum of the left wrist.

2. **De Quervain's tenosynovitis:**
    - **Affects:** Middle-aged
    - **Presents with:** Pain and/or swelling along the radial border of the wrist over the distal end of the radius and/anatomical snuffbox
    - **Pathologically:** Tenosynovitis of abductor pollicis longus and extensor pollicis brevis within the region of the first extensor compartment
    - **Clinically:** Tenderness present over the radial border of the wrist. Finkelstein and Eichhoff tests are positive
    - **Diagnosis:** X-rays are normal. USG or MRI can establish the diagnosis.
    - **Treatment:**
        - **Conservative:** Nonsteroidal anti-inflammatory drugs (NSAIDs), physiotherapy, local steroid injection, and thumb splint
        - **Surgical release** of the first extensor compartment, if conservative treatment fails.

3. **Dupuytren's contracture:**
    - **Affects:** Middle-aged to elderly. Men > female
    - **Risk factors:** Alcoholics, smokers, diabetics, and patients on antiepileptic medications
    - **Presents with:** Flexion contracture of the ring finger (most commonly) followed by the little finger
    - **Pathologically:** Contracture of palmar aponeurosis
    - **Clinically:**
        - MCP joint and PIP joint flexion deformity of little and ring finger (most commonly affected)
        - Visible and palpable cord-like palmar aponeurosis **(Fig. 6.21)** (*Note:* No wasting of muscles or neurological deficit unlike VIC).
    - **Diagnosis:** Clinical
    - **Treatment:** Mild cases respond by mobilization of contracture, bracing, and local injection of *Clostridium histolyticum* collagenase. Moderate- to-severe cases require needle aponeurotomy or palmar aponeurectomy.

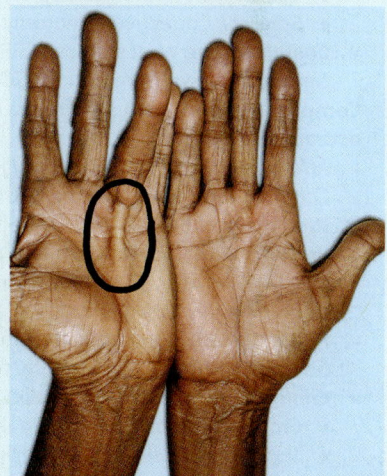

Fig. 6.21: Dupuytren's contracture of the left hand.

4. **Trigger finger:**
    - A condition characterized by extension of a finger with effort.
    - **Affects:** Middle-aged patients
    - **Risk factors:** Rheumatoid arthritis, diabetes, and gout
    - **Presents with:** Finger extends with effort and with a sudden trigger-like action. Early cases often present with pain over the palm around the MCP joint.
    - **Pathologically:** Stenosing tenosynovitis of the flexor tendon sheath wherein smooth tendon gliding is prevented at the level of A1 pulley.
    - **Clinically:** Commonly, middle or ring fingers are affected.
        - Extension of the flexed finger is not easy; the patient actively extends finger with a sudden release.
        - Often, a palpable nodule is felt along the flexor sheath of the finger. The nodule can be painful.
    - **Diagnosis:** Clinical, USG
    - **Treatment:** Early cases respond to observation, NSAIDs, treatment of the underlying condition, and local steroid injection. Surgical release of the A1 pulley (at the level of MCP joint) is required in resistant cases.
5. **Malunited Colles' fracture:** Patients with malunited Colles' fracture give a history of fall on an outstretched hand, following which they sustain a Colles' fracture. Typically, Colles' fracture has been managed with a below-elbow cast.
    - It is commonly observed in older patients. Colles' fracture is a fragility fracture signifying underlying osteoporosis.
    - **Presents with:** Deformity (manus valgus), restricted ROM, +/– pain
    - **Pathologically:** Malunited distal radius fracture
    - **Clinically:**
        - Manus valgus deformity
        - *Altered relation of two styloid processes*: The radial and ulnar styloid processes are at the same level, or radial styloid moves proximal to the ulnar styloid process.
        - Decreased wrist ROM
    - **Diagnosis:** X-ray
    - **Treatment:**
        - **Conservative:** Analgesics, physiotherapy
        - **Surgical:** Corrective osteotomy to correct deformity and functional disability, if any.
    - **Complications:** Wrist stiffness, CRPS, wrist osteoarthritis, rupture of extensor pollicis longus tendon, carpal tunnel syndrome, and TFCC injury
6. **Complex regional pain syndrome (CRPS) (Synonyms: Reflex sympathetic dystrophy/Sudeck's osteodystrophy):**
    - **Affects:** Any age. It can affect any joint but most commonly involves wrist-hand and ankle-foot.
    - Common after trauma to the wrist and hand. Sometimes even the shoulder becomes painful and stiff, which is known as "shoulder-hand syndrome."
    - **Presents with:** Disproportionate pain, stiffness in fingers and wrist, swelling of hand and wrist, discoloration of fingers, nail changes, and cold sweaty hand—occasional paraesthesia and tingling, especially with type 2 CRPS.
    - **Pathologically:** Idiopathic dysfunction of the sympathetic nervous system of the limb after the trauma (type 1 CRPS) or after the nerve injury (type 2 CRPS).
    - **Clinically:**
        - *Gross swelling of the hand and wrist*
        - Thin and shiny skin, hand and finger discoloration (mottled appearance), spindle-shaped fingers, nail changes

- *Diffuse tenderness over the hand and fingers*
- *Altered temperature and abnormal sweating pattern over the hand*
- *Loss of active and passive movements, excruciating pain during movements*
  ➢ **Diagnosis:** Primarily, a clinical diagnosis!
  - **X-ray of affected part:** Patchy osteoporosis; evidence of underlying injury, if any!
  - **Bone scan:** Increased uptake
  ➢ **Treatment:** Always conservative; pain control and physiotherapy are the essences of treatment. Occasionally, local sympathetic ganglion block may be required.
7. **Volkmann's ischemic contracture (VIC):**
   ➢ Sequelae of Volkmann's ischemia (compartment syndrome) of the forearm
   ➢ **Presents with:** Flexion contracture of fingers and wrist
   ➢ **Pathologically:** During the high pressures of compartment syndrome, the muscles and nerves of the forearm compartment bear the brunt of the ischemic damage. Ischemic damage to the flexor muscles results in fibrosis leading to shortening of the muscle-tendon complex
   ➢ **Clinically:**
   - Wasting of forearm and hand muscles **(Fig. 6.22)**
   - Scars of an old injury or surgery present over the forearm.
   - Forearm muscles feel like a cord
   - *Volkmann's sign:* In the wrist's neutral or palmar flexion position, the fingers remain in a lesser flexed or neutral position at MCP and IP joints. This flexion attitude at finger MCP and IP joints exaggerates when dorsiflexion

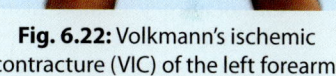

Fig. 6.22: Volkmann's ischemic contracture (VIC) of the left forearm.

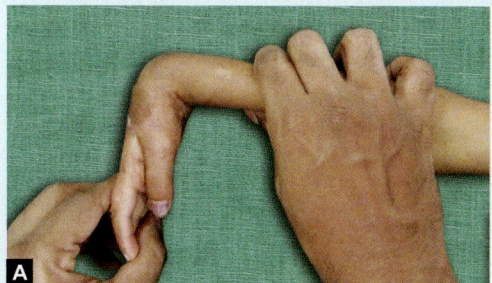 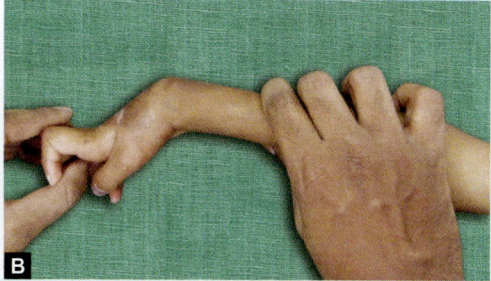

Figs. 6.23A and B: Volkmann's sign. (A) Finger joints are straight with wrist palmar flexed; (B) Finger joints flex with attempted dorsiflexion of the wrist.

is attempted at the wrist. Volkmann's sign is due to the "bowstringing effect" or a "constant length phenomena" of the fibrosed muscle-tendon complex **(Figs. 6.23A and B)**
- Neurological deficit in the forearm and hand in the median and ulnar nerve distribution
  ➢ **Diagnosis:** Clinical, X-ray, NCV
  ➢ **Treatment:** Early cases may respond to occupational therapy, bracing, and muscle stretching. Moderate-to-severe cases require muscle sliding surgery (Max Page procedure), bone shortening, neurolysis, free muscle transfer, flap coverage, or proximal row carpectomy.
8. **Mallet finger:**
   ➢ Persistent flexion deformity of the DIP joint **(Fig. 6.24)** and inability to actively extend the DIP.
   ➢ **Pathology:** Rupture of extensor tendon slip at the base of distal phalanx or avulsion fracture of the base of the distal phalanx.

- **Mechanism of injury:** Acute forceful passive flexion of the DIP joint during concomitant active joint extension. For example, while catching a ball with extended fingers.

9. **Jersey's finger:**
   - The reverse of mallet finger, usually in the ring finger
   - **Pathology:** Due to the rupture of the FDP tendon
   - Sweater finger sign: Due to ruptured FDP, the patient cannot actively flex the DIP of a finger while he/she is asked to make a fist.

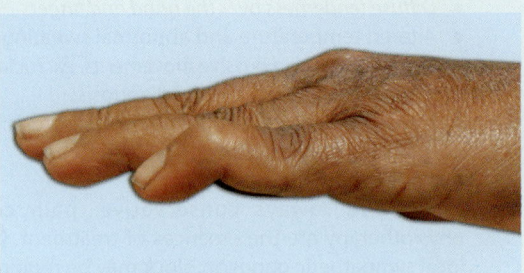

Fig. 6.24: Mallet little finger.

10. **Carpal tunnel syndrome:**
    - **Affects:** Middle-aged. Uni- or bilateral
    - **Risk factors:** Hypothyroid, rheumatoid arthritis, diabetics, malunited Colles' fracture, Smith's and Volar Barton, pregnancy, Cushing's syndrome
    - **Presents with:** Pain around the wrist and hand with associated tingling and numbness over the hand along median nerve distribution area. Pain is often severe at night. Features of the underlying condition (RA, hypothyroid).
    - **Pathologically:** Compression of the median nerve in the carpal tunnel
    - **Clinically:**
      - Phalen's test, reverse Phalen's test, and Durkan's test +
      - Sensory and motor assessment of the median nerve
    - **Diagnosis:** X-ray, NCV, USG, and MRI
    - **Treatment:** Most cases respond to conservative treatment (wrist brace, gabapentinoids, analgesics, treat the underlying condition). Severe cases require flexor retinaculum release (open/endoscopic).

11. **Congenital anomalies:**
    - **Syndactyly:** Webbing of fingers/sideways fused fingers **(Fig. 6.25)**
    - **Polydactyly:** Supernumerary fingers
    - **Camptodactyly:** Flexion deformity of the finger at PIP joint (usually little finger)
    - **Macrodactyly:** Overgrowth of fingers
    - **Radial clubhand:** Radial side tissues (radius bone, thumb, and scaphoid) are poorly/not developed.

12. **Madelung deformity:**
    - **Definition:** A congenital dyschondrosis of distal radius physis leading to disruption of the volar and ulnar aspect of physis, which results in volar and ulnarward tilted distal radial articular surface and *a dorsally prominent distal ulna* **(Fig. 6.26)**.
    - **Etiopathology:** Dysplastic, genetic (Turner's syndrome), post- traumatic, and rarely infective or metabolic.

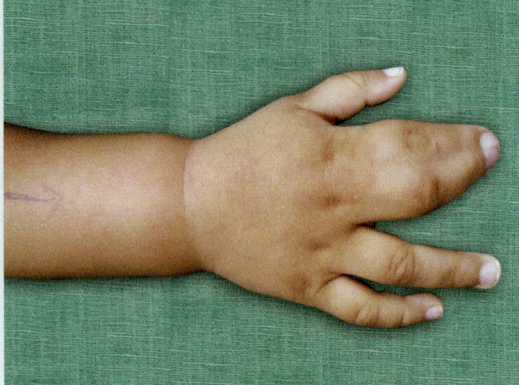

Fig. 6.25: Syndactyly.

    - **Clinical presentation:** Patient presents with wrist pain and deformity. There is radial deviation of the hand, and hand is translated volarly to the long axis of the forearm. There is Bayonet-like deformity of the distal radius and dorsal prominence of the distal ulna. Limited dorsiflexion of the wrist, and forearm rotations.

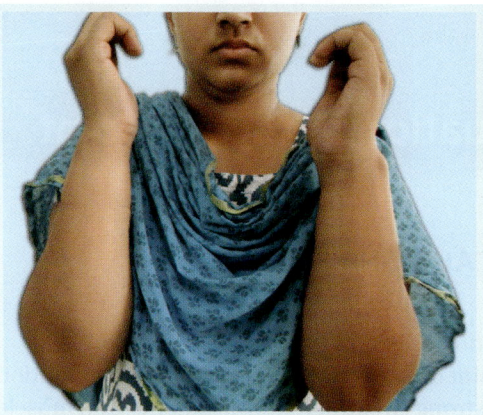

Fig. 6.26: Madelung deformity.

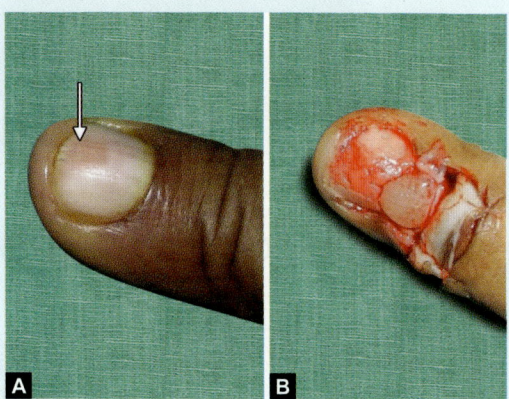

Figs. 6.27A and B: Glomus tumor.

Tumors
13. **Glomus tumor:**
    - ➢ **Affects:** Young adults
    - ➢ **Presents with:** Paroxysmal pain in the finger with cold intolerance and exquisite tenderness
    - ➢ **Pathologically:** Arteriovenous anastomosis incorporating the nerves
    - ➢ **Clinically:**
        - ♦ Red- or violet-colored pinhead size tumor under the nailbed **(Figs. 6.27A and B)**
        - ♦ Nail ridging is common.
        - ♦ **Love's pin test:** Pressure with pinhead over nail causes exquisite tenderness

CHAPTER 7

Clinical Evaluation of the Hip Joint

SURGICAL ANATOMY AND ITS CLINICAL SIGNIFICANCE

1. **Osteology**
   - The hip joint is formed by the acetabulum and the head of the femur **(Fig. 7.1A)**.
   - It is the most stable ball and socket type of joint due to the round structural configuration of the femoral head, deep acetabular socket, strong circumferential ligaments, and muscle cover.
2. **Vascularity of the femoral head:** About 85% of the blood supply to the femoral head in an adult is via the medial and lateral circumflex femoral vessels that are branches of the profunda femoris **(Fig. 7.1B)**. These circumflex vessels form a circumferential anastomosis around the greater trochanter, which gives rise to numerous radial sub- synovial intracapsular retinacular vessels traversing along the neck of the femur to supply the femoral head. About 10–15% of the blood supply to the femoral head is via the artery of the ligamentum teres.
3. **Stabilizing structures**
   - The acetabular margin is lined by the *acetabular labrum* **(Fig. 7.1A)**. The *capsule* surrounds the hip joint. Medially, capsule is attached to the acetabular margins. Laterally, the capsule is attached over the intertrochanteric line anteriorly and 1 cm medial to the intertrochanteric crest posteriorly. The inferior part of the acetabulum is lined by transverse ligament.
   - *Three ligaments stabilize the hip joint:* Iliofemoral (ligament of Bigelow), ischiofemoral, and pubofemoral. The iliofemoral ligament is strongest among the three **(Figs. 7.1C and D)**.
   - Ligamentum teres connects the femoral head to the acetabulum floor **(Fig. 7.1A)** and often carries a small vessel (artery of ligamentum teres) supplying the femoral head.
4. **Type of joint:** The hip joint is a deeply seated ball and socket synovial joint.
5. **Movements at the hip joint:** Flexion, extension, abduction, adduction, external, and internal rotation.
6. **Important muscles around the hip joint**

    The important muscles around the hip joint, their nerve supply, and action are mentioned in **Table 7.1**. Before we move on to understand the history taking and examination in hip pathologies, it is vital to recollect common conditions which affect the hip joint **(Box 7.1)**.

HISTORY AND ITS EVALUATION

Chief Complaints and History of Present Illness

The patients with hip pathology present with complaints such as:
- Pain
- Morning stiffness
- Deformity

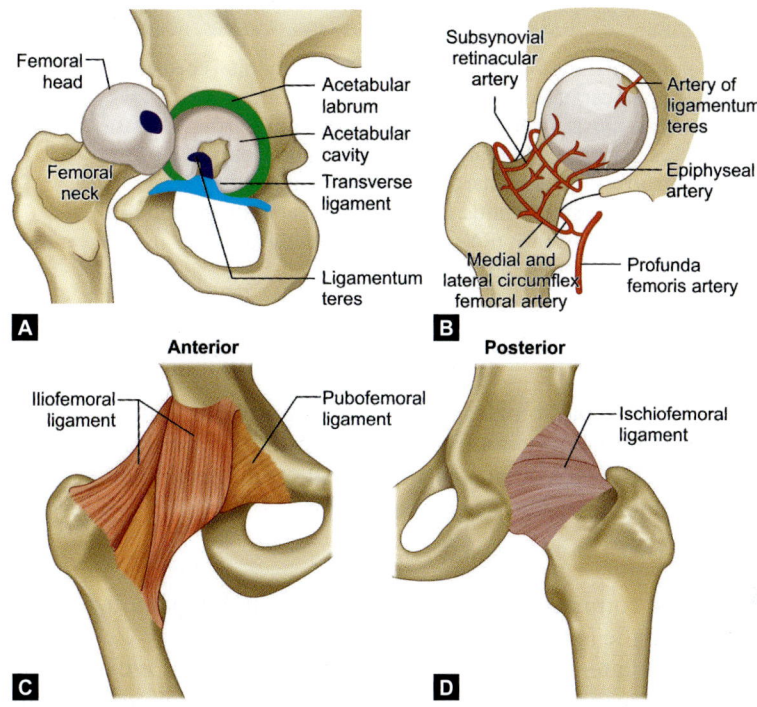

Figs. 7.1A to D: (A) Hip joint showing articulating bones, acetabular labrum, ligamentum teres and transverse ligament; (B) Blood supply of femoral head; (C and D) Ligaments of the hip joint.

TABLE 7.1: Important muscles around the hip joint, their insertion, nerve supply, and action.

Muscle	Insertion	Nerve supply	Principal action
Iliopsoas	Lesser trochanter	Femoral nerve and direct branch from lumbar plexus	Hip flexor
Gluteus maximus	Gluteal tuberosity of femur	Inferior gluteal nerve	Extensor, assists in external rotation
Gluteus medius, gluteus minimus	Lateral, anterior, and superior surfaces of the greater trochanter (GT)	Superior gluteal nerve	Abductor
Adductor longus, brevis, magnus, and gracilis	Medial aspect of femur shaft	Obturator nerve	Adductor
Anterior fibers of gluteus medius and minimus, tensor fascia lata	Greater trochanter	Superior gluteal nerve	Internal rotator
Piriformis, Gemellus superior and inferior, quadratus femoris, obturator externus and internus	Piriformis fossa, posterior aspect of the greater trochanter	Piriformis: *Nerve to piriformis* Obturator internus, Gemellus superior: *Nerve to: Obturator internus* Gemellus inferior, Quadratus femoris: *Nerve to: Quadratus femoris* Obturator externus: *Obturator nerve*	External rotator

> **BOX 7.1:** Common conditions affecting the hip joint.
> - **Congenital:** Developmental dysplasia of the hip (DDH), congenital coxa vara
> - **Developmental:** Slipped capital femoral epiphysis (SCFE)
> - **Idiopathic:** Avascular necrosis (AVN) of the head of the femur, Perthes' disease, transient synovitis
> - **Traumatic:** AVN, 2° osteoarthritis, fractures, dislocation, labral tears
> - **Infective:** Tom Smith arthritis, tubercular arthritis, pyogenic arthritis
> - **Degenerative:** Primary hip osteoarthritis, femoroacetabular impingement (FAI)
> - **Inflammatory:** Rheumatoid arthritis (RA), ankylosing spondylitis (AS)
> - **Hematological:** Sickle cell anemia causing AVN

- Limp
- Limb length discrepancy

While evaluating the hip pathologies during history and examination, a point must always be kept in mind that there can be an overlap of symptoms from the abdomen, pelvis, and lumbosacral structures. Hence, a detailed history and thorough examination help rule out other conditions, which can masquerade as a hip pathology.

Pain

Pain is one of the most common symptoms associated with hip pathology, and that must be evaluated in detail with the following questions:

- **Uni- or bilateral:** A bilateral hip pain may indicate more generalized or systemic pathology such as rheumatoid arthritis, avascular necrosis (due to systemic cause), or ankylosing spondylitis, whereas unilateral pain suggest a local pathology (post-traumatic osteoarthrosis, Perthes' disease, or infection).
- **Traumatic vs. non-traumatic origin:** The event of trauma to the hip joint can help differentiate from non-traumatic hip pathologies. For example, avascular necrosis of the hip following fracture neck femur whilst femoroacetabular impingement of the hip generally would not follow significant traumatic episode.
- **Onset of pain:** Acute (traumatic, septic) or insidious (OA, AVN, TB) help in differentiating between different pathologies.
- **Severity of pain:** Inflammatory and infective (TB, pyogenic) conditions result in moderate-to-severe pain, whereas mechanical causes (OA, FAI) result in mild-moderate pain.
- **Character of pain:** Dull aching pain is present in mechanical causes, whereas throbbing pain is felt in infection, inflammation, or tumor.
- **Radiation of pain:** The pain of the hip pathology can radiate along the femoral/obturator/sciatic nerve on the anterior/medial/posterior side of the thigh, respectively. Further, one must remember that the lumbosacral pathologies could also result in pain over anterior and posterior aspects of hip and thigh, whereas irritation of lateral cutaneous nerve of the thigh could result in pain over the lateral aspect of the thigh.
- **Referred pain:** Often, the pain due to hip pathology is referred to the knee due to a similar nerve supply of both joints. For example, the pain of Perthes' disease and SCFE often results in referred pain to the knee.
- **Diurnal variation:** Pain with activity indicates more of a mechanical hip pathology (labral or chondral tears, osteoarthritis, etc.), whereas inflammatory or infective pathologies hurt even at rest or night. *TB hip could result in a night cry (Refer to Chapter 1 for differences between mechanical and rest pain).*

- **Aggravating and relieving factors:** Pain due to osteoarthritis or FAI of the hip is more with activity, whereas pain due to inflammatory arthritis is more at night or rest and improves with activity.
- **Remission and exacerbation:** It is observed in inflammatory (RA) and metabolic arthritis (gout, pseudogout).

Morning Stiffness

It may indicate an inflammatory pathology in the hip (RA, AS). Patients with AS report increasing stiffness with rest and improvement with activity. They also report chronic low back pain with morning stiffness and night spasms.

Deformity

The deformity could be primary or secondary. Primary deformities arise out of conditions affecting the hip, such as *inflammatory* (RA, AS), *infective* (TB, septic arthritis), *post-traumatic* (fracture, dislocation) and *degenerative* (osteoarthritis). Secondary deformities arise from pathologies in the spine, pelvis, and the lower limb (excluding hip). One must probe the onset, duration, progression, associated symptoms, and any history of trauma or infection regarding deformity.

Limp

- Limp could be due to pain, stiffness, short limb, and weak/altered abductor mechanism of the hip.
- *Painless limp* is seen in limb length discrepancy, paralytic, or a congenital deformity (DDH, coxa vara), whereas *painful limp* is observed in Perthes, SCFE, traumatic, infective, inflammatory, or tumorous conditions.

Limb Length Discrepancy (LLD)

Onset (after trauma/infection/others), duration, progression of LLD must be evaluated. True LLD indicates inadequate development of bone (congenital or metabolic disorder), damage to the bone (infection, trauma, surgery), or loss of contact between articulating bones (dislocations).

Current Disability

An inquiry has to be made as to how the current problem has affected the activities of daily living, occupation, and sports, if any. These disabilities also indicate loss of movement in certain directions. For example, difficulty in squatting suggests restriction of extreme hip flexion, while difficulty in sitting cross-legged suggests the restriction of the flexion, abduction, and external rotation of the hip joint.

Use of Walking Aids, Shoe Raise

The use of a walking aid (axillary crutch, walking stick) may suggest a painful or unstable hip. A shoe raise indicates limb shortening.

Constitutional Features

Constitutional features such as fever, malaise, loss of weight and appetite are often present in infective (TB), inflammatory and malignant conditions.

Past History
Childhood history of DDH, Perthes' disease, and SCFE can predispose to 2° osteoarthritis of the hip at a later age.

Family History
The family history of DDH, TB, spondyloarthropathy, gout, rheumatoid arthritis, and hemoglobinopathies (sickle cell anemia) is important as they all carry possibility of familial transmission.

Treatment History
Treatment history can give a clue to the current diagnosis. Several examples are listed below.
- The treatment for any systemic disease involving prolonged steroid intake can cause AVN of the hip.
- Fracture neck femur of the hip could lead to complications like AVN or nonunion, whereas intertrochanteric femur can cause malunion.
- A surgical history around the hip may give a clue to the underlying pathology such as open surgical drainage in septic arthritis of the hip.

Personal, Menstrual, Allergy History
A habit of chronic alcohol intake or smoking can cause AVN of the hip.

At the end of history assessment, many common clinical hip conditions can be reasonably well diagnosed based upon a combination of age and key complaints. **Table 7.2** summarizes

TABLE 7.2: Hip Clinical diagnostic snippets.

Symptoms and/or signs	Most likely pathology/diagnosis
An 18-month-old female child walks with a painless limp. She has painless waddling gait and restricted abduction and internal rotation	Developmental dysplasia of the hip
A male child between 5–12 years of age hailing from the South West coast of India presents with painful restriction of hip movement	Perthes disease
An obese, adolescent child, may be having hypogonadism, presents with pain in the hip or knee, walks with externally rotated limb	Slipped capital femoral epiphysis
A neonate/infant with excessive crying, refusal to feed, and pseudoparalysis of the lower limb or an older child with inability to bear weight with a history of high-grade fever	Septic arthritis of the hip
A person of any age with poor nutritional status, hip pain with a history of night cry, and other constitutional symptoms	Tuberculosis of the hip
A young adult with dull aching groin/hip pain, without a significant trauma history. There may be a history of steroid intake/alcohol consumption	Idiopathic/secondary avascular necrosis
An elderly patient with the mechanical hip pain, walks with a stick with severe restriction of the range of hip movements	Primary or secondary hip arthritis

TABLE 7.3: Relevant general findings in case of hip disorders.

Skin	Rashes on face—SLE; psoriatic plaques—psoriasis. Both psoriasis and SLE cause hip OA
Eyes	Uveitis—ankylosing spondylitis; blue sclera— osteogenesis imperfecta
Pinna	Tophi—Gout; blackish discoloration—ochronosis. Gout can cause AVN hip, ochronosis can cause hip OA
Low set ears	Turner's and Down syndrome, which are associated with hip dysplasia
Low posterior hairline	Turner's syndrome, Down syndrome, Klippel-Feil syndrome
Nails	Pitting, onycholysis—psoriasis
Facial puffiness, lemon on stick appearance	Chronic steroid intake, which can cause AVN hip

the important snippets for the clinical diagnosis of common hip pathologies. However, all of them require confirmation with the specific examination.

EXAMINATION

General and Systemic Examination

Standard general and systemic examination must be performed as many hip disorders are a part of systemic disease such as RA, sickle cell anemia, TB, or AS. In all the patients with non-traumatic hip pathology, a thorough head-to-toe survey should be done as many clinical findings are part of systemic disease, syndrome, or chronic drug intake resulting in hip and spine disorder. Many such conditions with associated findings in the body are listed in **Table 7.3**.

Local Examination

After appropriate consent, privacy and chaperone, the patient should be suitably undressed, but private parts should be adequately covered. The presence of a female attender is a must if a female patient has to be examined.

Gait

Gait must be noted in an ambulatory patient. There are various types of gait such as antalgic gait, Trendelenburg gait, waddling gait, short-limb gait, and gluteus maximus gait. *(Refer to Chapter 14 on Gait to understand the nuances of each type of gait).*

Attitude

Typically, it is described in the supine position. The normal attitude is hip and knee in extension, ankle in plantar flexion, and lower limb in 10–15° of external rotation with patella facing outwards and laterally **(Fig. 7.2)**.

Inspection

It should be done in both standing followed by supine positions and, in a sequence *'proximal-to-distal'* to avoid missing any landmark/finding.

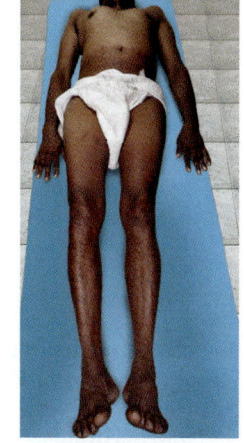

Fig. 7.2: Lower limb attitude.

General Findings

Swelling, scar, sinus anywhere should be described in a standard fashion. Typically, swelling in the hip region (Scarpa's triangle, gluteal) could be due to a cold abscess whose origin could be from the spine or an anteriorly dislocated femoral head.

Specific Findings

Observe patient both in standing and sitting.

Inspection in Standing

One must inspect patient from front, side, and behind:
a. **Inspection from the front (Fig. 7.3):** Observe for:
   1. *Level of both shoulders:* Shoulder levels could be different in limb length discrepancy/pelvic tilt.
   2. *Position of the anterior superior iliac spine (ASIS):* Lower/higher/same level must be noted as that may indicate the type of hip deformity or limb shortening.
   3. *Scarpa's triangle:* Scar/sinus/swellings should be noted in the Scarpa's triangle. The anatomy of Scarpa's triangle is mentioned in **Box 7.2**.
   4. *Level of the greater trochanter (GT):* The level of two GT must be compared. A higher GT level may be observed in a non-union neck femur, malunited intertrochanteric fracture femur, or a dislocated hip.
   5. *Thigh folds:* Asymmetric or prominent thigh folds are observed in the case of unilateral DDH.
   6. *Patella orientation:* With both lower limb parallel to each other in standing, the patella always faces slightly laterally. Excess lateral facing of the patella with respect to the normal side indicates external rotation deformity of the limb, whereas straight/inward facing patella indicates internally rotated limb.
   7. *Thigh and calf muscle wasting:* It indicates a chronic condition of the hip such as TB arthritis.
b. **Inspection from the side:** Observe for:
   1. *Spine:* Observe for natural thoracic kyphosis and lumbar lordosis. Note any attenuation or increase in curves.
   2. *Trochanteric region:* Swelling, scar, and sinus.
   3. *Hip* (Neutral/flexed); *knee* (extended/flexed/recurvatum); and *heel level* (plantigrade/equinus/calcaneus)

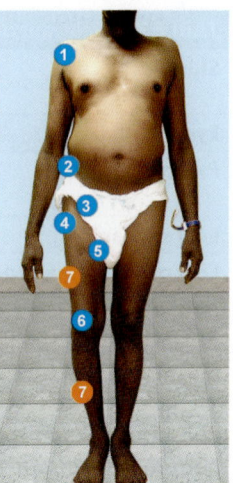

Fig. 7.3: Inspection from the front (check point 1–7; Point 7 in orange circle suggests thigh and calf muscle wasting.

Note: Level of ASIS indicating the type of deformity at the index hip joint.
A lower level of ASIS of index side: May indicate abduction deformity at the hip.
Higher level of ASIS of index side: May indicate adduction deformity at the hip.

BOX 7.2: Anatomy and content of the Scarpa's triangle.

- **Scarpa's (femoral) triangle:** It is a triangle in the upper part of the thigh bounded superiorly by the inguinal ligament, laterally by the medial border of the sartorius, and medially by the medial border of the adductor longus. The floor is formed laterally by the iliopsoas and medially by the pectineus.
- **Contents (from lateral to medial):** Femoral nerve, artery, and vein, lymph nodes
- **Causes of swelling/fullness in scarpa's triangle:** Anterior dislocation hip, psoas abscess, enlarged lymph nodes, saphena varix

c. **Inspection from behind (Fig. 7.4):** Observe for:
   1. *Level of shoulder:* The shoulder level may differ, especially in patients with limb length discrepancy.
   2. *Spine:* Look for deformities in the spine (scoliosis).
   3. *Level of posterior superior iliac spine (PSIS,* "Dimple of Venus")
   4. *Gluteal muscle wasting:* Underlying gluteal wasting indicates long-standing hip pathology.
   5. *Popliteal fossa:* Look for any swelling.
   6. *Thigh and calf muscle wasting:* Wasting indicates long-standing disuse of the limb.
   7. *Heel status:* Plantigrade/equinus/calcaneus/varus/valgus.

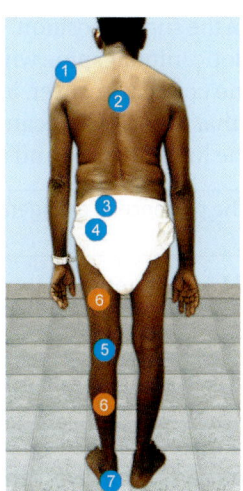

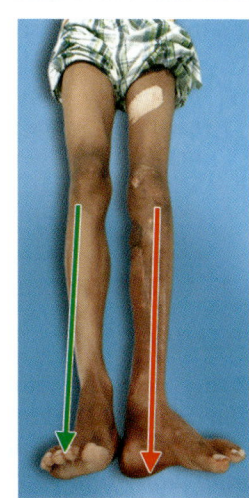

Fig. 7.4: Inspection from behind (check points 1–7). Point 6 in orange circle suggests thigh and calf muscle wasting.

Fig. 7.5: Normal rotational alignment of the right lower limb (green arrow) while abnormal external rotation of the left lower limb (red arrow).

Inspection in Supine Position

It should always be performed on a hard bed. The supine examination should commence once the patient seems to be lying straight. To ensure that patient is lying straight without any spino-pelvic-lower limb tilt, the clinician can hold both ankles of the patient and gently tug patient downwards to make patient straight.

a. **Inspection from the front:** The findings are similar to those in standing. However, limb length discrepancy is easily noted in the supine position by comparing the heel or medial malleolus level. Typical findings to be noted are:
   1. *Level of both ASIS:* Both the ASIS can be on the same or different levels. A higher or lower level of index ASIS indicates adduction or abduction deformity of the hip, respectively.
   2. *Rotational deformities of the lower limb:* In a normally aligned lower limb, the patella faces slightly laterally and upwards and the lower limbs are 10–15° externally rotated. Further, if one draws an imaginary line from the center of the patella to the shaft of the tibia, the line passes through the second toe. In any rotational deformity, the line will not be in alignment with the 2nd toe **(Fig. 7.5)**.
   3. *Scarpa's or femoral triangle:* Observe for 'any abnormal fullness', swelling, scars, or sinuses. The normal fullness may be lost in a posteriorly dislocated hip, whereas it is increased in the presence of swelling.
   4. *Level of the greater trochanter (GT):* Level of the affected GT and compare with the normal side, whether it is higher/lower or at the same level.
   5. *Thigh folds:* Observe any asymmetry.
   6. *Thigh (quadriceps) and calf muscle wasting, if any*
   7. *Limb length discrepancy:* Assessed by checking the level of both ASIS, lower pole of the patella, medial malleolus, or the heel.
b. **Inspection from the side:** Typical findings to be noted are:
   1. *Lumbar lordosis:* It is best examined from the side in the supine position (ALWAYS on a hard bed).

In a normal person in the supine position, there is no space between the examination couch and the normal lordotic lumbar spine when the clinician brings his eyeline parallel to the lumbar spine and the couch. However, in the case of exaggerated lumbar lordosis, there is enough space so that the clinician can view the other side of the wall or can insinuate his hand between the lumbar spine and the couch **(Fig. 7.6)**.

> **Note:** In most cases, the presence of exaggerated lumbar lordosis indicates fixed flexion deformity of the hip.

2. *Attitude of hip and knee:* Whether it is in neutral or flexion.

Palpation

During palpation from the front, side, and behind, several key findings, such as *rise in local temperature, tenderness over joint lines and major bony and soft tissue landmarks*, and assessment of the *deformities* at the hip in all three planes are ascertained from front, side and back.

The **rise in local temperature** should be felt over anterior, lateral, and posterior aspects of the hip joint. Although not readily appreciated in a deeply seated hip joint, any temperature rise indicates infective or inflammatory pathology.

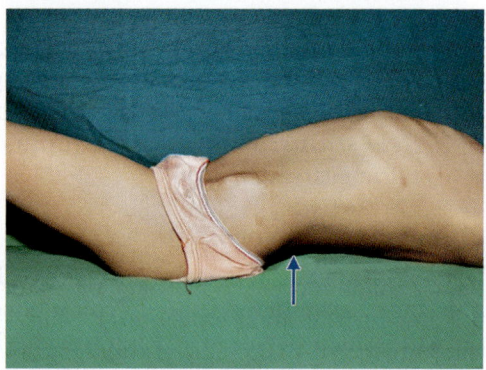

Fig. 7.6: Exaggerated lumbar lordosis (blue arrow).

Palpation from the Front

1. **Level of both ASIS:** ASIS is the first bony prominence palpated at the lateral end of the inguinal ligament while the clinician runs his thumb along the inguinal ligament. Confirm the level of ASIS; high, low, or same as compared to the contralateral side.
2. **Tenderness:** Tenderness must be checked over the joint line, important bony and soft tissue landmarks such as pubic tubercle, symphysis pubis, and both greater trochanters.
   Method to palpate anterior hip joint line: The anterior hip joint line is located 2–3 cm below and lateral to the mid-inguinal point **(Fig. 7.7)**.

> Note that the mid-inguinal point is the mid-point between the ASIS and pubic symphysis, while the mid-point of the inguinal ligament is the middle of the inguinal ligament, which stretches between pubic tubercle and ASIS.

3. **Palpation of greater trochanter:** Compare both the greater trochanters for level, broadening, thickening, and tenderness. Always palpate the normal GT followed by index one for comparison.

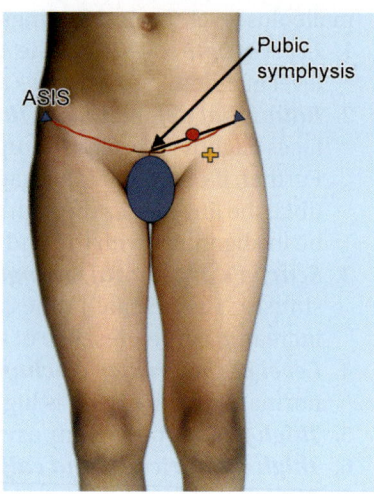

Fig. 7.7: Location of the anterior hip joint line (yellow cross). The red circle indicates mid-inguinal point (Note that it is not the mid-point of the inguinal ligament).

Palpation from the Side
Lumbar lordosis: Normally, the lumbar spine touches the couch, and the clinician cannot insinuate his/her fingers underneath the lumbar spine. However, in the case of exaggerated lumbar lordosis, the clinician will easily pass his fingers through the gap between the lumbar spine and couch.

Palpation from Behind
1. **Tenderness:** Tenderness must be felt over spine, PSIS, SIJ, ischial tuberosity (IT), and the rest of the gluteal region. The landmark/technique to palpate important bony prominences is mentioned below.
   PSIS: The dimples in the gluteal region on either side of the sacrum indicate PSIS.
   SI joint: SIJ can be palpated about 2.5 cm inferomedial to the PSIS and further straight downwards.
   Ischial tuberosity: It is felt midway between the lower sacrum and the tip of the GT. To make IT more prominent, the patient can turn in the lateral position and flex the hip and knee to 90°.
2. **Palpate for any abnormal mass or swelling in the gluteal region:** The presence of a globular bony mass which moves with femoral rotation could be the femoral head (in case of the posteriorly dislocated femoral head).

Assessment of Deformity
The deformities of the hip can be in the sagittal (flexion), coronal (abduction-adduction), or axial (rotation) plane.

The assessment of deformities in the sagittal, coronal and axial plane is discussed below.
1. **Deformity in the sagittal plane:** The typical sagittal plane deformity is a fixed flexion deformity of the hip (FFDH). Its presence is indirectly indicated by "exaggerated lumbar lordosis." FFDH is masked by anterior tilting of the pelvis, which is hidden by exaggerated lumbar lordosis. Therefore, to unmask the FFDH, one must obliterate the exaggerated lumbar lordosis.
   Test for unilateral flexion deformity: Thomas Hip Flexion Test
   Method: The patient lies supine over a hard couch with both lower limbs parallel to each other. In an exaggerated lumbar lordosis, the clinician can easily insinuate his fingers between the lumbar spine and the couch. Keeping one hand under the exaggerated lordotic lumbar spine, the unaffected hip is gradually flexed by the other hand of the clinician while keeping the knee in flexion till the lumbar lordosis is just obliterated and the clinician feels his/her fingers being tightly gripped between the couch and the lumbar spine. At the same time, the index/affected hip moves in 'further' flexion. Now ask the patient to hold the unaffected flexed knee with his/her both hands clasped together, and measure the 'angle of flexion' of the affected hip from the horizontal plane with the goniometer **(Figs. 7.8A and B)**. Note that the hand cannot be insinuated between the couch and the lumbar spine once the lumbar lordosis is obliterated.

   The methods to detect bilateral FFD are out of scope of the chapter for undergraduates.

The Rationale of Thomas Hip Flexion Test
Typically, with gradual flexion deformity of the hip, the ipsilateral foot will move away from the ground, and the patient would require ankle in equinus to keep the foot in contact with the ground for ambulation. However, the pelvis gradually starts tilting anteriorly for ambulation with plantigrade

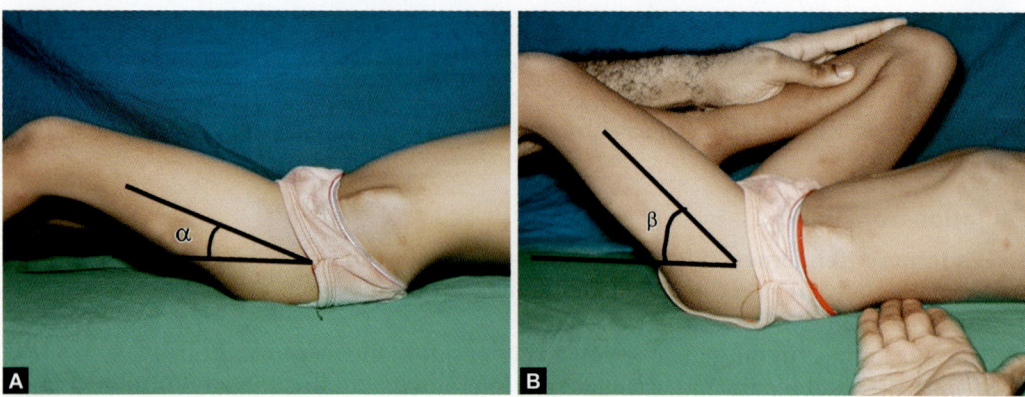

Figs. 7.8A and B: Thomas hip flexion test for unilateral fixed flexion deformity of the hip. (A) Exaggerated lumbar lordosis with an apparent flexion deformity of left hip indicated by α angle; (B) Normal (right) hip is flexed until lumbar lordosis is obliterated, which is indicated by inability to insinuate the fingers under the lumbar spine. The exact flexion deformity of the left hip is indicated by β angle.

feet (ankle in neutral). Further, as the pelvis tilts anteriorly, lumbar lordosis also increases to keep the spine straight in the sagittal plane. Therefore, the whole process of anterior tilt of the pelvis and concomitant exaggerated lordosis is to keep the foot plantigrade while simultaneously conceal the flexion deformity of the hip. During hip flexion (of Thomas test), the femoral shaft hitches against the anterior acetabular margin and tilts the pelvis posteriorly (or normal position), exposing the hip's 'concealed' flexion deformity.

2. **Deformity in the coronal plane (ABduction or ADduction):** In a normal person standing or lying supine, the two ASIS remain at the same horizontal level. In abduction or adduction deformity of the hip, there is a compensatory coronal tilting of the pelvis (for plantigrade ambulation), resulting in different levels of the ASIS. *Therefore, ASIS at the different levels indicates coronal plane deformity at the hip joint.* The coronal plane deformity could be unilateral or bilateral. Before we understand the assessment of coronal plane deformity, it is important to understand several terminologies of coronal plane deformity as well as the rationale behind ASIS titling during coronal plane deformity.
Terminologies in coronal plane deformity assessment:
- *Squared pelvis:* When both ASIS are brought to the same level, it is called squared pelvis.
- *Unsquared pelvis:* When both ASIS are not at the same level, it is called unsquared pelvis.

> **Position of ASIS in abduction and adduction deformity**
> - When the index side ASIS is lower than the normal side, one must suspect **abduction deformity** of the index hip joint.
> - When the index side ASIS higher than the normal side, one must suspect **adduction deformity** of the index hip joint.

The rationale of ASIS tilting downward or upward in Abduction/Adduction deformity, respectively: In a patient who gradually develops abduction deformity of the hip over weeks and months due to any underlying pathology, the foot would be off the ground and the patient would be unable to ambulate in a plantigrade fashion. Hence, to bring the foot back onto the

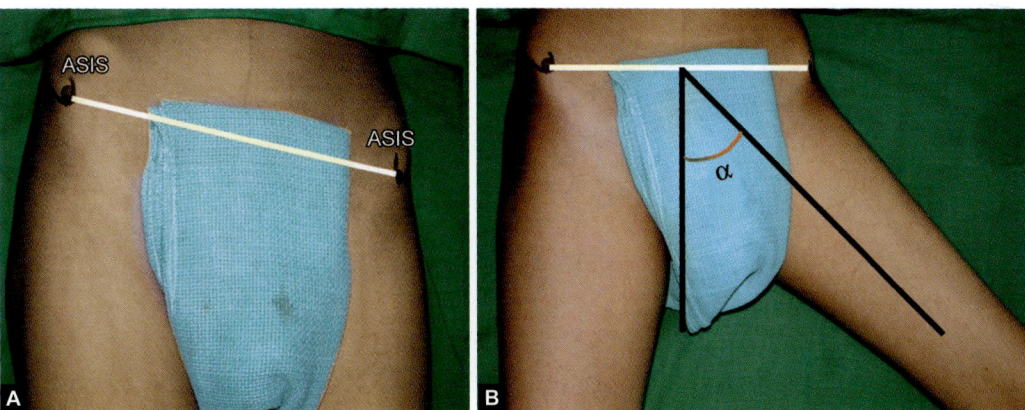

Figs. 7.9A and B: Measurement of hip abduction deformity after squaring the pelvis. (A) Left (index) anterior-superior iliac spine (ASIS) is at a lower level; (B) Both ASIS are at the same level (squared pelvis) after abducting the left hip. α denotes the amount of abduction deformity in the left hip.

ground, the pelvis on the affected side tilts downwards in the coronal plane (lowered ASIS) as a compensatory mechanism of the body, enabling the patient to walk in a plantigrade fashion.

Similarly, in a gradually developing adduction deformity, the affected limb crosses the midline, making walking difficult. Hence, the pelvis tilts upwards (ASIS moving upwards), bringing back the affected limb in a neutral position and enabling the patient to walk in a plantigrade fashion.

Coronal plane deformity assessment: Perkin's method is deployed to assess the unilateral coronal plane deformity where the pelvis is squarable whereas Kothari's method is utilized if the pelvis is not squared or squarable. Note that discussion regarding the Kothari's method and bilateral coronal plane deformity is out of scope for this chapter (for undergraduates).

Perkin's method to assess the unilateral coronal plane deformities in a pelvis that can be squared.

Method: With the patient supine and limbs parallel, the clinician keeps his thumb and middle finger over the two ASIS and gently moves the affected hip by holding the limb near the ankle. If the ASIS is higher, move the hip in further ADduction to bring the ASIS at the same level of the contralateral side. If the ASIS is at the lower level, move the hip in further ABduction to get the ASIS at the same level of the contralateral side. Once both ASIS are at the same level, the angle of the deformity (adduction or abduction) should be measured from the midline with a goniometer **(Figs. 7.9A and B)**.

3. **Deformity in the axial plane (rotational deformity):** Rotational deformities (internal and external rotation) are *revealed deformities* and are not concealed (hidden) by the movements or compensated by the pelvis or the spine. Rotational deformities can be detected with the patient in a supine or prone position.

Movement

While assessing the ROM of the hip joint, one must note several important points as mentioned below.

1. **Always check the deformities before commenting upon the range of motion (ROM).**
   If the joint has a deformity, the ROM must be described with fixed deformity and further

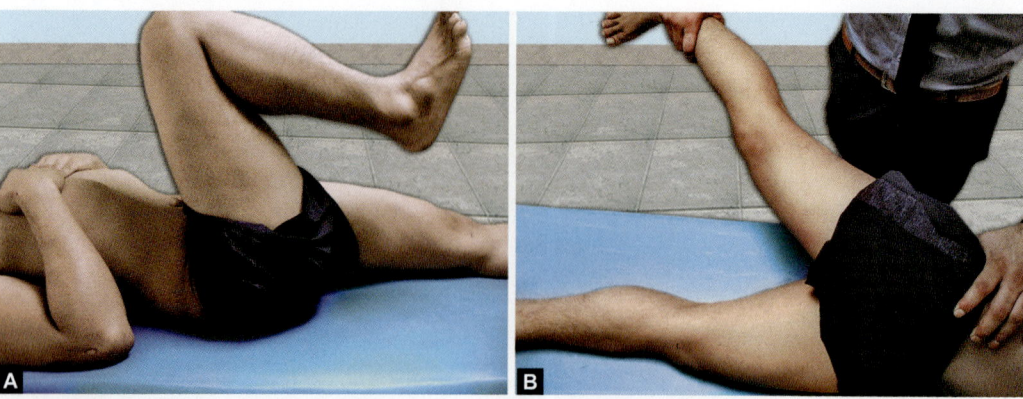

Figs. 7.10A and B: *Hip movement:* Flexion (pelvis stabilization not shown) and extension (with pelvis stabilized).

movements. For example, 20° flexion deformity with further free flexion up to 80°. Then the ROM of flexion is 20–80°.

2. **Stabilize the pelvis while assessing movements.** *Active movements must be assessed first followed by passive ROM. Always compare with contralateral side.*
3. **Always comment upon characteristics of movement, such as total range, painless or painful, and associated crepitus.**

The method to check hip ROM (for right side) is described below **(Figs. 7.10 to 7.12)**.

a. **Hip flexion:** The hip flexion ROM is assessed with the knee in flexion **(Fig. 7.10A)**. One must stop flexing hip just when pelvis starts tilting posteriorly due to the pressure of thighs over the front of the pelvis. The normal hip flexion is 120°.
b. **Hip extension:** This can be tested in two ways; either in a lateral position **(Fig. 7.10B)** till movement of pelvis is detected or in a prone position, with the knee in flexion. The latter method is better as the pelvis remains more stable, and the slightest movement of the pelvis is detected earlier than in the lateral position. The normal hip extension is 10°.
c. **ABduction:** To assess ABduction of the right hip, the clinician holds the right leg near the ankle by his right hand while his left-hand thumb and the middle finger are kept over the ASIS to detect any pelvic movement. Now, the hip is abducted gradually till the upward movement of ASIS is first detected **(Fig. 7.11A)**. The angle between the imaginary midline and the abducted thigh measures the abduction. The normal hip abduction is 40°.
d. **ADduction:** To assess ADduction of the right hip, the clinician holds the leg by the right hand while the left-hand thumb and the middle finger are kept over the ASIS to detect any pelvic movement. Now, the hip is adducted gradually until the downward movement of ASIS is first detected **(Fig. 7.11B)**. Usually, the thigh can cross the proximal-third/middle-third of the contralateral thigh in the adducted position. The angle between the imaginary midline and the adducted limb measures adduction. The normal hip adduction is 10°.
e. **Hip rotations:** The rotation ROM should be assessed both in extended hip-knee and flexed hip-knee **(Figs. 7.12A to C)**. Typically, the hip rotations in flexion are 5–10° more than an extended hip as the hip joint capsule is relaxed in a flexed position.

> **How to measure the angle of ROM during hip movements using a goniometer?**
> Place one of the arms of the goniometer parallel to the flexed/abducted/adducted/rotated limb whereas the other arm of the goniometer is kept parallel to the imaginary midline of the body. The angle between the two arms of the goniometer is the angle of movement in that plane **(Fig. 7.13)**.

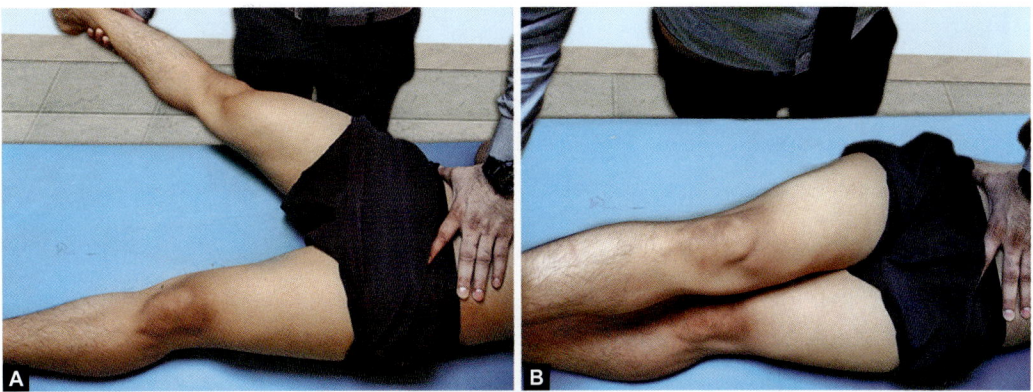

Figs. 7.11A and B: *Hip movement:* Abduction and adduction (with pelvis stabilized).

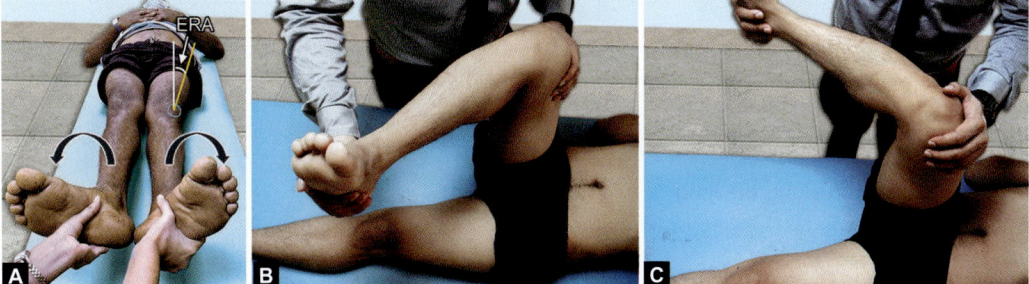

Figs. 7.12A to C: *Hip movement:* (A) External rotation with hips in extension is indicated by curved blue arrows *(Note—internal rotation not shown here)*. White line indicates imaginary vertical and yellow line indicates imaginary perpendicular over the patella. ERA is external rotation angle between the two lines; (B) External rotation in 90° flexion; (C) Internal rotation in 90° flexion of the hip. *Note:* Fingers should be over both ASIS to detect movement of the pelvis during rotation assessment (not shown in figures B and C).

Measurements

Important parameters to be measured during hip examination are limb length and muscle wasting.

A. **Limb length measurements** encompass assessment of apparent and true limb length, Bryant triangle, and Galeazzi test. Bryant triangle assessment concludes whether the shortening of the femur is supra- or infra-trochanteric. The Galeazzi test is a simple method to assess whether the shortening of the lower limb is in the femur or tibia.
B. **Wasting of thigh and calf muscles** is assessed by measuring the thigh and calf girth, respectively.
   a. **Limb length measurement:** The lower limb, especially thigh length, varies in a tilted pelvis as thigh measurements are from a point on the pelvis (ASIS) to the medial joint line. Since a tilted pelvis affects ASIS level (up or down), it affects the 'measured length of thigh.'

   Therefore, when thigh length is measured without correcting the pelvic tilt (unsquared pelvis- ASIS at different level), it is known as *apparent length*, while thigh length obtained after correcting pelvic tilt (squared pelvis- ASIS at same level) is known as *true length*.

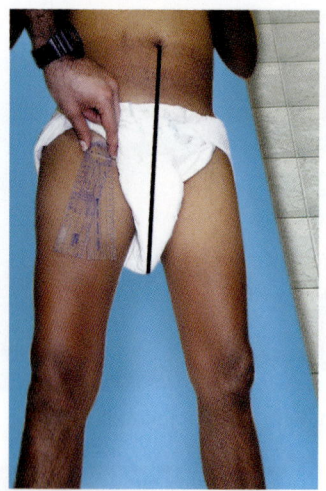 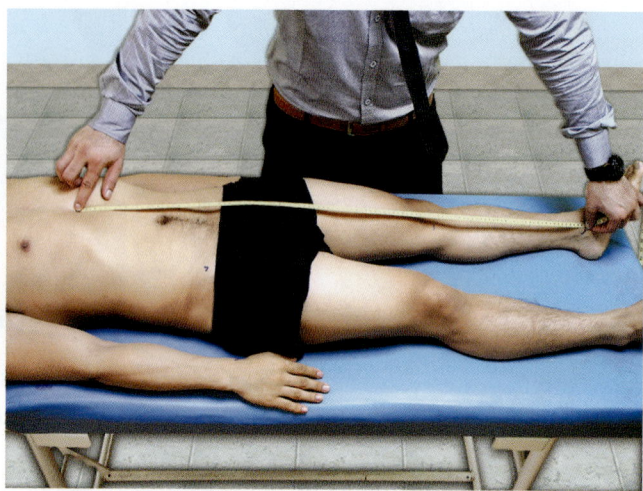

Fig. 7.13: Measurement of the hip abduction ROM with a goniometer (Black line represents the imaginary midline along which static limb of goniometer is kept parallel while dynamic limb is placed along the long axis of the thigh).

Fig. 7.14: Technique to measure the apparent length of the lower limb without pelvis being squared.

1. ***Apparent limb length:*** The lower limbs should be kept parallel to measure the apparent limb length discrepancy. *The squaring of the pelvis is not required. Method*: With the patient supine, hold both the ankles and gently tug the patient downwards by a few inches as that corrects any truncal tilt or pelvic obliquity. Keep both lower limbs in the same position and measure the apparent length from the *Xiphisternum to the tip of the medial malleolus* on both sides *(Note:* Always mark these bony land- marks with skin marking pencil before the measurement) **(Fig. 7.14)**.
2. ***True limb length:*** It should be measured *only after squaring the pelvis*. The method of pelvis squaring has been discussed during assessment of abduction and adduction deformity of the hip (vide supra).
   Method: With the patient supine and squared pelvis, both limbs are placed in an identical position. *The distance between the ASIS and the medial joint line of the knee* and between the *medial joint line and the tip of the medial malleolus* **(Figs. 7.15A and B)** gives a measure of the segmental length of the thigh and leg, respectively. It also reveals the exact site (thigh/leg/both) of limb length discrepancy.

> **Example of 'Squaring the Pelvis' and Measuring the Limb Length**
> - *If there is a 20° adduction deformity* in the left hip, the left ASIS will be at a higher level than the right. To square the pelvis, the left lower limb is gradually adducted by 20°. This brings 'ASIS of affected side' at the level of 'ASIS of normal side'. After squaring the pelvis, the right limb should also be kept in 20° adduction. Now, sequentially measure the true length of the limb, keeping both limbs in 20° adduction.

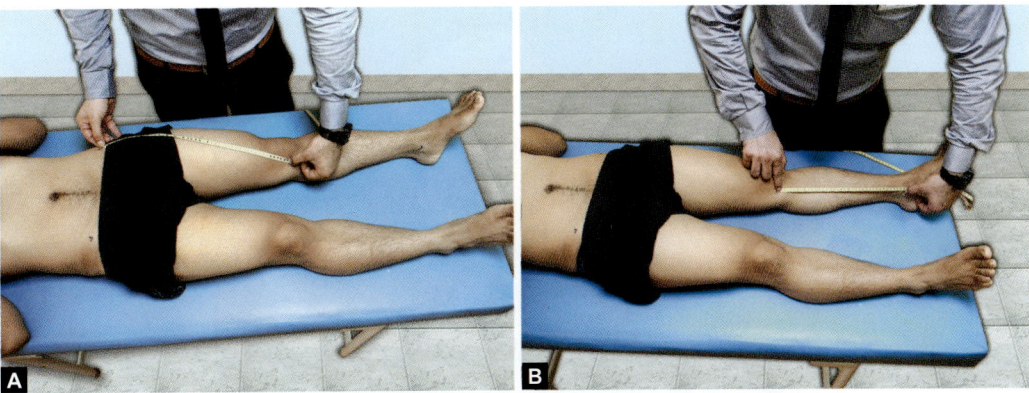

Figs. 7.15A and B: Technique to measure the true length of the lower limb after squaring the pelvis. (A) Measurement of the femur component; (B) Measurement of the tibial component.

> • If there is a 30° abduction deformity in the right hip, the right ASIS will be lower than the left. To square the pelvis, the right lower limb is abducted by 30°. This brings 'ASIS of affected side' at the level of 'ASIS of normal side'. After squaring the pelvis, the left (normal) hip should also be kept in 30° abduction. Now, sequentially measure the true length of the limb, keeping both limbs in 30° abduction.

3. **Bryant's triangle measurement:** Bryant's triangle measurement is done to ascertain whether shortening in the femur is supratrochanteric or infratrochanteric **(Fig. 7.16)**. Of note— *Bryant's triangle measurement can be done only in a squared pelvis*.
   Method: The patient lies *supine* with the *pelvis squared* and the *limbs are in an identical position in coronal and sagittal planes*. Mark the ASIS and the tip of the greater trochanter

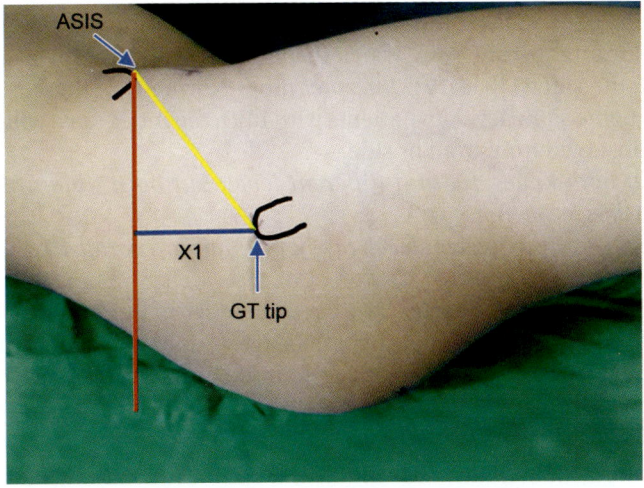

Fig. 7.16: Measurement of Bryant's triangle. Red line: perpendicular towards the floor; Blue line: base of the triangle; Yellow line: hypotenuse of the triangle. X1 is the supratrochanteric length.
(GT: greater trochanter; ASIS, anterior superior iliac spine).

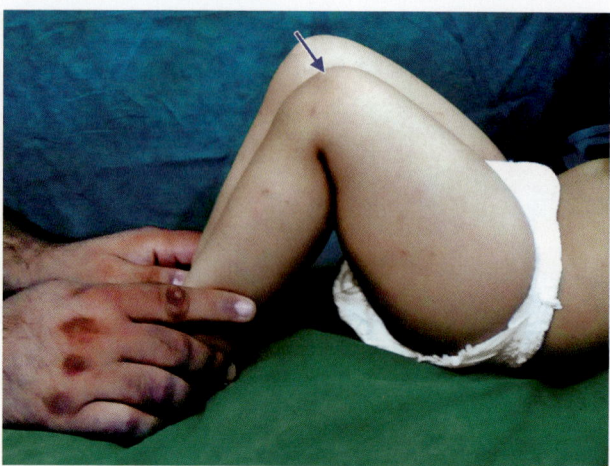

Fig. 7.17: Galeazzi test. Blue arrow indicates the level of the knee (lower).

(TGT) and join them by a straight line (yellow line). Next, a plumb line is dropped from the ASIS toward the floor (red line). Further, a perpendicular line (X1) is drawn from the TGT to the plumb line (blue line). The length of the perpendicular line (X1) is measured. A similar triangle is drawn on the normal side where X2 would denote length of the base of the triangle.

Interpretation of Bryant's triangle:
- *Supratrochanteric shortening*: The discrepancy in limb length will equal X2–X1.
- *Infratrochanteric shortening*: There will be no discrepancy in X1 and X2.

4. ***Galeazzi test/Allis sign:*** To assess the location (thigh/leg) of unilateral limb length discrepancy LLD.
   Method: The patient lies supine with both hips flexed at 45° and knee at 90°. Watch the knee level from the front. Also, watch the knee level and parallelism of the femur and tibia from the side **(Fig. 7.17)**. *Interpretation:* Normally, if there is no LLD, both the knees are at the same level. In patients with LLD, the index knee will be at a lower level whether observed from front or side.
   Further, *If both knees are at a different level, but both tibia are parallel:* Length discrepancy is in the tibia.
   If both knees are at a different level, but both femur are parallel: Length discrepancy is in the femur

b. **Wasting of thigh and calf muscles:** The circumference of thigh (site of maximum girth or 15 cm proximal to the superior pole of patella in an adult) and calf (at the maximum girth of calf or 10 cm distal to the tibia tuberosity) should be measured in every case **(Fig. 7.18)**.

Neurovascular Examination

It should be performed in the standard fashion.

Special Tests

Many special tests are performed to detect hip stability, muscle contracture, and femoroacetabular impingement.

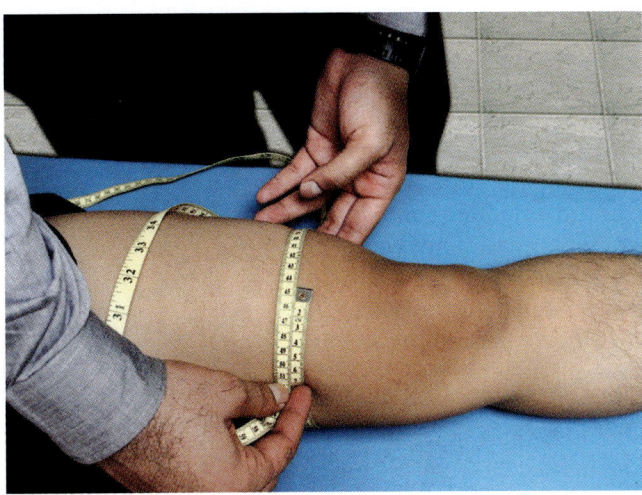

Fig. 7.18: Measurement of thigh wasting.

a. **Hip stability:** Telescopy test, Trendelenburg test, vascular sign of Narath, and test for DDH.
b. **Muscle contracture:** Ely's test
c. **Hip impingement:** FADDIR test.

Test for Hip Stability

There are several tests to assess hip stability, such as the Telescopy test, Trendelenburg test, vascular sign of Narath, and tests for DDH (Ortolani, Barlow's).

1. **Telescopy test:** It is performed when the lever arm of the hip (neck) is suspected to be broken (fracture neck femur) or the fulcrum is disturbed (dislocated head).
   Method: With the patient in a supine position, the hip and knee joints are flexed to 90° and the hip is adducted by 10°. For the left side, the clinician keeps the right thumb over the ASIS to stabilize the pelvis while the other fingers of the right hand are kept over the tip of GT to feel the excursion of the femur. Next, the clinician's left hand holds the patient's knee, applies gentle repeated push and pull force along the line of the femur and feels the trochanteric excursion with his fingers **(Fig. 7.19)**.
   Interpretation: The excursion (movements) of the GT in a normal hip is less than 1 cm. In telescopy positive cases, an excursion up to 4–5 cm is felt.
   Positive telescopy test observed in:
   - Nonunion femoral neck fracture or inter-trochanteric fracture
   - Chronic posterior dislocation of the hip
   - Developmental dysplasia of the hip

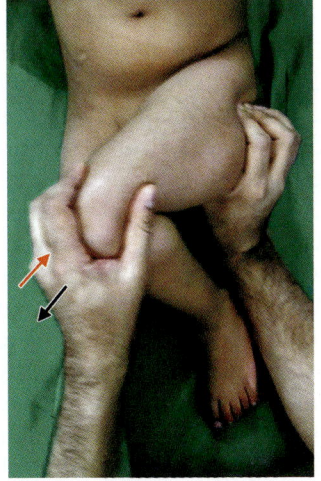

Fig. 7.19: Telescopy test. Orange and black arrows indicates push-pull direction, respectively.

2. **Trendelenburg test:** It was described by Friedrich Trendelenburg in 1894. It is performed to assess the integrity of the abductor mechanism of the hip in a single leg stance, i.e., when the patient is standing on a single limb, his/her abductor mechanism of the same side swings in action to keep the unsupported contralateral hemipelvis from drooping down. Any condition disrupting the hip abductor mechanism would result in a positive Trendelenburg test (*Read the description of the abductor mechanism on Page 140*).

    Prerequisites for the Trendelenburg test:
    - ❏ The patient should be able to stand on the affected side for at least 30 seconds.
    - ❏ At least 15° free adduction and abduction on the index side should be possible.

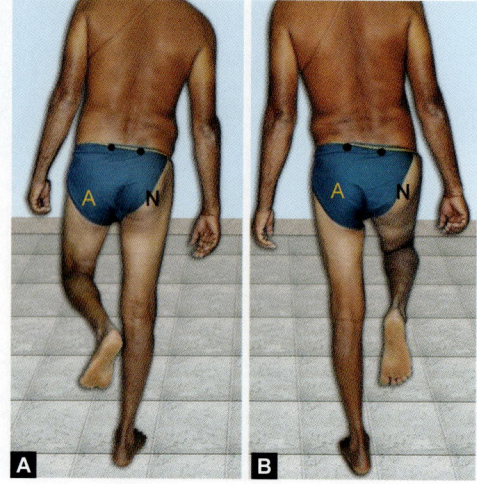

Figs. 7.20A and B: Trendelenburg test. (A) Negative Trendelenburg test for right hip; (B) Positive Trendelenburg test for left hip.

(A: Affected hip-left; N: Normal hip-right).

    Before performing the test on the patient, the clinician should ideally demonstrate to the patient to understand and perform accordingly.

    Method of standard Trendelenburg test: With the patient standing, the clinician stands behind the patient. Both PSIS are exposed. The patient is first asked to stand for at least 30 seconds on the normal side (N) with the affected side (A) foot off the ground with the knee in 60–70° flexion and hip 15–30° flexion. The PSIS on the affected side (observe two black circles in **Fig. 7.20A**) should move upwards or at least stay at the same level (normal). Next, ask the patient to stand for at least 30 seconds on the affected side with the normal side foot off the ground (**Fig. 7.20B**).

    Interpretation: The test is positive if the PSIS of the normal side dips down within 30 seconds while weight bearing on the affected side.

    Common conditions with positive Trendelenburg test:
    - ❏ Dislocation of the hip—anterior, posterior or central
    - ❏ Developmental dysplasia of the hip
    - ❏ Fracture neck of the femur/nonunion
    - ❏ Paralysis of hip abductors
    - ❏ Developmental coxa vara or coxa valga

3. **Vascular sign of Narath:** It is performed to assess whether the femoral head is articulating with acetabulum or 'dislocated'.

    Method: The patient lies supine on a couch. The femoral artery is palpated against the head of the femur, which lies 1–2 cm inferolateral to the mid-inguinal point (mid-point of the symphysis pubis and the ASIS).

    Interpretation: In an anatomically articulated hip joint, normal pulsation of the femoral artery is well palpable against the femoral head, whereas femoral artery pulsations are either feeble or not palpable in a posteriorly dislocated or subluxated head.

4. **Test for developmental dysplasia of the hip (DDH):**
    i. **Barlow test:** It is performed in a patient with suspected DDH *to assess whether the hip is dislocatable or not.*

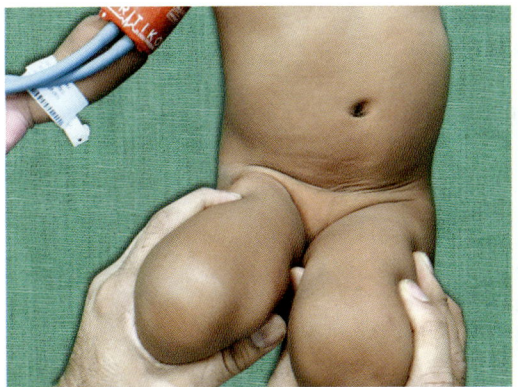

Fig. 7.21: Barlow test (for dislocatable hip).

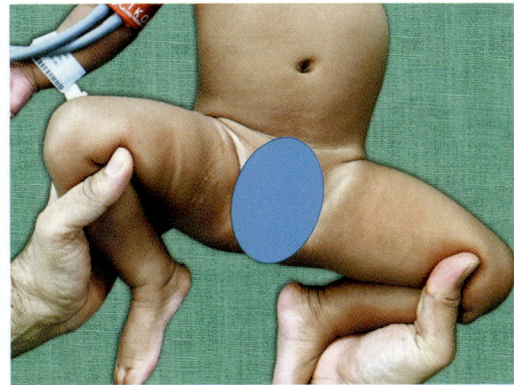

Fig. 7.22: Ortolani test (for relocatable hip).

Method: With the patient lying supine, the clinician flexes patient's hips to 90° by holding the thighs. The thumb is placed on the medial aspect of the thigh, whereas the index and middle fingers are placed over the GT. Next, the hip is adducted with gentle downward pressure along the long axis of the femur; simultaneously, lateral pressure is exerted by the thumb on the medial aspect of the thigh **(Fig. 7.21)**.

Interpretation: The test is positive if the femoral head can be pushed out of the acetabulum.

ii. **Ortolani test:** It was described by Marino Ortolani in 1936 to detect DDH, especially whether the *hip is relocatable (reducible)* or not.

Method: The clinician holds both thighs with his hands with the patient's hips and knees 90° flexed. The thumb is placed on the medial aspect of the thigh, whereas the index and middle fingers are placed over the GT. The hip is abducted with gentle traction, and simultaneously the trochanter is gently levered upward and forward **(Fig. 7.22)**.

Interpretation: The test is positive if the femoral head reduces into the acetabulum with a "click."

Tests for Muscle Contracture

Ely's test: ***For Rectus femoris contracture***
Method: The patient is made to lie prone on the couch. With the hip in extension, the knee is gradually flexed. In a normal patient, the knee can be flexed such that heel touches the buttocks without any hip flexion. In a patient with rectus femoris contracture, as the knee is flexed, the hip appears to flex gradually before the heel touches the buttock **(Fig. 7.23)**.

Tests for Hip (Femoroacetabular) Impingement

There is pain, loss of hip rotation, and flexion with occasional clicks in patients with hip impingement.

Impingement test: FADDIR (flexion, adduction, internal rotation) test.

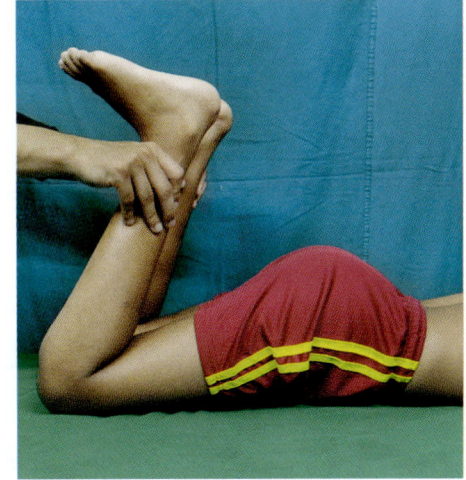

Fig. 7.23: Ely's test (for Rectus femoris contracture).

Method and interpretation: With the patient supine, the index hip is flexed to 90°, adducted, and internally rotated **(Fig. 7.24)**. Pain in the anterior part of the hip/groin indicates anterior impingement. It is a highly sensitive test but not specific.

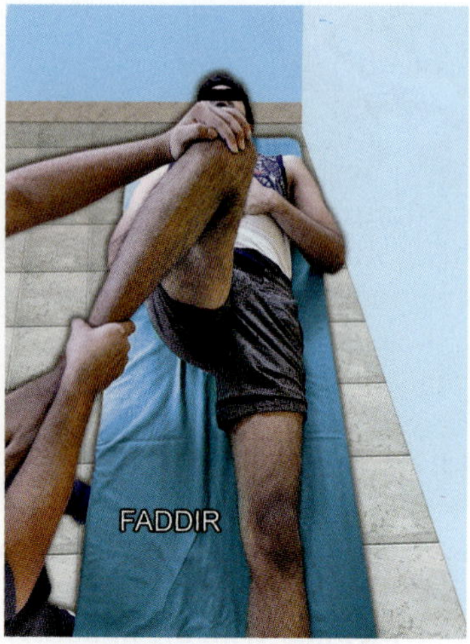

Examination of Joints Above and Below

One must always examine both sacroiliac joints and spine in all cases of hip pathology as the referral pattern of pain is similar in these areas. Apart from the spine and SIJ, one must also quickly examine both knees and ipsilateral ankle.

Lymph Node Examination

Local inguinal lymph nodes must be examined especially when one suspects infective and tumor conditions.

Fig. 7.24: Tests for hip impingement. FADDIR with adducted hip.

A NOTE ON ABDUCTOR MECHANISM AND TRENDELENBURG TEST

The Trendelenburg test is performed to assess the integrity of the abductor mechanism of the hip. So the question is "What is the abductor mechanism of the hip?" "Is it merely about the abductor muscle of the hip?"

The hip abductor mechanism is not merely about abductor muscle function, but it is a class one lever mechanism comprising the fulcrum, the lever arm, and forces on either end of the lever **(Fig. 7.25)**. This "intact" lever mechanism involves balancing the weight of the body, which passes via the unsupported hemipelvis during the swing phase of the gait without letting the pelvis drop.

The abductor mechanism comprises:
- *Fulcrum:* Acetabulum
- *Lever arm:* Head, neck, and trochanter

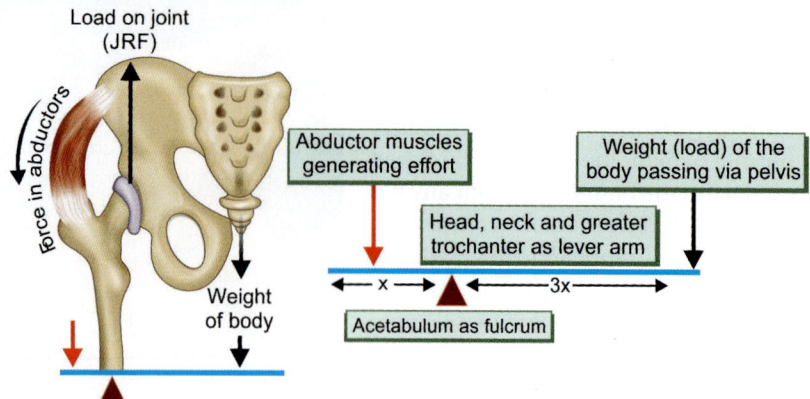

Fig. 7.25: Abductor mechanism of the hip (Left image). The right image depicts various components of the lever mechanism and forces acting on the hip.

(JRF: joint reaction force).

- **Force:** Generated by hip abductors (gluteus medius and gluteus minimus)
- **Load (weight) of the body.**

The normal response of the abductor mechanism: When one of the legs is off the ground (swing side), the ipsilateral unsupported hemipelvis 'tends' to drop due to the effect of gravity. However, the pelvis is balanced and lifted by the "intact abductor mechanism" of the contra-lateral side (stance side) **(Fig. 7.26A)**.

Abnormal response of abductor mechanism: In case of a faulty "abductor mechanism of the stance side," the unsupported hemipelvis on the swing side tends to drop **(Fig. 7.26B)**. This is known as a '*positive Trendelenburg test*'.

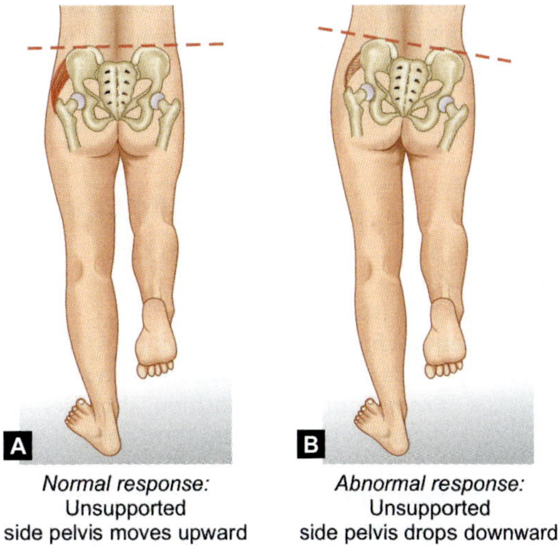

A Normal response: Unsupported side pelvis moves upward

B Abnormal response: Unsupported side pelvis drops downward

Figs. 7.26A and B: Normal and abnormal responses of abductor mechanism.

However, to avoid excess drooping down of the hemipelvis during walking, the compensatory mechanisms of the body responds by tilting/lurching to the stance/affected side using the trunk muscle resulting in uplifting of the drooping hemipelvis. This is known as the Trendelenburg gait, with the pelvis 'rocking up and down' and the trunk lurching to the affected side.

The abnormal response (positive Trendelenburg) can happen due to:
1. **Fulcrum issues:** *Lever is not on the fulcrum in* the dislocated hip (congenital/traumatic, post-septic), central fracture-dislocations.
2. **Broken or altered lever length:** Fracture neck femur, intertrochanteric femur fracture, slipped capital femoral epiphysis.
3. **Ineffective force generation in abductors due to:**
   - *Neuromuscular affections of abductors:* Superior gluteal nerve injury/affections leading to palsy of abductors and myopathies affecting hip abductors.
   - *Post-surgery weakness of abductors:* Any surgery that could damage the abductors during exposure of the pelvis or the hip can affect the function of the abductors.
   - *Altered length of abductor muscles in coxa vara or coxa valga:* In cases with coxa vara/valga, the length of the abductor muscle and lever arm decreases or increases respectively, which alters muscle contraction function. Together, this affects the normal functioning of the abductor mechanism.

USE OF CANE IN HIP DISEASES

To balance the faulty abductor mechanism with the drooping pelvis on the opposite side, the body tends to lurch on the same side. However, this energy-consuming mechanism creates a sizeable joint reaction force (JRF). Therefore, painful hip conditions (diseased or postoperative) require an alternative mechanism to reduce the JRF for comfortable walking.

The reduction in abnormally high JRF can be accomplished by using a cane on the unaffected side. A 'vertical ground reaction force' is generated when the cane touches the ground with minimal force, adding up to the abductor mechanism's forces, which reduces JRF by almost 50%, even with a mere 15% of the body weight is applied to the ground with a cane. The use of cane can produce more ground reaction force with little weight application as it increases the lever arm distance, providing more mechanical advantage by reducing the force of the abductor mechanism.

Hip Examination Proforma

1. **Gait**
2. **Attitude**
3. **Inspection (standing, supine):**
   - **General findings:** Skin overlying, swelling, scar, sinus
   - **Specifics findings in inspection on standing:**
     a. *From front:* Head position, shoulder level, shape of the chest, position of ASIS, rotational deformity (if any), Scarpa's triangle, GT level, thigh fold, patella orientation, thigh, and calf muscle wasting
     b. *From side:* Lumbar lordosis, flexed attitude of hip and knee, trochanteric region
     c. *From back:* Level of scapula, a rib hump, spine (overlying skin, deformity, swelling), PSIS level, gluteal wasting, gluteal fold, thigh and calf wasting, popliteal fossa, and heel status
   - **Specifics findings of inspection in the supine position:**
     a. *From front:* ASIS level, rotational deformity, Scarpa's triangle, GT level, thigh fold, thigh and calf muscle wasting, limb length discrepancy
     b. *From side:* Lumbar lordosis, flexed attitude of hip and knee (if any)
4. **Palpation:**
   a. *From front:*
      - A local rise in temperature
      - *Tenderness:* Soft tissue and bony landmarks, anterior hip joint line, GT (level, broadening, tenderness)
   b. *From side:* Lumbar lordosis
   c. *From back:* Spine, SIJ, PSIS, gluteal region, ischial tuberosity
   d. *Deformity assessment:*
      - **Sagittal plane deformity:** Hip flexion deformity
        - Thomas hip flexion test
      - **Coronal plane deformity:** Abduction/adduction deformity
      - **Rotational deformity of femur, tibia and foot**
   e. *Confirmation of palpatory characteristics of swelling, scar, sinus*
5. **Movements**: Active and passive
   - Flexion, extension, abduction, adduction, external and internal rotation
   - Crepitus, spasm; if any
6. **Measurements:** Limb length (apparent and true), thigh-calf circumference, Bryant's triangle, Galeazzi sign
7. **Neurovascular examination**
8. **Special tests:**
   a. *Test for stability:* Telescopy test, Trendelenburg test, vascular sign of Narath, and test for DDH—Barlow and Ortolani test
   b. *Tests for muscle contracture:* Ely's test
   c. *Test for hip impingement and arthritis:* FADDIR
9. **Joint above (spine) and below (knee, ankle), contralateral hip, knee, and ankle**
10. **Lymph node examination**

Common Conditions Affecting Hip and their Salient Features

1. **Developmental dysplasia of the hip:**
    - **Affects:** First born, female
    - **Pathology:** Dysplastic, shallow acetabulum; small, subluxated femoral head; increased neck-shaft angle; hypertrophied ligamentum teres; inverted labrum; hourglass shape contracted capsule.
    - **Clinical features:**
        - Painless limp, abduction restricted, whereas both rotations are exaggerated.
        - Supratrochanteric shortening
        - Trendelenburg, and telescopy test positive
        - *Vascular sign of Narath*: Positive
        - Barlow's and Ortolani's ± (depending upon age)

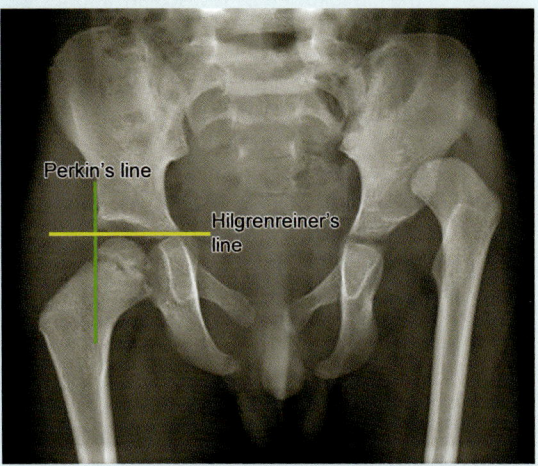

Fig. 7.27: Developmental dysplasia of the left hip.

   - **Diagnosis:** X-ray—subluxated/dislocated femoral head (out of the inferomedial quadrant formed by Perkin and Hilgenreiner line) dysplastic acetabulum **(Fig. 7.27)**. USG is useful till six months of age when the femoral head is not well-formed (α angle decreases with severity, while β angle increases with severity).
   - **Treatment:** Options vary according to the reducibility of the hip and age of the patient—closed reduction, bracing (Pavlik harness), open reduction, hip spica application, varus derotation osteotomy, pelvic osteotomy.

2. **Tuberculosis of the hip:**
    - **Affects:** Any age
    - **Presents with:** Painful limp, deformity, history of fever, night cries. There may be a history of contact with patients suffering from TB
    - **Pathologically:** TB of the hip; stage of synovitis/arthritis/deformity
    - **Clinically:** Deformity according to the stage
    Stage of synovitis: Flexion, abduction, external rotation; apparent lengthening
    Stage of arthritis: Flexion, adduction, internal rotation; apparent shortening
    Stage of advanced arthritis: Flexion, adduction, internal rotation; true shortening. There may be dislocation, subluxation, gross destruction of head of femur, protrusio in this age:
        - Thigh muscle wasting ++
        - Supratrochanteric shortening (depends on stage)
        - **Vascular sign of Narath:** Negative (except during dislocation); **Trendelenburg sign:** Caution while testing due to fixed deformities; **Telescopy:** Negative (even in case of subluxation due to fibrosis)
    - **Diagnosis:** X-ray, biopsy, other tests for TB
    - **Treatment:** ATT, treatment according to the pathological stage (synovectomy, arthrodesis, joint replacement)

3. **Perthes' disease (Legg–Calve–Perthes disease, pseudo-coxalgia):**
    - **Affects:** Age 5–11 years, common in South West region of India
    - **Presents with:** Painful limp, mechanical hip pain, occasionally presents with knee pain (referred pain).

- **Pathologically:** Idiopathic avascular necrosis of the hip followed by revascularization and reformation—remodeling of the head of the femur.
- **Clinically:** Abduction and internal rotation restricted, occasionally all ROM restricted.
    - *Vascular sign of Narath:* Negative
    - *Supratrochanteric shortening:* Later stage
    - *Trendelenburg sign:* Positive; *Telescopic sign:* Negative
- **Diagnosis:** X-ray **(Fig. 7.28)**
- **Treatment:** According to age of the patient and stage of the disease. Options vary from conservative treatment to varus derotation osteotomy, pelvic osteotomy (containment surgery).

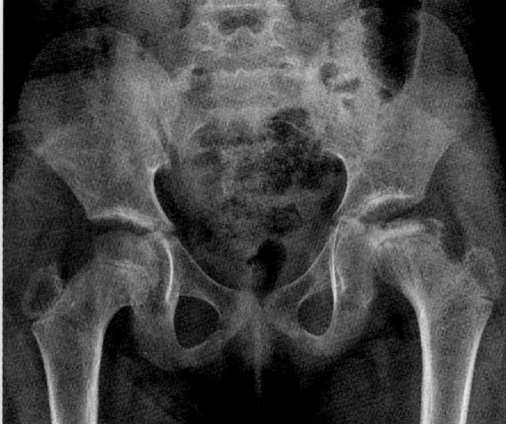

Fig. 7.28: Perthes' disease—left hip.

4. **Slipped capital femoral epiphysis (adolescent coxa vara):**
   - **Affects:** Obese adolescents; may be associated with endocrinal abnormality (hypothyroidism, growth hormone treatment).
   - **Presents with:** Painful limp, mechanical hip pain, occasionally presents with knee pain (radiation).
   - **Pathologically:** Disease of proximal femoral physis leading to slip of the femoral meta- physis with respect to the femoral epiphysis, often bilateral.
   - **Clinically:**
      - Adduction and external rotation deformity
      - Flexion, abduction, and internal rotation are restricted
      - *Trendelenburg sign:* Positive
      - *Vascular sign of Narath:* Negative
   - **Diagnosis:** X-ray **(Fig. 7.29)**, a hormonal workup may be required to rule out hypogonadism.
   - **Treatment:** Observation, in situ pinning of the femoral epiphysis, proximal femur osteotomy.

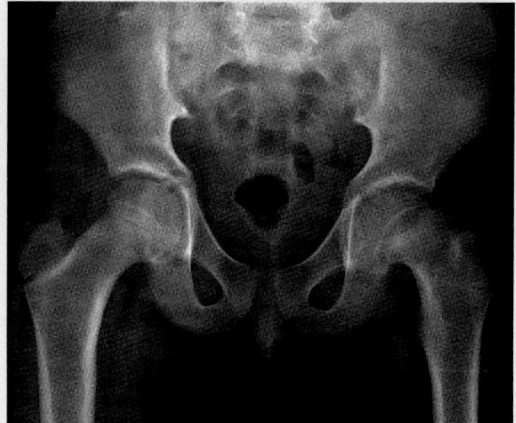

Fig. 7.29: Slipped capital femoral epiphysis—left hip.

5. **Avascular necrosis of the hip:**
   - **Affects:** Mostly young adults
   - **Presents with:** Painful limp, mechanical pain at the hip, history of trauma (hip dislocation, fracture neck femur), chronic alcoholism, steroid intake, chronic gout, Caisson's disease, Goucher's disease, sickle cell anemia.
   - **Pathologically:** Due to the above- said etiology(s), avascularity of the subchondral bone leads to necrosis and collapse of the subchondral bone followed by damage to the overlying cartilage leading to 2° hip osteoarthritis.
   - **Clinically:**
      - Tender hip joint line
      - Painful ROM (active and passive), limited abduction, and internal rotation
   - **Diagnosis:** X-ray **(Fig. 7.30)**, MRI (Diagnostic)
   - **Treatment:** Core decompression (with or without fibula graft), hip replacement.

6. **Primary osteoarthrosis of the hip:**
   - **Affects:** Older age >50–55 years
   - **Presents with:** Mechanical hip pain
   - **Pathologically:** Femoral and acetabular cartilage degeneration, osteophytes, synovitis, capsular contractures, subchondral cysts
   - **Clinically:**
   - **Deformity:** Flexion, adduction, external rotation
     - All ROM restricted and painful, Stinchfield test positive.
     - *Vascular sign of Narath:* Negative
     - *Supratrochanteric shortening:* Minimal or none
     - *Trendelenburg and telescopic sign:* Negative
   - **Diagnosis:** X-ray
   - **Treatment:** Conservative, total hip replacement

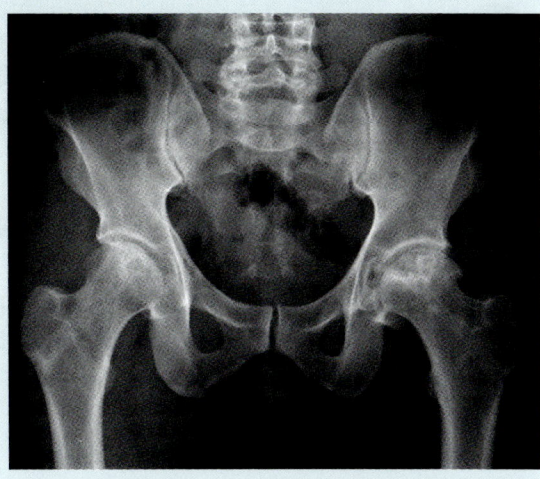

Fig. 7.30: Avascular necrosis of the left hip.

7. **Femoroacetabular impingement (FAI):**
   - **Affects:** Young men and women
   - **Presents with:** Pain in the hip during walking, prolonged sitting, sporting activity, C-sign
   - **Pathology:** There are two types of FAI—Pincer and Cam type (**Fig. 7.31**). In pincer type, there is excessive coverage of femoral head by acetabular rim resulting in damage to the labrum and cartilage (**Fig. 7.31A**). The cam type is characterized by excess bone near femoral head neck junction resulting in damage to the labrum and cartilage (**Fig. 7.31B**). Occasionally, there are combined pincer and cam lesions (**Fig. 7.31C**).
   - **Clinically:** Internal rotation painful and limited, positive impingement tests
   - **Diagnosis:** X-ray, MRI
   - **Treatment:** Conservative treatment—analgesics, physiotherapy, activity modification. Surgical options—debridement of cam lesion, labral debridement and repair, chondroplasty.

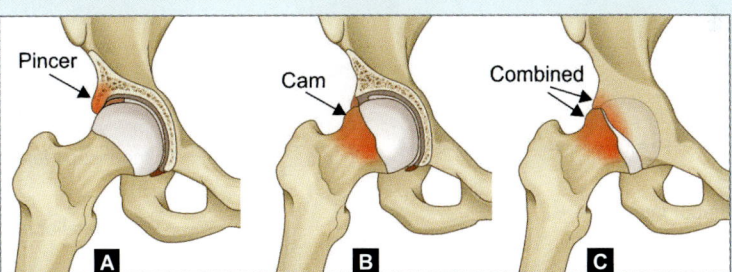

Figs. 7.31A to C: Types of femoroacetabular lesion.

CHAPTER 8

Clinical Evaluation of the Knee Joint

SURGICAL ANATOMY AND FUNCTION OF THE KNEE JOINT

1. **Osteology:**
   - ❑ *The knee joint* is formed by the lower end of the femur, the upper end of the tibia, and the patella **(Figs. 8.1A and B)**. So, it is a combination of two joints namely:
     i. Tibiofemoral joint
     ii. Patellofemoral joint

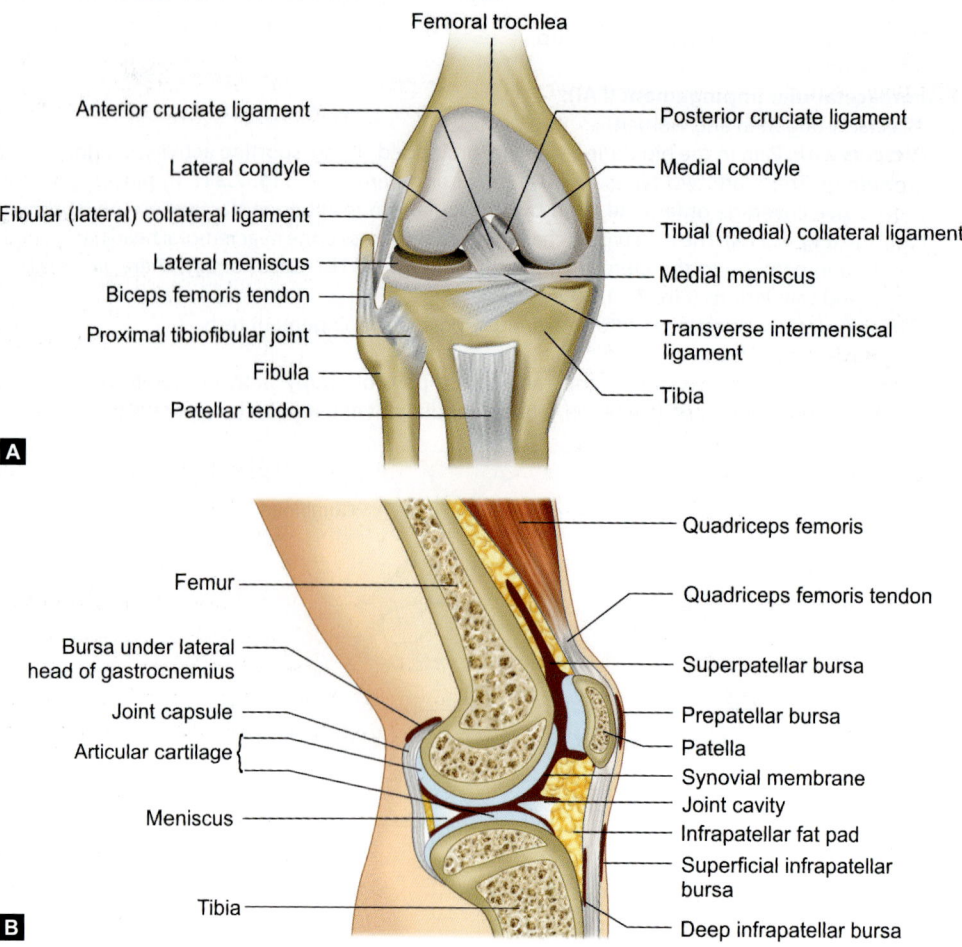

Figs. 8.1A and B: Anatomy of the knee joint in coronal (A) and sagittal (B) sections.

- **Tibial condyles:** The *tibial condyles are* relatively flat, while femoral condyles are convex, and that *makes the tibiofemoral articulation shallow.* To deepen the tibial plateau and enhance the knee joint congruency, the meniscus plays an important role.
- **Femoral condyles:** There are two femoral condyles—medial and lateral. The medial femoral condyle (MFC) is larger and projects more inferiorly. For adequate articulation of the larger MFC with smaller medial tibial plateau during terminal 20° extension, MFC undergoes 10° internal rotation over a fixed tibia, or the tibia externally rotates over a fixed femur. This is known as *"physiological locking of the knee"* or *"screw home mechanism." The screw home mechanism is assisted by adequate strength of the quadriceps, especially vastus medialis and also by cruciate ligaments.* A screw-homed/locked knee during standing decreases the work performed by the quadriceps. *The unlocking of the knee, i.e., external rotation of the MFC over a fixed tibia, is assisted by the popliteus muscle.* The lateral femoral condyle (LFC) is smaller and projects more anteriorly. The anterior projection of LFC is responsible for an adequate deepening of the femoral trochlea, which imparts lateral stability to the patella. In patients with anteroposteriorly flat lateral femoral condyle, the trochlear groove turns shallow (trochlear dysplasia), resulting in lateral patellar instability.
- **Patella:** It is the largest sesamoid bone in the body and an integral part of the quadriceps apparatus. Patella *increases the lever arm of the quadriceps by almost 35-50%,* enhancing the extension power of the quadriceps. The proximal 2/3rd of the posterior surface of the patella is covered with 4-5 mm thick hyaline cartilage and articulates with the femoral trochlea to form the patellofemoral joint (PFJ).
  Activities requiring flexion beyond 15-20° (sitting on a chair, squatting, kneeling, or cross-leg sitting) or stair ascent/descent result in increased contact forces across the PFJ. An increased contact force in a patient with PFJ cartilage damage (osteoarthrosis, chondromalacia) results in pain during the above activities (*cf. Tibiofemoral OA wherein pain is more while standing, walking, and running as tibiofemoral compartment is more loaded during activities requiring vertical position*).

2. **Ligaments of the knee:** There are several stabilizing structures of the knee such as cruciates, collaterals, menisci, MPFL, and capsule.
   i. **Anterior cruciate ligament (ACL):** ACL is distally attached to the tibia, just anterior to the intercondyloid eminence of the tibia, and proximally onto the medial wall of the lateral femoral condyle, over and behind the intercondylar ridge **(Fig. 8.2A)**. Anatomically, it has two bundles—larger anteromedial (AM) and smaller posterolateral (PL) based upon their attachment to the tibia. Both bundles have different functions. *AM bundle is taut in flexion, whereas PL bundle is taut in extension.*
      - *Function of ACL:* Primarily, ACL prevents the excess anterior translation of the tibia over the femur. Further, AM bundle is responsible for anteroposterior stability of the knee, whereas the PL bundle provides rotational stability to the knee during pivoting activities.
   ii. **Posterior cruciate ligament (PCL):** PCL is attached proximally onto the lateral wall of the MFC and distally to the posterior tibia 1-1.5 cm below the tibial plateau in the midline **(Fig. 8.2B)**. Anatomically, it has two bundles—a larger anterolateral bundle (ALB) and a smaller posteromedial bundle (PMB) based on their tibial attachment. Both bundles have different functions. *During knee flexion, ALB becomes taut and PMB is lax whilst during knee extension, ALB is lax and PLB is taut.*

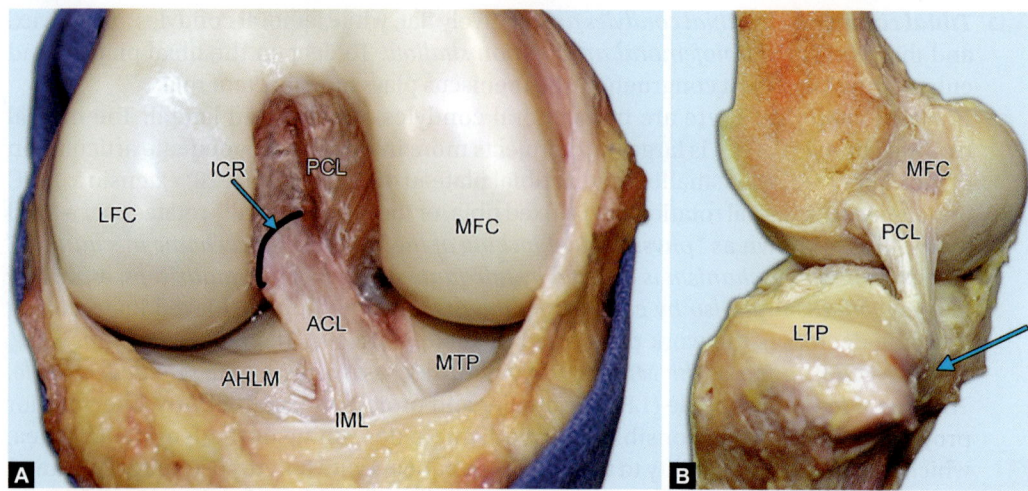

Figs. 8.2A and B: (A) Coronal view of the 90° flexed cadaveric knee with ACL and PCL. Black curved line on medial wall of LFC denoted intercondylar ridge; (B) Sagittal section of the cadaveric knee with attachment of the PCL (blue arrow shows PCL attachment is below and behind the tibial plateau).

(ACL: anterior cruciate ligament; LFC: lateral femoral condyle; LTP: lateral tibial plateau; PCL: posterior cruciate ligament; MFC: medial femoral condyle; IML: intermeniscal ligament; AHLM: anterior horn of lateral meniscus; MTP: medial tibial plateau; ICR: Intercondylar ridge). *Image courtesy:* Dr Charley Brown, UAE.

- *Function of PCL:* Primarily, PCL serves to prevent the excessive posterior translation of the tibia over the femur. Further, PCL also helps in the screw-home mechanism of the knee.
iii. **Medial side stabilizers of the knee:** It comprises medial collateral ligament (MCL), posterior oblique ligament (POL), and posteromedial capsule **(Fig. 8.3)**. The POL, posteromedial capsule, semimembranosus tendon and medial meniscus root are known as the posteromedial corner (PMC) of the knee. Further description of PMC is out of scope of this chapter.
   a. *Medial collateral ligament* has two components: (1) superficial MCL (sMCL), and (2) deep MCL (dMCL). Proximally, the sMCL attaches slightly proximal and posterior to the medial epicondyle on the femur. Distally, sMCL attaches 6 cm distal to the joint line over proximal medial tibia. The dMCL has two parts—the meniscofemoral and meniscotibial (coronary ligament), which attach close to the articular cartilage margin of the femur and tibia, respectively.
   Function: sMCL provides 85% valgus stability to the knee joint and dMCL aids 10–15% of valgus stability in flexion.

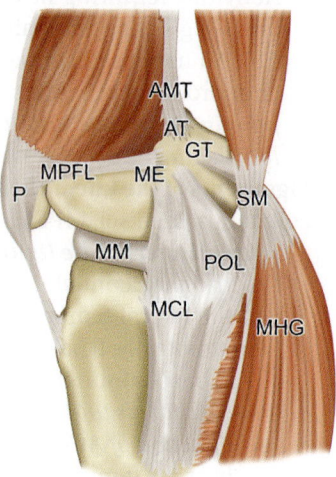

Fig. 8.3: Illustrated view of the medial side of the knee.

(MPFL: medial patellofemoral ligament; MM: medial meniscus; AMT: adductor magnus tendon; ME: medial epicondyle; P: Patella; GT: gastrocnemius tubercle; AT: adductor tubercle; POL: posterior oblique ligament; MCL: medial collateral ligament; SM: semimembranosus; MHG: medial head of the gastrocnemius).

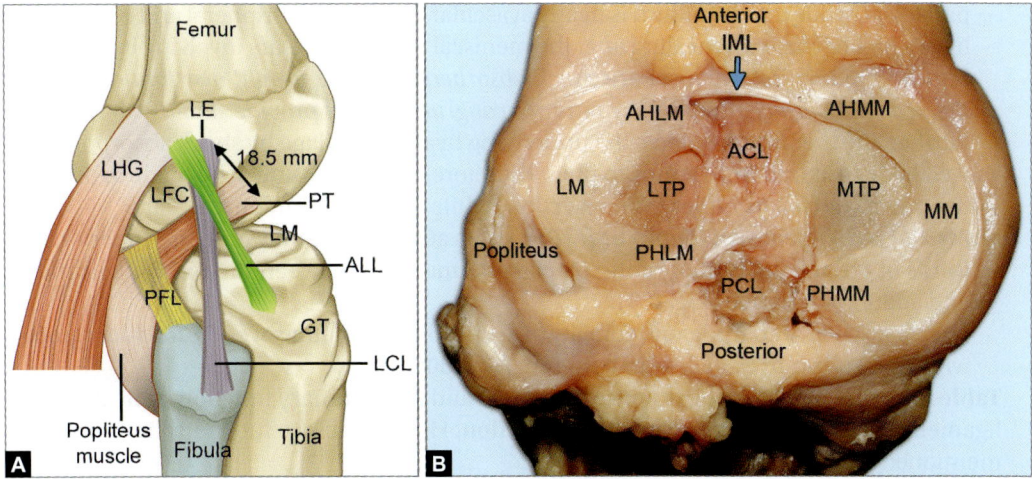

Figs. 8.4A and B: (A) Illustrated representation of the lateral side of the knee; (B) Cadaveric axial view of the tibial plateau with both menisci.

(PFL: popliteofibular ligament; LCL: lateral collateral ligament; LFC: lateral femoral condyle; LHG: lateral head of the gastrocnemius; LE: lateral epicondyle; LM: lateral meniscus; AHLM: anterior horn of the lateral meniscus; AHMM: anterior horn of the medial meniscus; PCL: posterior cruciate ligament; ACL: anterior cruciate ligament; PHLM: posterior horn of the lateral meniscus; LTP: lateral tibial plateau; MM: medial meniscus; MTP: medial tibial plateau; P: popliteus; PT: popliteus tendon; GT: Gerdy's tubercle; ALL: anterolateral ligament; IML: intermeniscal ligament; PHMM: posterior horn of medial meniscus). *Image courtesy:* Dr Charley Brown, UAE.

b. *Posterior oblique ligament (POL) and posteromedial capsule* are the primary valgus restraint of the knee at or near full extension, along with cruciates.
iv. **Lateral side stabilizers of the knee:** Major lateral side stabilizers are lateral collateral ligament (LCL), popliteofibular ligament (PFL), and popliteus muscle. The popliteus, PFL, IT band, biceps femoris, and posterolateral capsule are part of the posterolateral corner (PLC) of the knee. Further description of PLC is out of scope of this chapter.
   a. *Lateral collateral ligament:* Superiorly, LCL is attached slightly proximal and posterior to the lateral epicondyle and inferiorly over the anterolateral part of the fibular head **(Fig. 8.4A)**. *Function:* LCL provides varus stability to the knee joint between 5 and 30° of flexion.
   b. *Popliteus tendon* is inserted 18.5 mm anterior and distal to the attachment of the LCL in the popliteal sulcus **(Figs. 8.4A and B)**. After its insertion into the popliteal sulcus, it courses posterodistally in an oblique fashion to be inserted onto the posteromedial tibia. PFL attaches to the back of the fibular head.
   Function of popliteus and PFL: They act as important external rotation stabilizers of the knee.
v. **Menisci:** There are two menisci, medial and lateral; which are crescent-shaped, triangular in cross-section, and fibrocartilaginous structures **(Fig. 8.4B)**. Menisci are attached to the tibial plateau via anterior and posterior horn, and over the periphery of the tibial and femoral condyles via meniscotibial (coronary) ligaments and meniscofemoral ligaments, respectively. In contrast to the medial meniscus, which is firmly attached to the tibial plateau, the lateral meniscus is loosely attached to the tibial plateau, especially around the popliteus tendon (no capsular attachment). *Due to the firm attachment of the medial meniscus to the tibia and femur, medial meniscus is more prone to injury compared to the lateral meniscus.* Regarding meniscal vascularity, the periphery of the meniscus is quite vascular, the central

part lesser, while the inner third is nearly avascular. Hence, the peripheral and central tears have a higher chance of healing after the meniscal repair than tears involving inner third.
Function of menisci: Menisci are *shock absorbers, improve weight distribution, deepen the articular surface and thereby improve congruence, and provide stability* to the knee. Further, the meniscus protects the underlying hyaline cartilage by shock absorption and weight distribution from femur to tibia. Therefore, all attempts must be made to preserve the meniscus (repair rather than resection) while treating the meniscal tears.

vi. *Medial patellofemoral ligament (MPFL):* It is attached laterally onto the superior two-thirds of the medial border of the patella and medially between the medial epicondyle and adductor tubercle **(Fig. 8.3)**.
Function: MPFL imparts lateral stability to the patella articulating over the trochlear groove, while the knee moves in flexion between 0 and 30°.

Table 8.1 summarizes the ligaments of the knee and their primary function. Note that most ligaments do have a secondary restraint function. However, those functions have not been mentioned to avoid confusion.

3. **Type of joint:** The knee joint is a modified hinge-type bicondylar synovial joint. It is a combination of tibiofemoral and patellofemoral joint.
4. **Movements:** Predominantly flexion–extension occurs in the knee joint, which is visibly measurable by goniometer. Further, a small degree of external and internal rotations along with abduction and adduction do happen in the knee joint but they are not accurately measurable by naked eye, and hence are not mentioned in the routine examination.
5. **Other relevant facts:**
   - **'Q'-angle or quadriceps angle:** 'Q'-angle or quadriceps angle is a measure of quadriceps force vector acting laterally over the patella. Hence, an increased 'Q'-angle can predispose to lateral patella dislocation due to increased lateral quadriceps force vector. Normal Q-angle is 10–13° in males and 15–17° in females. Increased femoral anteversion, external tibial torsion, and genu valgum increase 'Q'-angle, and, thereby, contributing to patellar instability.
   - **Popliteal fossa:** It is a diamond-shaped fossa at the back of the knee. Its boundaries are: Biceps femoris tendon (superolateral), semimembranosus, and semitendinosus (superomedial), while medial and lateral heads of gastrocnemius form the inferomedial

TABLE 8.1 : Summary of function and tests of various ligaments of the knee.

Ligament		Standard function as primary restraint	Tests
ACL		Anterior stability to the knee by preventing excess anterior movement of the tibia in relation to the femur	Anterior drawer, Lachman, Pivot shift test
PCL		Posterior stability to the knee by preventing excess posterior movement of tibia relative to the femur	Posterior drawer, sag sign, quadriceps active test
Medial side of the knee	sMCL	85% valgus stability to the knee in 0–30° flexion 15% valgus stability to the knee in 0–30° flexion	Valgus stress test in 30° flexion
	dMCL		
Lateral side of the knee	LCL	Varus stability to the knee from 5–30° flexion	Varus stress test in 30° flexion
Medial patellofemoral ligament		Prevents excess lateral patella movement in 0–30° flexion of the knee	Apprehension (Fairbank) test
Menisci		Shock absorption, load transfer, lubrication, joint stability and congruency, proprioception	McMurray, Thessaly, Apley grinding test

and inferolateral boundaries, respectively. The major contents of the fossa are the popliteal artery, vein, tibial and common peroneal nerve.
6. **Major bursae around the knee:** Prepatellar, infrapatellar, suprapatellar, pes anserine, and semimembranosus bursa.
7. **Vascular supply to the knee joint:** The knee joint blood supply is derived from a rich anastomosis of the five genicular arteries, namely, the superior medial and lateral, the middle (posterior), and the inferior medial and lateral genicular arteries.
8. **Nerve supply to the knee:** Various structures in and around the knee are supplied by articular branches of femoral, common peroneal, and tibial nerve.
9. **Sensory innervation around the knee:** The front of the knee is by cutaneous branches of the femoral nerve, medially and inferiorly by saphenous nerve and infrapatellar branches of the saphenous nerve, respectively, posteriorly by the posterior cutaneous nerve of thigh, and laterally by the lateral sural cutaneous nerve (branch of the sciatic nerve).
10. **Muscles around the knee joint:** The clinically relevant muscles are mentioned in **Table 8.2**. Before proceeding for history taking and examination of the knee, one must know the common conditions affecting the knee joint as that makes the history taking easier **(Box 8.1)**.

TABLE 8.2: Important muscles around knee joint, their insertion, nerve supply, and action.

Muscles	Insertion	Nerve supply	Action
Quadriceps (rectus femoris, vastus lateralis, vastus intermedius, and vastus medialis)	Over the superior pole, medial, and lateral border of the patella	Femoral nerve	Knee extension. Vastus medialis obliquus (VMO) is also responsible for the terminal extension of the knee
Hamstrings (biceps femoris, semitendinosus, and semimembranosus)	Semitendinosus and semimembranosus over medial tibia, and biceps femoris over the fibular head	Sciatic nerve	Knee flexion

BOX 8.1: Common conditions affecting the knee joint.

- **Congenital:**
  - Congenital dislocation of the knee, discoid meniscus
- **Traumatic:**
  - *Ligament injuries:* ACL, PCL, MCL, and LCL—in isolation or combination
  - *Recurrent dislocation patella (RDP)*
  - *Post-traumatic:* Stiffness, arthritis, and deformity
  - *Meniscal tears*
  - *Intra-articular fractures, patella fracture*
- **Infections:** Tuberculosis of knee, pyogenic arthritis
- **Inflammatory:** Rheumatoid arthritis, Reiter's arthritis
- **Metabolic:** Gout, pseudogout, rickets
- **Degenerative:** Primary osteoarthritis, Baker'scyst
- **Others:**
  - Chondromalacia patellae
  - *Various bursitis:* Semimembranosus, prepatellar, and infrapatellar
  - Osgood–Schlatter disease
  - Synovial chondromatosis

(MCL: medial collateral ligament; PCL: posterior cruciate ligament; ACL: anterior cruciate ligament; LCL: lateral collateral ligament)

HISTORY AND ITS EVALUATION

Chief Complaints

The common complaints in patients with knee affection are—
- Pain
- Swelling
- Instability
- Difficulty in movement
- Locking, clicks/thuds
- Malalignment (deformity) or limb-length discrepancy

Note: Two essential questions remain the key to initiate the evaluation of complaints. One, when were you apparently all right, and two, how did it start?

History of Present Illness

Pain

It is the most common complaint, which could be acute or chronic. While most conditions cause chronic pain, acute pain is observed in:
a. **Acute trauma:** History of fall/RTA/sports injury (major /minor) could lead to injury to various structures.
b. **Acute infection:** Septic arthritis
c. Exacerbation of chronic condition (inflammatory/degenerative/metabolic)

One must assess various characteristics of pain such as onset, duration, progression, radiation, nature, timing of pain and associated stiffness. It is important to differentiate whether the nature of pain is mechanical or occurs at rest as etiologies vary in these two types **(Box 8.2)**.

BOX 8.2: Mechanical versus rest pain.

An important objective of musculoskeletal pain assessment is to understand the nature of pain, i.e., whether it is *mechanical pain* or *rest pain*, as both have different etiologies *(Refer to Chapter 1, Page 4)*:
a. **Mechanical pain** is observed in degenerative diseases/mechanical pathologies such as meniscal tears/cartilage injury/osteoarthritis. Due to degenerative/mechanical pathologies, knee pain is typically associated with activities or while the joint is loaded and relieved while resting. For example, chondromalacia patellae or patellofemoral arthritis causes pain on climbing stairs; tibiofemoral arthritis causes pain during walking and standing, and meniscal tears or cartilage injury result in pain during walking/squatting.
b. **Rest pain** is observed in inflammation/infection/tumorous conditions. For example, rheumatoid arthritis (RA), tuberculosis, and osteosarcoma.

Swelling

It could arise within the joint or from an extra-articular structure (bone, muscle, tendon, nerve, vessels, skin, and subcutaneous tissue). The reasons for "swelling arising within the joint" are synovial hypertrophy, effusion, or both.
a. **Effusion:** Effusion occurs due to excess synovial fluid/hemarthrosis/pus.
b. **Synovial hypertrophy:** Classically observed in infective and inflammatory pathologies.

It is also important to note the onset of swelling, which could help understand the pathology **(Box 8.3)**.

Note: Hemarthrosis is due to intra-articular fracture (#) or injury of intra-articular structures that are vascular such as ACL/PCL/periphery of meniscus. Rarely, it is due to bleeding diathesis (Hemophilia).

> **BOX 8.3:** Importance of timing of swelling onset (immediate/after several hours) in the knee pathology.
> - Swelling, which appears immediately or within a few hours after the trauma, indicates hemarthrosis.
> - Swelling, which appears after 12–24 hours of the trauma, indicates effusion due to the synovial reaction resulting from injury to the lesser vascular or avascular structures of the joint (meniscus or cartilage).
> - Chronic swelling could be due to effusion/synovial hypertrophy or both.

Instability

A complaint such as "my knee gives way" or "I cannot trust my knee" while running, jumping, turning, stair climbing, walking on uneven ground indicates an unstable joint. Typically, instability happens after a twisting injury during a sporting activity or a major trauma such as a road traffic accident. However, patella dislocation could be atraumatic or even with minimal trauma during running, climbing a stool, and dancing.

Difficulty in Movement

Often, difficulty in moving a joint or loss of motion is another complaint, which occurs due to pain, swelling, deformity, mechanical block, or other causes of joint stiffness. One must try to ascertain the cause of stiffness; extrinsic or intrinsic or both *(Refer to Chapter 1)*.

Locking

It is a pathological condition wherein the patient is suddenly unable to move the knee in any direction, flexion/extension (*Note:* cf. physiological locking, which occurs during terminal extension of the knee while walking).

Most common cause of a locked knee is *bucket-handle tear of the meniscus or loose body in the joint*. The common source of loose body in the joint is cartilaginous or osteocartilaginous fragment (traumatic, osteochondritis dessicans) or synovial chondromatosis (multiple loose bodies). *(Refer to Chapter 1, Page 9 for further details about locking)*.

Clicks, Thuds

Audible clicks are singular short noise occurring during one cycle of flexion-extension. It is a common feature of the loose body or meniscal tear. Thud is a singular loud pop occurring during flexion-extension, which is a typical feature of the discoid lateral meniscus.

Malalignment (deformity) or Limb-length Discrepancy

Traumatic, metabolic (rickets), infective, degenerative, or congenital conditions can cause an alignment disturbance (deformity) or limb-length discrepancy. Various common deformities observed in the knee are:

a. **Genu varum:** It is common at birth but resolves gradually to normal knee alignment. Commonly, genu varum is observed in osteoarthritis (OA), rickets.
b. **Genu valgum:** It is also physiological (common in 2–4 years of age) and tends to resolve by 6 years. It is more frequent in females and may be a contributory factor in recurrent dislocation of the patella (due to increased Q-angle). It is frequently observed in rickets and rheumatoid arthritis.
c. **Genu recurvatum:** A bilateral recurvatum is often due to the physiological laxity of tissues. However, unilateral recurvatum is always pathological, which frequently occurs due to posterior capsular tear of the knee in combination with PCL and PLC tears.
d. **Flexion deformity:** It is always pathological.

Constitutional Symptoms

Symptoms such as fever, malaise, loss of weight and appetite may indicate an underlying infective, inflammatory, or tumor disorder.

Effect on Activities of Daily Living (ADL)/Professional Activities

It is important to understand how current complaints have affected the ADLs and professional activities, which may help plan the treatment.

Past History

- DM, thyroid disorder may have a bearing on the current complaints. For example, diabetics are prone to infections, poor wound healing, and delayed/non-union. Hypothyroid patients may present with knee pain as a part of polyarthralgia.
- History of chronic gout/any surgical intervention may explain the current complaints.

Personal History

History of smoking, diet, alcohol intake, sleep, and bowel-bladder habits.

Treatment History

A detail of treatment history can unfold the clues about the current diagnosis.

Family History

It may be positive in RA, hemophilia, osteoarthritis and other congenital disorders.

Other Relevant History: Drug Intake, Menstrual History and Allergies

At the end of history assessment, many common clinical conditions of the knee can be reasonably well diagnosed based upon a combination of age and key complaints. **Table 8.3** summarizes the important snippets for the clinical diagnosis of common knee pathologies. However, all of them require confirmation with the specific examination.

TABLE 8.3: Clinical diagnostic snippets of the knee.

A 19-year-old man who sustained an injury to the knee due to a tackle while playing football or road traffic accident, and is now complaining of instability during running, jumping, walking on uneven ground, or pivoting sports	Consider *ligament injuries*, especially ACL
Any patient who walks into the clinic with a limp and knee pain after sustaining a dashboard injury to the knee/fall from a scooty with a direct hit over the knee!	Consider a *PCL tear* Patients with PCL tear may not directly complain of instability, but when further probed, they say that descending stair/ramp makes the knee feel unstable!
An adolescent girl who did not sustain any significant trauma to her knee but complaints of 'giving away' feeling on activities like dancing, playing, or climbing stool	Consider *patella instability*
A 28-year-old lady presents with pain in the anterior aspect of the knee, which aggravates after prolonged sitting, squatting, or on climbing stairs	Consider *chondromalacia patellae*

Contd...

Contd...

A 48-year-old lady who has had knee pain for several months or years presents with a swelling in the posterior aspect of the knee	Consider a **Morant–Baker cyst** A ruptured Baker's cyst presents with acute onset pain and swelling in the calf, mimicking deep vein thrombosis
An 58-year-old overweight lady presents with knee pain, which worsens with activity with/without progressive deformity (varus) of the legs	Think of **primary osteoarthritis** Note: Valgus deformity is common in inflammatory arthropathy

EXAMINATION

General and Systemic Examination

Meticulous general and systemic examination must be performed, especially if the disease is known to have a systemic effect. For example, rheumatoid arthritis, tuberculosis, etc.

Local Examination

The entire lower limb should be completely exposed from the pelvis and below after ensuring adequate privacy, and chaperone. The private parts must be suitably covered.

Gait

Gait pattern should be noted. Details of various type of gait pattern is described in chapter 14.

Attitude

Usually, knee examinations are performed in the supine position. The attitude of both lower limbs can be described in a standard fashion.

Inspection: From Front, Side, and Behind

It is done in standing and supine positions from front, side, and back of the knee. Observe for following—
a. **Standing:** Patient must be examined from front and back.
   From Front: Observe for lower limb alignment (varus, valgus) and ankle-foot for flatfoot/cavus (*Note:* A foot deformity such as flat foot can also result in knee pain).
   From behind: Examine popliteal fossa for any swelling/dilated veins.
b. **Inspection in the supine position:**
   i. **General findings:** Look for swelling, scar, sinus, ulcer and describe in standard fashion.
   ii. **Specific findings:** From front and side, observe for any deformity, muscle wasting, swelling, and limb length discrepancy.
      1. *Deformity:* Common deformities are observed in coronal and sagittal planes.
         ○ *Coronal plane deformities:* Coronal plane deformities are genu varum and valgum, which should be observed from the front of the patient both in standing and supine. The clinician holds both the ankles together and gradually brings both lower limbs parallel to each other. In a normal lower limb alignment, there is little space between two MFCs (about 1–2 fingers), and both malleoli touch each other **(Fig. 8.5A)**.
         In genu varum: Both medial malleoli touch each other, but both MFCs stay apart by more than 2–3 finger breadth **(Fig. 8.5B)**.

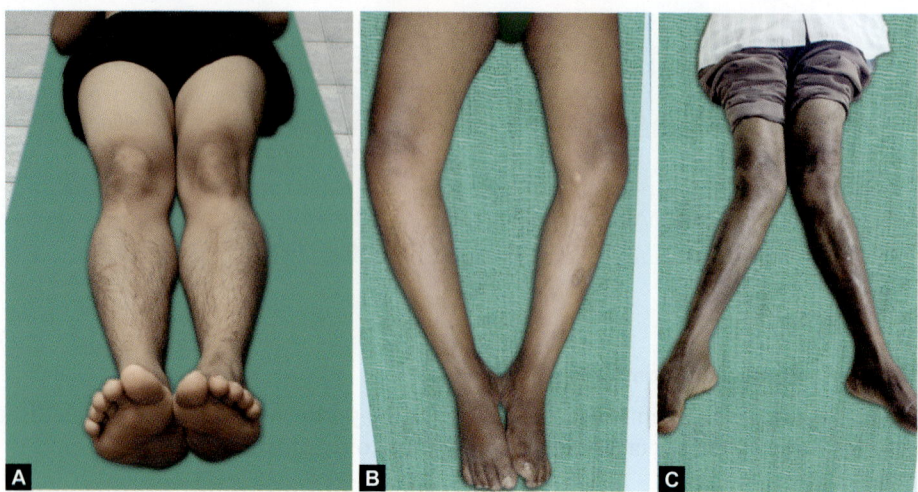

Figs. 8.5A to C: (A) Normal alignment of the lower limb; (B) Genu varum; (C) Genu valgum.

In genu valgum: Both MFC touch each other while both medial malleoli stay apart **(Fig. 8.5C)**.

> **Important note about genu varum and valgum** *(Salenius curve)*
> A child is born with bilateral physiologic genu varum (10–15°), which gradually progresses to neutral alignment by two years. From 2–4 years of age, it progresses to physiologic genu valgum (10–20°). Then, by the end of seven years, it becomes neutral or remains in slight valgum (5–7°).

- *Sagittal plane deformity:* Sagittal plane deformities are flexion deformity and genu recurvatum, which should be observed from the side of the patient. The clinician stands on the side of the patient and observes the relationship between the popliteal fossa (back of the knee) and the couch. In a normal knee, there is no gap between the couch and popliteal fossa **(Fig. 8.6A)**. In flexion deformity of the knee, the popliteal fossa does not touch the couch, and there remains a gap between the couch and the popliteal fossa **(Fig. 8.6B)**. Flexion deformity commonly occurs due to contracted posterior structures, pain/spasm, or effusion.

   Recurvatum knee or knee hyperextension is best confirmed with patient either in standing or during palpation in supine (*read palpatory assessment of recurvatum in movement section*). In a normal knee during standing, the weight-bearing axis passes through center of hip-knee and ankle in both anteroposterior (AP) and lateral planes **(Fig. 8.6C)**. However, in genu recurvatum, the axis on lateral (side) view passes in front of the knee **(Fig. 8.6C)**. Note that *bilateral, symmetrical genu recurvatum is physiological for that person and indicates laxity of tissues (ligaments, capsule) or rarely bony anomaly. However, unilateral recurvatum is almost always pathological*, indicating injury to the posterior ligaments (PCL and PLC) and posterior capsule, or malunited fractures around the knee.

2. **Muscle wasting:** Note the wasting in the thigh muscles, especially of the vastus medialis obliquus (VMO), and in the calf.
3. **Swelling:** Typically, the para-patellar recess/gutter are hollow and there is no suprapatellar fullness. Swelling around the knee joint could be intra- or extra-articular. Mild intra-

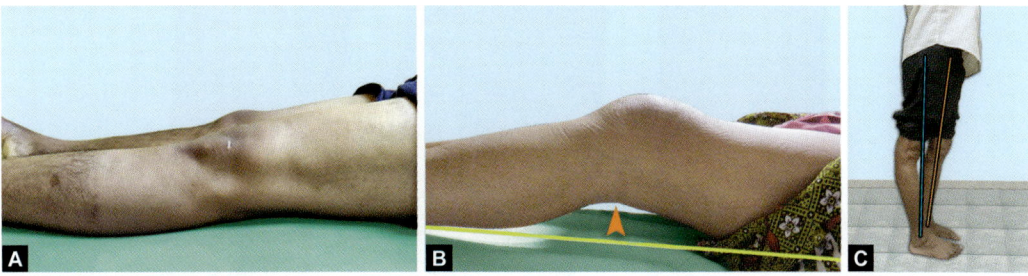

Figs. 8.6A to C: (A) Normal knee from the side in supine with popliteal fossa touching the couch; (B) Flexion deformity of the left knee where popliteal fossa fails to touch couch (orange arrow shows the gap between popliteal fossa and yellow line depicts the horizontal plane of the couch); (C) The weight-bearing axis of left lower limb (orange line) is passing through the center of the knee while the weight-bearing axis of the recurvatum right knee (blue line) is passing from the front of the knee (genu recurvatum).

articular effusion results in obliteration of the parapatellar recess (or hollows), while moderate-to-large effusion may give rise to a horseshoe-shaped swelling indicating fullness of suprapatellar and parapatellar areas (**Fig. 8.7**). Other swellings in front and on the sides of the knee are pre-patellar (Housemaid's bursa) (**Fig. 8.8A**), infrapatellar (Clergyman's knee), and pes anserinus area [pes anserinus bursitis (**Fig. 8.8B**)].

4. **Limb length discrepancy:** Observe level of both medial malleoli and heel with both limbs parallel to each other. Look for any shortening or lengthening of the limb, which can be assessed with the level of heels and malleolus.

c. **Inspection in the prone position:** Never forget to examine the patient in prone, especially the popliteal fossa.
- *Examination of the popliteal fossa:* Observe for any swelling [Baker's cyst (**Fig. 8.8C**)], visible pulsation *(popliteal artery aneurysm),* or *varicose veins.*

Note: Pes anserinus ("goose's foot" in Latin) is the anatomic term used to identify the insertion of the conjoined medial knee tendons (sartorius, gracilis and semitendinosus) over the anteromedial proximal tibia superficial to the MCL; the name derives from the conjoined tendon's webbed, foot-like structure. Pes anserinus tendons are enveloped by the pes anserinus bursa.

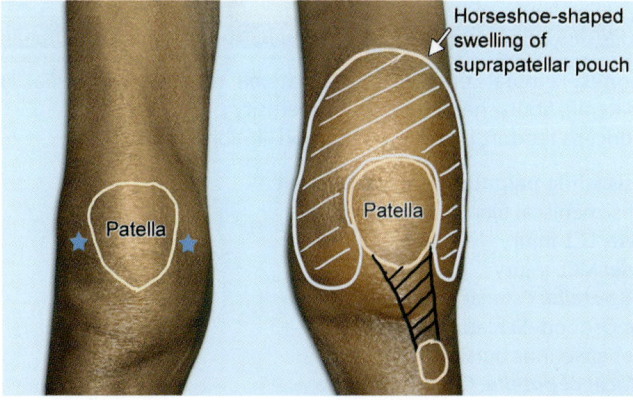

Fig. 8.7: Horseshoe-shaped swelling of the left knee. Blue star on the either side of right knee patella denotes parapatellar hollows/recess.

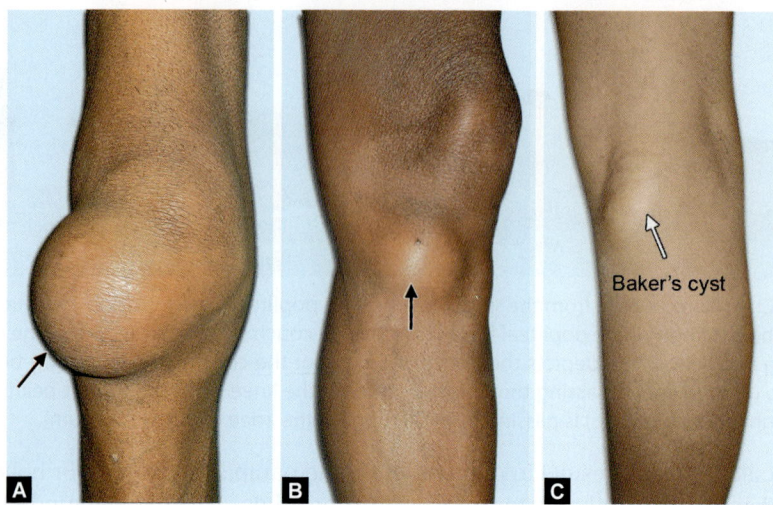

Figs. 8.8A to C: (A) Prepatellar bursa; (B) Pes anserinus bursitis; (C) Baker's cyst.

Palpation

The knee and surrounding area must be palpated for local rise in temperature, bony and soft tissue tenderness, and other specific findings such as swelling, joint line tenderness, effusion, synovial hypertrophy, patellofemoral cartilage status, clicks, thuds, loose bodies, popliteal fossa, and ligament laxity.

a. **The local rise in temperature:** A rise in local temperature indicates underlying inflammatory, infective, or tumor-related disorders.
b. **Tenderness:** Always palpate in a sequence (clock- or anti-clockwise) to feel for tenderness over various bony and soft-tissue landmarks. Some important bony and soft tissue landmarks are mentioned in **Box 8.4** and shown in **Figure 8.9**.
c. **Specific assessments during knee palpation:**
   I. *Swelling:* It could be intra- or extra-articular.
      i. The extra-articular swelling around the knee should be described as per the standard description of swelling during palpation.

BOX 8.4: Several important bony and soft tissue landmarks to be palpated around the knee.

- **Joint line and bones:** Femoral condyles (medial, lateral), epicondyles (medial, lateral), patella, tibial plateau (medial, lateral), fibular head, and tibial tuberosity
- **Soft tissue:** Quadriceps tendon, patellar tendon, and iliotibial band (ITB)

Clue to the diagnosis while palpating the tender spot
- *Joint line:* Arthritis, meniscal tear
- *Lateral epicondyle:* LCL injury
- *Medial epicondyle:* MCL injury
- *Lower pole of the patella:* Patellar tendinosis
- *Tibial tuberosity:* Osgood–Schlatter disease
- *Pes anserinus:* Pes anserinus bursitis
- *Facet (undersurface) of patella:* Chondromalacia
- *Fibular neck:* For common peroneal nerve tenderness and thickening in Hansen's disease

ii. Intra-articular swelling is usually due to joint effusion, synovial hypertrophy, or both. Assessment of both is mentioned below after joint line assessment.

II. *Joint line tenderness:*
   Method: While the patient is supine, the knee is flexed to 90°. The clinician palpates the tibial tuberosity (TT) using the thumb. For the medial joint line, the thumb is advanced proximal to the TT, just adjacent to the medial side of the patella tendon until it dips into a soft (which denotes the joint space/line) and continues to move in the medial direction to palpate the medial joint line **(Figs. 8.10A and B)**. Similarly, the joint line is palpated on the lateral side.
   Interpretation: A tender knee joint line indicates arthritis, meniscal tear, or mid-substance collateral ligament injury.

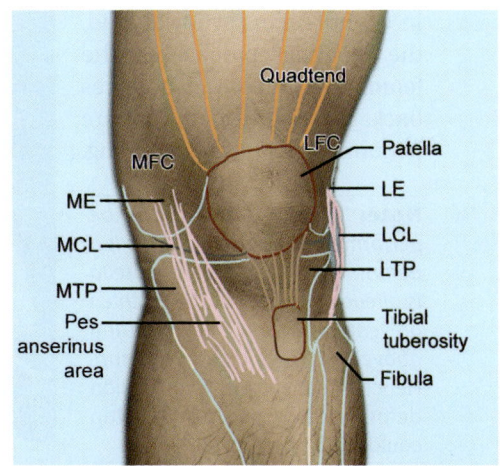

Fig. 8.9: Major soft tissue and bony landmarks around the knee for palpation.

(ME: medial epicondyle; LE: lateral epicondyle; MCL: medial collateral ligament; LCL: lateral collateral ligament; MTP: medial tibial plateau; LTP: lateral tibial plateau; LFC: lateral femoral condyle; MFC: medial femoral condyle).

III. *Patellar tap/ballottement test:* It is performed to ascertain an excess of synovial or other fluid (blood, pus) in the joint, which results in a 'floating patella'.
   Method: The patient lies supine with the *knee in extension*. For the right knee of the patient, the clinician uses his left hand to gently squeeze the excess fluid in the suprapatellar pouch from proximal to the distal direction, and the hand is placed just above the patella to retain the squeezed fluid in the pouch (*Note: In an adult, the suprapatellar pouch extends four fingerbreadths above the superior border of patella*). Then, the thumb and tip of all the fingers of the right hand are placed together on the anterior aspect of the patella and the patella is pushed toward the femoral trochlea with a "jerk" **(Fig. 8.11)**.

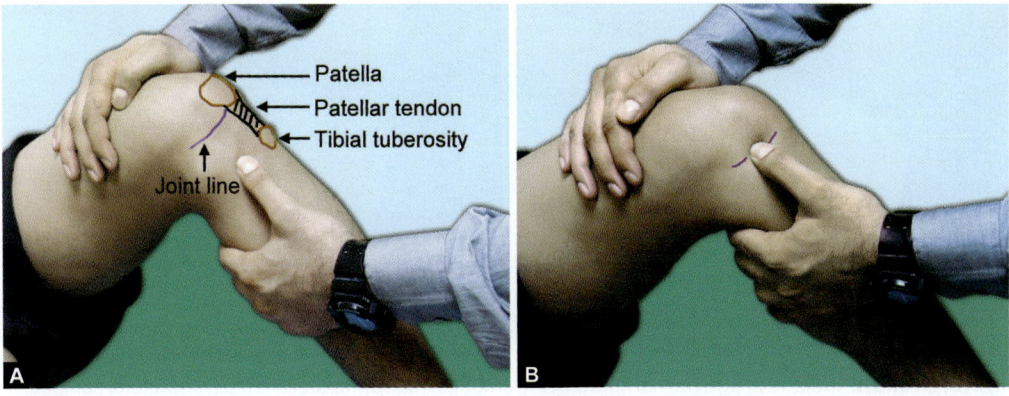

Figs. 8.10A and B: (A) Thumb is adjacent to patellar tendon over the proximal tibia; (B) Thumb over left knee medial joint line (observe the indented skin).

In case of excess synovial fluid, the "floating" patella hits the femoral trochlea and bounces back. Multiple repetitions are performed to confirm the finding.

Note: *Patella tap cannot be performed in a knee with flexion deformity >10–15° as the patella is already engaged in the trochlea preventing it from freely floating above the trochlea for the tap. Hence, in patient with fixed flexion deformity, one can say that tap could not be performed.*

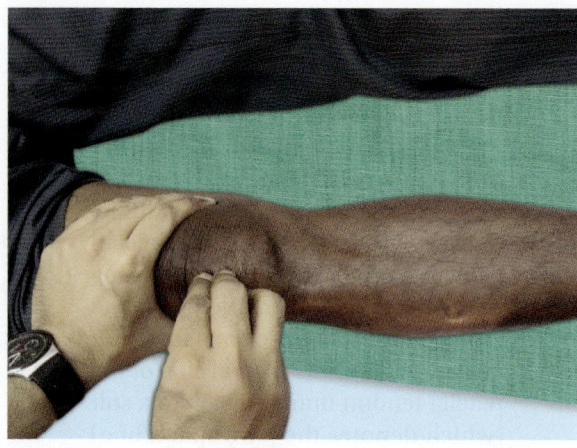

Fig. 8.11: Patellar tap.

Interpretation: A positive patellar tap is pathognomonic of excess fluid in the joint. The standard patellar tap technique is not valuable for severe effusion as floating patella cannot displace the excess fluid during downward jerk. In the case of mild effusion, the "patella tap" is negative as minimal fluid is insufficient to enable the patella to float over the trochlea (*Normal amount of synovial fluid in an adult knee joint* is 5 mL). Stroke or bulge test is used to assess minimal knee joint effusion (**Box 8.5**).

IV. **Synovial hypertrophy:** Synovial hypertrophy is merely a sign indicating the reaction of the synovium to underlying existing intra-articular pathology (infection, arthritis,

---

BOX 8.5: Techniques to assess minimal fluid in the knee joint.

Stroke/bulge test for effusion: With patient supine and knee in extension, the clinician performs upwards strokes with his fingers on the medial parapatellar hollow/gutter to milk the fluid into the superior and lateral compartment. The test is positive if fluid returns into the medial side of the knee, leading to a bulge in the medial parapatellar hollow **(Figs. 8.12A and B)**.

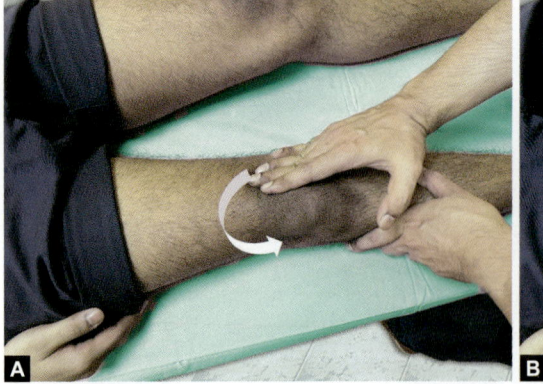 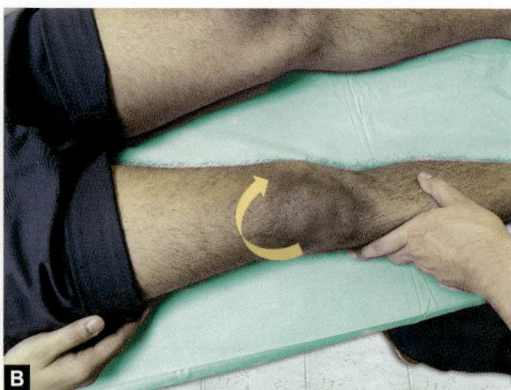

Figs. 8.12A and B: Stroke test. (A) Synovial fluid is being emptied into suprapatellar pouch and lateral parapatellar hollow/gutter; (B) Once hand is removed, gradual bulging of medial parapatellar gutter is noted as fluid moves back towards medial side (yellow arrow).

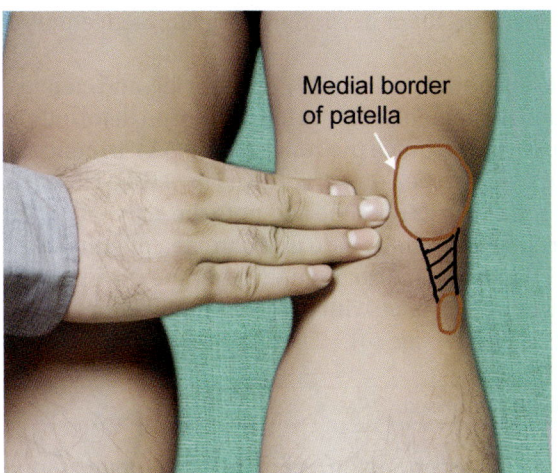
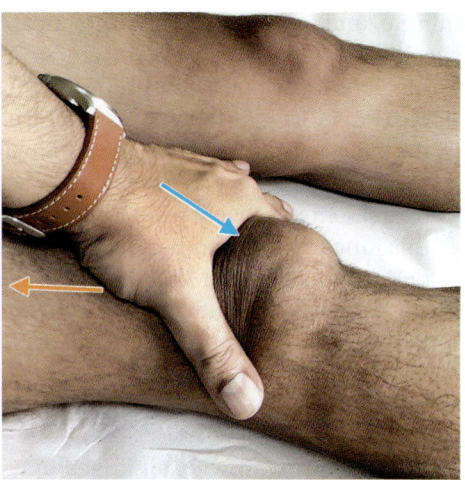

Fig. 8.13: Palpation of synovial hypertrophy.

Fig. 8.14: Patella grind or Clarke test. Blue arrow indicates downward pressure over the superior pole of the patella while orange arrow indicates contracting quadriceps.

meniscal tear, loose body, or pigmented villonodular synovitis). However, it does not indicate the underlying etiology.

Method: With the patient supine and knee extended, the hypertrophied synovium is palpated with the pulp of the index, middle, and ring finger by gentle rotatory movement over the medial femoral condyle (MFC), medial to the medial border of the patella **(Fig. 8.13)**. Hypertrophied synovium is felt as a boggy swelling.

V. ***Retropatellar tenderness (Patellar grind or Clarke's test):*** It is performed to ascertain the integrity of the patellofemoral cartilage.

The patient lies supine with the knee extended. The clinician places the web-space of his hand against the superior border of the patella and pushes the patella downwards while the patient is asked to contract their quadriceps by pushing the knee down towards the couch. If the patient's pain is reproduced during test performance (within 2 seconds), then the test is considered positive **(Fig. 8.14)** and is indicative of patellofemoral cartilage lesion.

VI. ***Palpate popliteal fossa:*** Palpate for swellings such as Baker's cyst (in the midline, below the joint line), semimembranosus bursa (medially located, above the joint line). Abnormal pulsations would be felt in the case of the popliteal artery aneurysm. Occasionally, there can be varicosities of small saphenous vein. Flexion of the knee greatly facilitates the palpation of deeper structures of the popliteal fossa.

VII. ***Common peroneal nerve over the neck of the fibula:*** It may be thickened and tender in patients with Hansen's disease.

VIII. ***Assess ligament laxity by checking Beighton score (refer chapter 4):*** A higher score indicates ligament laxity which is relevant in patients with patella dislocation.

Movements

The knee joint exhibits flexion/extension, internal/external rotation, and varus/valgus angulations. However, other than flexion–extension, most movements are composite and minute, and therefore, it is not practical to measure them in routine clinical practice unless specific restraints are damaged.

Also, one must look for the presence of fixed flexion deformity (FFD), extensor lag, and crepitus.

- **Flexion movement:** Before assessing flexion movement, observe for any flexion deformity in the knee. In a normal knee, the popliteal fossa would touch the couch **(Fig. 8.6A)**. In contrast, there is a gap between popliteal fossa and couch in flexion deformity **(Fig. 8.6B)**. Now, ask the patient to actively bend his index knee as much as possible and note the active ROM. At this juncture, the comparative level of both heel from the side gives an idea of equality or deficit of flexion ROM on the index side **(Fig. 8.15A)**. Also, note whether the flexion ROM was painless or painful, throughout or terminally. A knee with barely any movement is said to be *ankylosed* [fibrous/bony] (*Refer to Chapter 1, page 14*).

> **Note:** Always look for a deformity before the ROM is assessed.

- **Hyperextension:** Not all knees may have hyperextension/recurvatum. However, one must check the presence of hyperextension by holding the thigh against the couch with one hand and lifting the ankle with the other hand **(Fig. 8.15B)**. This maneuver reveals hyperextension, if any. Usually, hyperextension is 0°, but occasionally it could be up to 10–15° in lax individuals.
- **Extensor lag:** With the patient sitting, ask him/her to extend the knee against gravity. Note that extensor lag, if any, is judged by the inability of the patient to actively extend the knee to the neutral position of the knee or starting point of the flexion **(Box 8.6)**. Compare with the normal side **(Fig. 8.15C)**.
- **Crepitus:** Crepitus/grating is a continuous scratchy feel/noise appreciated by keeping the palm over the knee while patient's knee is actively/passively flexed and extended several times. It is elicited to ascertain the condition of the tibiofemoral or patellofemoral cartilage. The crepitus is felt in patients with cartilage damage due to underlying arthritis or chondromalacia or in the presence of loose bodies.

Method: It is assessed by keeping the palm over the knee while moving the knee through the available ROM. The crepitus (fixed/mobile) is felt over the palmar aspect of the hand.

Measurement

1. **Length of the limb:** With pelvis squared, the length of the lower limb is measured in the standard fashion [anterior superior iliac spine (ASIS) to the medial joint line (relative length of the femur); medial joint line to tip of the medial malleolus (length of the tibia)] **(Figs. 8.16A and B)**.
2. **Wasting of thigh and calf muscles:** Circumferential thigh muscle girth is measured over maximal thigh (approximately, 15 cm above the superior pole of patella in a young adult) and maximal calf girth (approximately, 10 cm distal to the tibial tuberosity in a young adult) and compared with the normal side.
3. **Q-angle:** It is the angle between the quadriceps tendon and the patellar tendon. Biomechanically, it is a measure of the lateral pull exerted on the patella by the quadriceps muscle.

Method: Patient lies supine with both lower limbs parallel to each other and quadriceps relaxed. With a skin marking pencil, mark ASIS, the center of the patella, and the tibial tuberosity (TT). Join ASIS and center of the patella with a straight line and another line joining

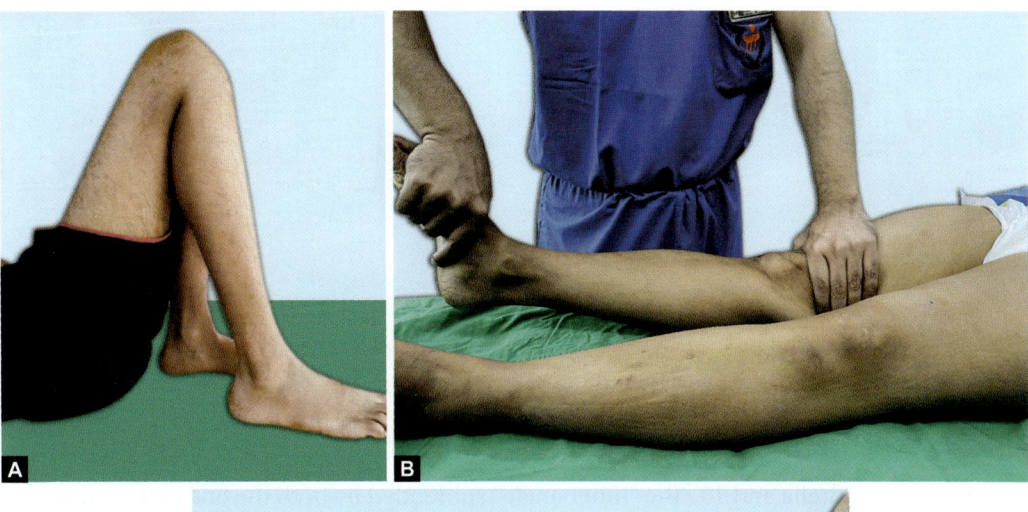

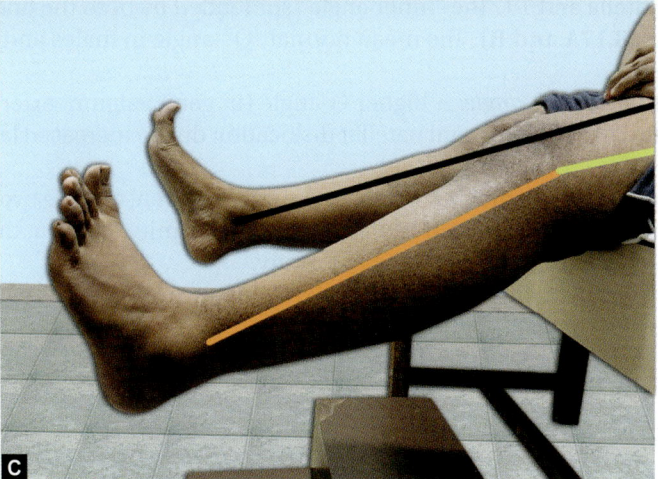

Figs. 8.15A to C: (A) Limited flexion movement of the right knee (Observe the difference in heel positions); (B) Demonstration of right knee hyperextension or recurvatum; (C) Extensor lag in the left knee compared to the right knee (The black line shows the thigh and leg axis of the right lower limb in one line, whereas the yellow-orange lines representing the thigh and leg axis of the left lower limb, respectively, are not in a straight line indicating extensor lag).

BOX 8.6: Extensor lag.

Extensor lag is a condition wherein the patient knee lags in extension, i.e., he/she is unable to actively extend the knee up to the neutral position of the knee or to the point of starting of flexion (in case of flexion deformity). Unlike the flexion deformity wherein both passive or active extension of the knee to the neutral position is not possible, the passive extension of the knee to the neutral or to the starting point of flexion is possible in extensor lag. Usually, extensor lag is due to a disuse-related or postoperative (not paralyzed) weakness of the quadriceps muscle.

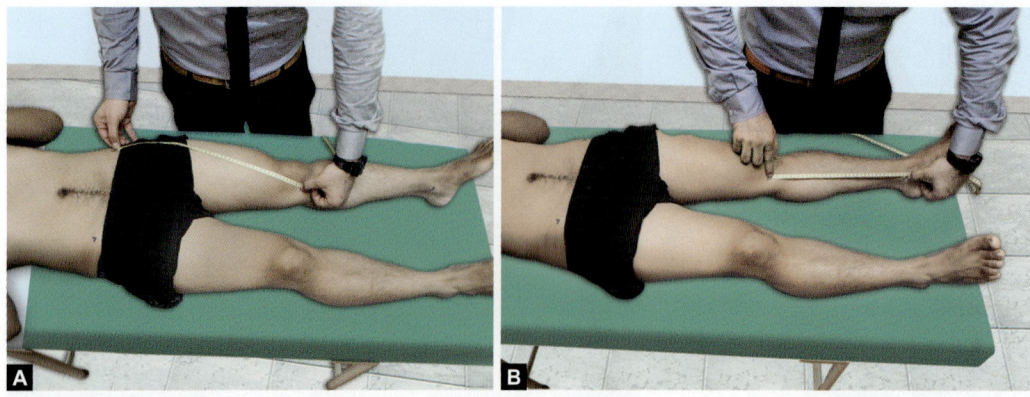

Figs. 8.16A and B: Measurement technique of segmental length of the lower limb.

center of the patella and TT. The "inner angle" subtended by both the lines is known as the 'Q'-angle **(Figs. 8.17A and B)**. The mean normal "Q"-angle in males and females is 14 and 17°, respectively.

Clinical importance of Q-angle: A higher Q-angle (in genu valgum, external tibial torsion) can predispose a patient for lateral patellar dislocation due to increased lateral pull over the patella.

4. **Intercondylar and intermalleolar distance:** The measurement of these two distances provide insight into the degree of genu varum and valgum deformity. Further, these distances are useful in monitoring the progress of the deformity.

   Method: By holding both the ankles, the clinician brings two lower limbs parallel to each other and starts closing the gap between both MFCs and medial malleolus. In varum, both malleoli touch each other, whereas MFCs stay apart. In valgum, both malleoli stay apart, whereas MFCs touch each other.
   - *For genu varum*—Measure the intercondylar distance (ICD) between the two MFCs.
   - *For genu valgum*—Measure the intermalleolar distance (IMD) between two medial malleolus.

Neurovascular Examination of Lower Limbs

It should be performed in the standard fashion.

Special Tests

1. Stability test for anterior cruciate ligament (ACL)

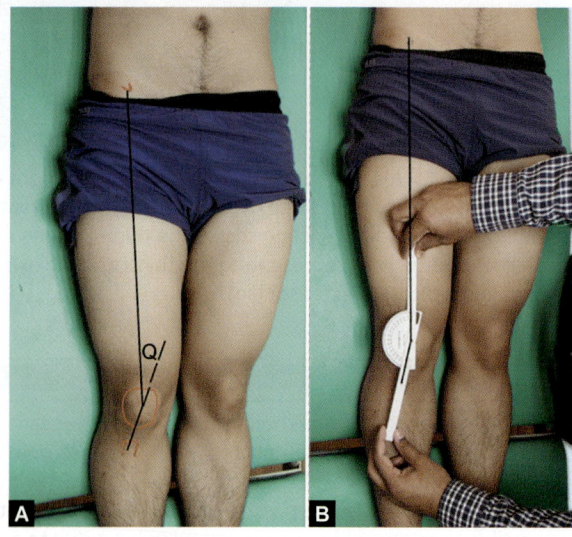

Figs. 8.17A and B: (A) Inner angle between the line from ASIS to the center of the patella and from the center of patella to the tip of tibial tuberosity; (B) Goniometer over these lines to measure the 'Q'-angle.

2. Stability test for posterior cruciate ligament (PCL)
3. Stability test for medial collateral ligament (MCL)
4. Stability test for lateral collateral ligament (LCL)
5. Meniscal tests
6. Patella stability tests

Stability Test for ACL

There are three tests that are commonly performed to test the integrity of ACL; Anterior drawer, Lachman, and Pivot shift test.

1. **Anterior drawer's test:**
   Prerequisite: The knee joint flexion should be possible up to a minimum of 90°.
   Method: With the patient supine on a couch, the hip is flexed to 45° and the knee is flexed to 90°. Now, the clinician sits on the patient's forefoot and stabilizes it. Further, the clinician places both his hands around the upper end of the tibia, palpates the hamstring tendons (on lower end of the thigh-knee junction on either side) with the fingers of both hands, and feels for hamstring tightness. If the hamstrings are found to be taut, the patient is asked to relax the hamstrings, or a gentle massage with fingers over the hamstring for several seconds helps relax the hamstrings. It is essential that hamstrings are relaxed, as tight hamstrings resists the forward movement of the tibia required for the anterior drawer test.

   Once the hamstrings are relaxed, the clinician places *both the thumbs over the anterior joint line on either side of the patellar tendon*. The purpose of the thumb over the joint line is to feel the normal step off of 1 cm between the anterior margin of the tibial plateau and femoral condyles, and further relative forward movement of the tibia with respect to the femoral condyle when anterior drawer is performed. Now, with thumbs over the joint line, the upper-end of the tibia is pulled anteriorly to feel the *"extent" of anterior movement of the tibia with respect to the femoral condyles along with "feel of endpoint"* (**Fig. 8.18**). This step is repeated a few times to confirm the extent of anterior movement and endpoint feel. A hard endpoint indicates an intact ACL, whereas a soft or mushy endpoint indicates torn ACL.
   Interpretation: In a normal knee with an intact ACL, the tibia cannot be pulled forward >1–2 mm beyond the normal step-off. *The test is considered positive if there is a soft endpoint feel and the tibial forward movement >3 mm*. Note that 'endpoint feel' is crucial in ligament integrity assessment as 'increased drawer movement' is often present in 'hyperlax individuals' or a reconstructed ligament. However, a 'hard' endpoint feel with increased drawer may suggest the presence of a lax joint with normal ACL. Further, always compare it with the contralateral side.

2. **Lachman test:** It is a *more sensitive* test for ACL tear than the anterior drawer test. Further, it is more useful in acute injuries of the knee where the knee cannot be flexed up to 90°.
   Method: The patient lies supine on the couch with the knee extended. For the right knee, the

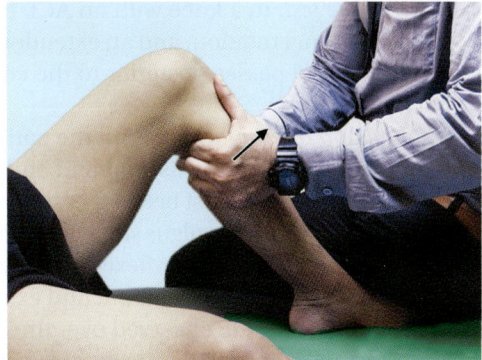

Fig. 8.18: Anterior drawer test (black arrow depicts anterior pull of the tibia).

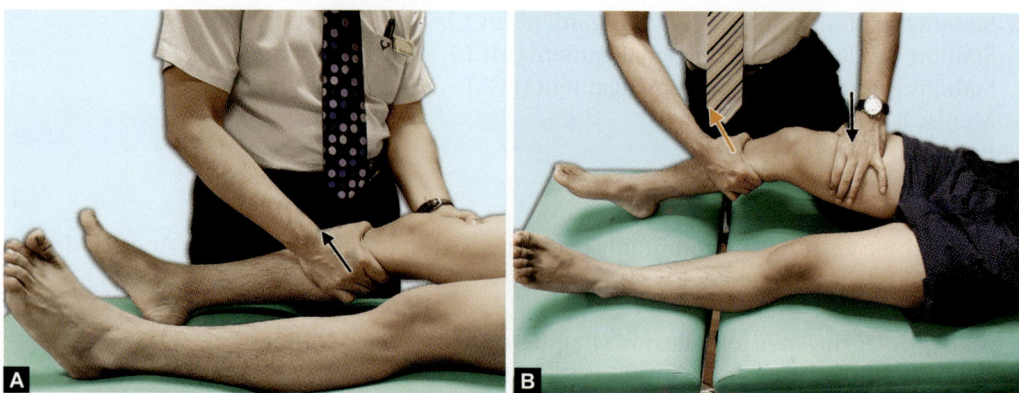

Figs. 8.19A and B: (A) Lachman test (black arrow indicates anterior/forward pull of the tibia); (B) Modified Lachman test (orange arrow indicates forward pull of the tibia, while black arrow indicates anchoring of the patient's femur over clinician's thigh).

clinician holds the lower end of the patient's thigh with his left hand and the upper end of the leg just below the tibial tuberosity by the right hand and the knee is gradually brought into 15–20° of flexion. Now, the clinician stabilizes the lower thigh with his left hand while the right hand pulls the leg forward and then lets loose repeatedly to determine the extent of forward movement of the tibia with respect to the femur and endpoint feel (soft/hard) **(Fig. 8.19A)**.
Interpretation: The test is considered positive if the anterior translation is > 3 mm and the endpoint feel is soft. If anterior translation <3 mm or the endpoint is hard, the Lachman test is negative.
Modified Lachman test: It is often difficult to hold the thigh and leg of obese patients or those who are in pain. In such a situation, supporting the thigh of the patient over the clinician's thigh spontaneously provides 15–20° flexion at the knee. Now, clinician places one hand over the patient's thigh to anchor it firmly against his thigh (black arrow in **Fig. 8.19B**) and the other hand pulls the tibia forward (orange arrow in **Fig. 8.19B**) to perform the Lachman test.
3. **Pivot shift test (MacIntosh):** It is the *most specific test for the ACL tear*. Theoretically, the pivot shift test detects the tear of the PL bundle of ACL (assessing rotational stability), while anterior drawer and Lachman detects tear of the AM bundle.
Basis of the test: In a knee with an ACL tear, the lateral tibial plateau *subluxes anteriorly* in valgus, internal rotation, and an extended position, and *reduces posteriorly* in 20–30° flexion as the IT band passes posterior to the center of rotation of the knee pushing tibial plateau backward.
Method and interpretation: With the patient supine, for the left knee, the clinician holds the patient's left ankle with his left hand and holds the upper end of the leg with the right hand keeping index finger just below the upper end of the fibula. Now, the leg is internally rotated with the left hand and valgus stress is provided while the right hand gives a counter for valgus. Now, the knee is gradually flexed. The tibial plateau subluxation, which appeared with the knee in valgus, internal rotation, and extension, reduces to normal at 20–30° of flexion by a click, jump, or a glide observed over the anterolateral aspect of the knee **(Fig. 8.20)**.

O'Donoghue triad: Triad of acute ACL, MCL and medial meniscus tear. However, in acute injuries, lateral meniscus injury is more common than medial.

Stability Tests for PCL

There are several tests to assess the integrity of PCL in the knee, such as sag sign, posterior drawer, and quadriceps active test.

Always start PCL assessment with the sag sign, which can be confirmed on inspection.

1. **Posterior sag sign:** Always start PCL integrity assessment by looking for a sag sign as that is one of the first and simplest clues for a PCL tear.
   Method: The patient lies supine on the couch with both knees flexed to 90° and hips to 45°. Now, the clinician stays on the side of the patient, and tangentially watches the alignment of the tibia to the knee on the index and normal side by drawing an imaginary line from the shin of the tibia toward the patella. In a normal knee, the imaginary line (blue line in **Fig. 8.21**) does not touch the patella and passes a few millimeters anterior to it, whereas the imaginary line (dark red line in **Fig. 8.21**) touches the anterior surface of the patella or passes through the patella in patients with PCL tear **(Fig. 8.21)**. In a *modified sag sign*, place a pen over the tibial shin to assess the posterior sag. In a normal knee, the pen placed over the shin does not touch the patella, whereas pen does touch the lower pole of the patella in patients with PCL tear as a result of posterior tibial sag **(Figs. 8.22A and B)**.

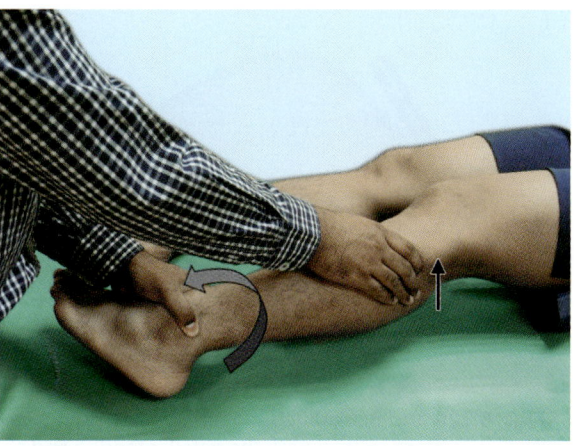

Fig. 8.20: Pivot shift test. Curved arrow indicates internal rotation of tibia, while black straight arrow indicates hand under fibula head.

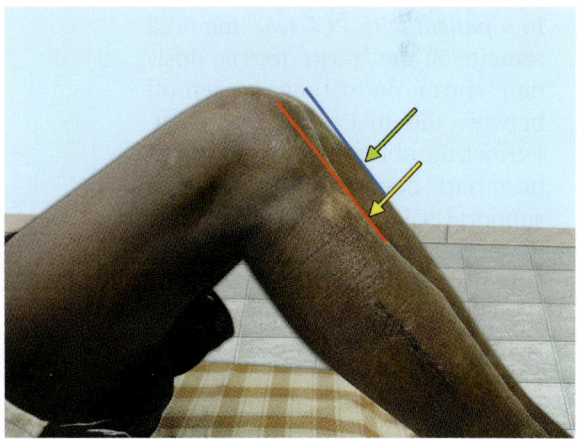

Fig. 8.21: Sag sign. Sag sign in PCL tear. Green and yellow arrow indicate normal knee (intact PCL) without a sag and a sagging knee with PCL tear, respectively.

   Interpretation: In the patient with PCL tear, the tibia sags posteriorly behind the plane of the patella, resulting in the imaginary line or the pen touching the patellar tendon and patella.

2. **Posterior drawer's test:**
   Method: With the patient supine, hip and knee flexed to 45° and 90°, respectively, the clinician sits on the patient's forefoot and stabilizes it. Then, the clinician places both his hands around the upper end of the tibia, *keeps both thumbs over the joint line*, pushes the tibia backward, and pulls it forward **(Fig. 8.23)**. Repeat the step of push-pull several times to assess 'posterior translation' and 'endpoint feel'.
   Interpretation: In a person with intact PCL, the thumb over the joint line can simultaneously feel the tibia, femur, and the normal 1 cm anterior step-off between the anterior surface of

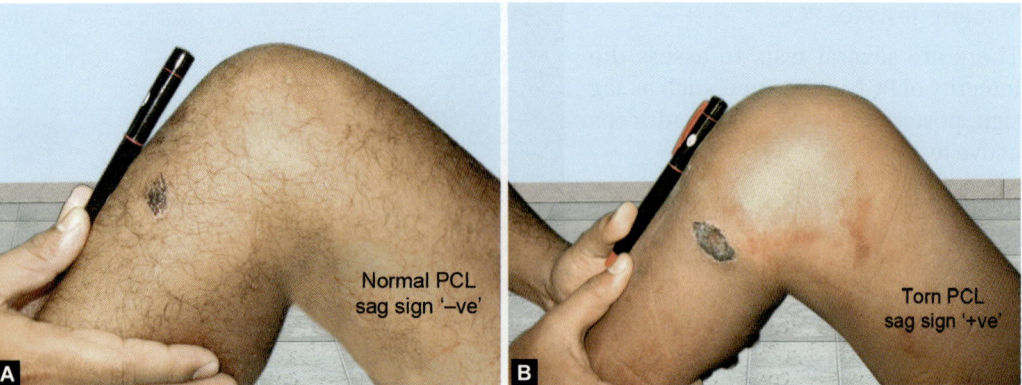

Figs. 8.22A and B: Modified sag sign. (A) Pen stays away from the patella with intact PCL; (B) Pen is in close contact with the patellar tendon and patella in the patient with a PCL tear.

the femoral condyle and anterior tibia border.

In a patient with PCL tear, the tibia remains in the "posterior sag position," and the normal anterior step-off between the tibia and femur is lost. Further, the tibia can be pushed more posteriorly due to a lack of posterior support (PCL tear). Also, always feel for an endpoint, soft or hard.

3. **Quadriceps active test:**
   Basis of the test: A posteriorly sagged tibia due to PCL tear moves anteriorly when quadriceps is activated to extend the knee against the fixed foot.
   Method: The patient lies supine with

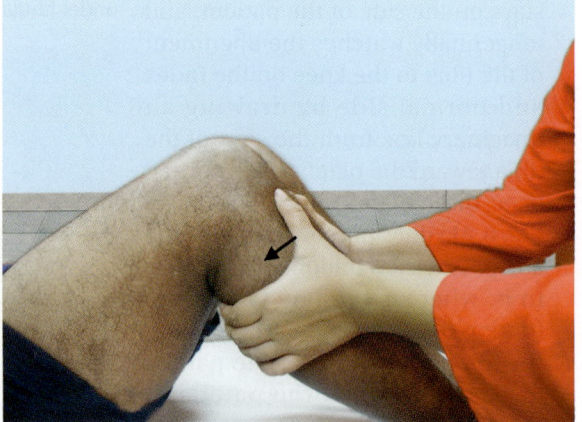

Fig. 8.23: Posterior drawer test (black arrow indicates posterior push).

the knee flexed to 90° and hips at 45°. The clinician holds and anchors the patient's foot to the examination couch and asks the patient to repeatedly attempt an active extension of the knee, which activates patient's quadriceps **(Figs. 8.24A and B)**. Observe any significant anterior tibial plateau movement from the side at the level of joint line.

Interpretation: In a knee with intact PCL without any posterior sag, quadriceps contraction will not lead to any noticeable anterior movement of the tibia (observed at the anterior knee joint line). However, in the case of a PCL tear with posterior tibia sag, the quadriceps activation leads to a noticeable tibia movement. Repeated quadriceps activation makes anterior tibial movement quite obvious.

Stability Tests for Medial Collateral Ligament (MCL)

1. **Valgus stress test:** For MCL integrity
   Method (for right knee): With the patient supine on the couch and index knee extended, the clinician stands on the lateral side of the index leg and holds the right leg just above the

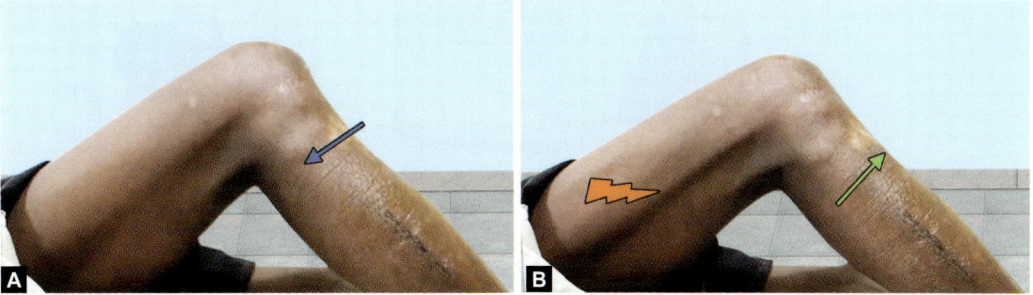

Figs. 8.24A and B: Quadriceps active test. (A) Sagging tibia (blue arrow); (B) Forward pushed tibia (green arrow) when quadriceps is actively contracted (orange lightening bolt symbol) with foot supported.

> **BOX 8.7:** Interpretation of valgus stress test in 30° flexion and 0° extension.
>
> - If there is a significant valgus opening only in 30° flexion, it indicates isolated MCL tear.
> - If there is a significant valgus opening (of the medial joint line) in 0° extension, it indicates tear in the cruciate ligaments as well as the posteromedial corner (posteromedial capsule, posterior oblique ligament).

malleolus with his right hand while the left hand is kept at the level of the lateral aspect of the knee (over the lateral femoral condyle), with the middle finger over the medial joint line. Now, valgus stress is applied using the hand holding the ankle, whereas the left hand at the level of femoral condyle acts as a fulcrum and the middle finger over the joint line feels for the extent of medial joint line opening. ***Remember that valgus (and varus) stress test should be performed in 0° extension and 30° flexion to assess the integrity of collateral and other posteromedial structures*** **(Box 8.7)**.

Another 'easy' method for valgus stress test: For the right knee, the clinician holds the right ankle of the patient in his/her right axilla between the chest wall and the arm while the index, middle, and ring fingers of the right hand are kept over the medial joint line and the left hand is kept over the lateral femoral condyle to act as a fulcrum during valgus stress **(Fig. 8.25)**. Next, the patient's leg is drawn into valgus, while the left hand of the clinician (over the lateral femoral condyle) acts as a fulcrum, while fingers of the right hand feel the extent of the medial joint line opening to assess the integrity of MCL and other medial structures **(Fig. 8.25)**.

Interpretation: An abnormal medial opening is felt in an MCL tear by the clinician's fingers placed over the medial joint line.

Stability Tests for Lateral Collateral Ligament

1. **Varus stress test:** For LCL tear
   Method (for right knee): The patient lies supine on the couch with the index knee extended. The clinician holds the right leg with right hand while the left hand holds the upper end of the leg. The left hand's thumb is kept over the lateral joint line and the remaining fingers are placed on the medial side of the knee. A varus stress is applied using the hand holding the ankle, whereas the fingers on the medial side of the knee act as a fulcrum **(Fig. 8.26)**. Like the valgus stress test, the varus stress test is performed in 0° extension and 30° flexion **(Box 8.8)**.

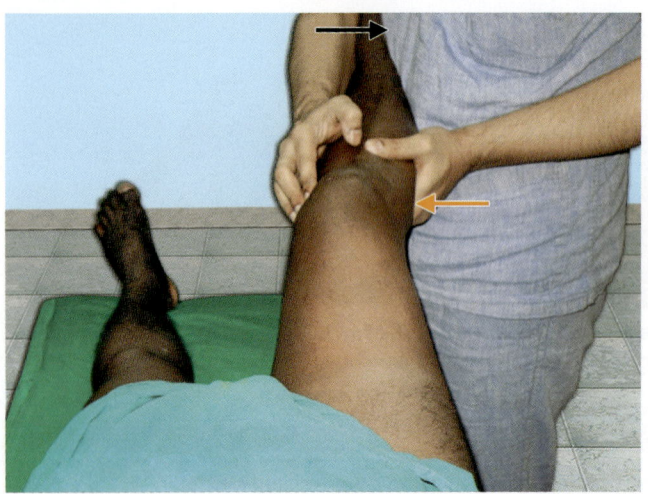
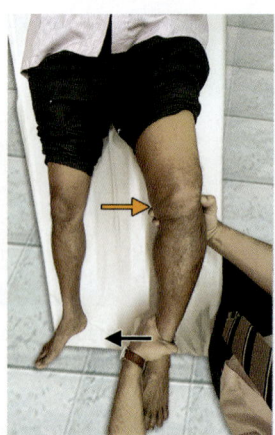

Fig. 8.25: Valgus stress test for the medial collateral ligament (black arrow indicates valgus pull on the tibia and orange arrow indicates fulcrum provided by the other hand).

Fig. 8.26: Varus stress test for the lateral collateral ligament (black arrow indicates varus stress on the tibia while orange arrow indicates fulcrum over the medial side of the knee).

> **BOX 8.8:** Interpretation of varus stress test in 30° flexion and 0° extension.
>
> - If there is a significant varus opening only in 30° flexion, it indicates LCL tear alone.
> - If there is a significant varus opening in 0° extension, it indicates a tear of cruciate ligaments as well as the LCL and posterolateral corner structures (posterolateral capsule, popliteus).

Interpretation: In the case of an LCL tear, there is an abnormal lateral opening felt by the thumb placed over the lateral joint line. Always compare the joint line opening with the normal side.

2. **Reverse pivot shift test:** It is a dynamic test performed to diagnose posterolateral corner (PLC) injuries. Other test to detect PLC injury is ***dial test***. However, the details of dial test is out of the scope of the chapter for undergraduates. (*Watch Video of Dial test*).

Meniscal Tests

Many tests such as McMurray, Apley's grinding, and Thessaly test are performed to diagnose meniscal tear. These tests are more specific compared to joint line tenderness, which is more sensitive.

1. **McMurray's test:**
    i. *McMurray for medial meniscus:*
    Method *(for the left knee)*: The patient lies supine on the couch with the knee extended. The *patient is asked to actively flex their index knee as much as possible.*

> **Of Note:** The clinician must not forcibly flex the knee, as patients with posterior-third meniscal tear may experience severe pain on forcible deep flexion.

The clinician holds the patient's left heel with his/her left hand while the right hand holds the distal end of the femur. Now, the clinician's left hand holding the heel externally rotates patient's leg, simultaneously pulls the leg outwards (valgus stress) and gradually extends the knee, while clinician's right-hand acts like a fulcrum over the knee resisting valgus **(Fig. 8.27)**. Repeat the maneuver several times.

Interpretation: In case of MM tear, the patient will wince with pain or there may be a click over the joint line or both.

ii. ***McMurray for lateral meniscus:***
Method (for the left knee): The patient lies supine on the couch with the knee extended. The *patient is asked to flex his/her index knee as much as possible*. The clinician holds the patient's left heel with the left hand while the right hand holds the distal end of the femur. Now, the clinician's left hand holding the heel *internally rotates* patient's leg, provides varus stress and gradually extends the knee, while the clinician's right hand acts like a fulcrum over the knee resisting varus. Repeat the maneuver several times.

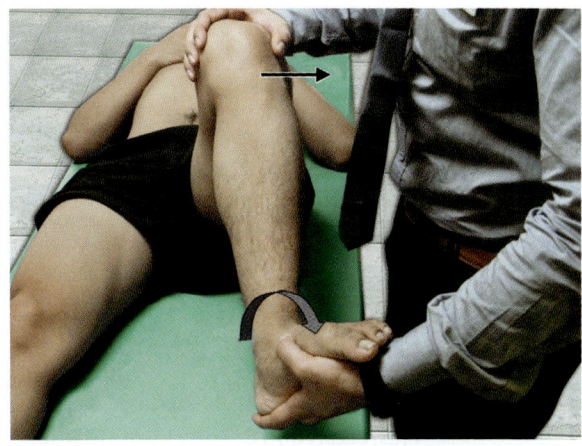

Fig. 8.27: McMurray test for medial meniscus. The gray arrow indicates external rotation force exerted by the left hand over the leg, while the black arrow indicates valgus stress imparted over the leg during the knee extension.

Interpretation: In case of LM tear, the patient will wince with pain or there may be a click over the joint line.

Note: Mnemonics for McMurray medial meniscus—VALER [valgus, external rotation]; McMurray lateral meniscus—VARIN [varus, internal rotation].

2. **Apley's grinding test:** It is a *useful test to differentiate between meniscal and ligamentous* (collateral and cruciates) injuries.
   However, Apley's grinding test *is not routinely performed* as there is an element of grinding involved in the test, which may "theoretically" damage the meniscus.
   This test *has two parts*: **Apley's compression test** and **Apley's distraction test**.
   Method: The patient lies prone on the couch, with the affected knee flexed to 90°. The patient's thigh is then anchored to the examination couch by the clinician's knee, and the clinician holds the patient's affected leg just below the ankle level.
   Apley's distraction test: While patient's thigh remains anchored to the couch by the clinician's knee, the patient's leg is distracted and rotated internally and externally. A painful distraction test is *suggestive of ligamentous injury* (collateral and cruciate) as the injured ligament(s) is/are stretched in "distraction" **(Fig. 8.28A)**.
   Apley's compression test: The clinician applies downward force on foot, and the leg is rotated internally and externally, which relaxes the ligaments (collaterals and cruciates) and compresses the menisci. A painful compression test *suggests the meniscal tear*, not the ligaments **(Fig. 8.28B)**.
3. **Thessaly test:** It is the *most sensitive and specific test for a meniscal tear*.
   Method: The patient stands on one leg while the clinician supports him/her by holding their palms with his hands. Now the patient flexes his knee to 20° and rotates the thigh and body internally and externally three times while maintaining the knee flexion **(Figs. 8.29A and B)**.

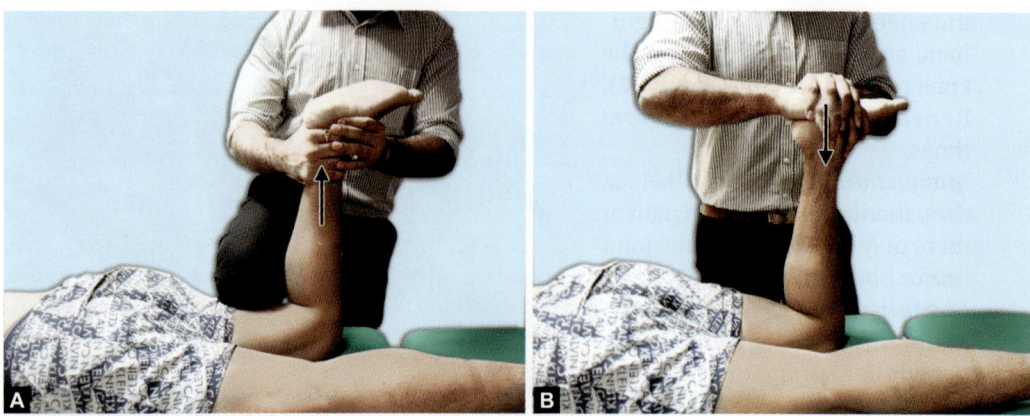

Figs. 8.28A and B: Apley's test. (A) Distraction test; (B) Compression test.

Interpretation: The patient experiencing pain or a popping sensation over the medial or lateral joint line while rotating their thigh indicates a meniscal tear.

Assessment of the Patella Stability

1. **Fairbank's apprehension test:** It is performed in patients with suspected lateral patella dislocation (LPD).
   Method: The patient lies supine, and the knee is kept in extension. The clinician keeps his/her thumb over the medial border of the patella, other fingers along the lateral femoral condyle. The patella is pushed laterally by the thumb, while the knee is gradually flexed from 0° to 30° and extended back to neutral. This step is repeated a few times between full extension and 30° flexion **(Fig. 8.30)**.

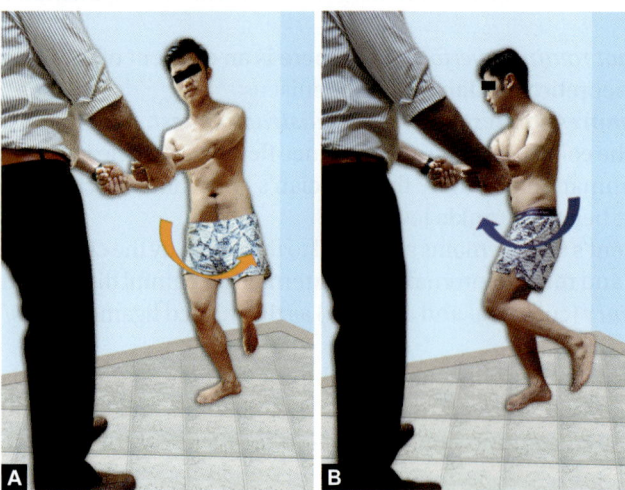

Figs. 8.29A to B: Thessaly test. (A) Internal rotation of the body (orange arrow) with respect to the affected knee; (B) External rotation of the body (blue arrow) with respect to the affected knee.

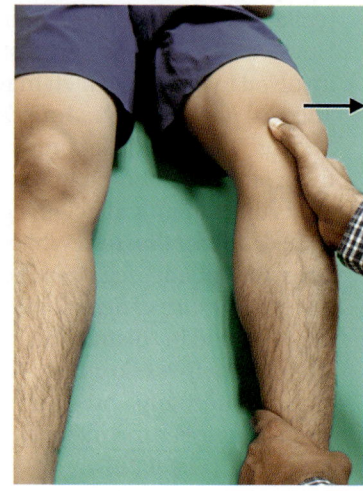

Fig. 8.30: Apprehension test. Black arrow indicates lateral push over patella while is being flexed.

Interpretation: In a patient with LPD, the patient shows apprehension (of impending dislocation) on his/her face, and often stops the clinician from continuing to push the patella laterally.

Examination of the Joint Above and Below

The hip and ankle-foot complex assessments should be done in a standard fashion. It is crucial to understand that the hip (e.g., Perthes') and ankle-foot complex (e.g., flat foot) pathologies result in knee pain either due to referred pain or by altering the biomechanical axis. Therefore, joints above and below must be examined, especially if clinical examination of the knee appears to be normal. A quick examination of the spine is also helpful as radiating pain often masquerades as knee pain.

Lymph Node Examination

Inguinal and popliteal lymph nodes should be palpated especially in infection and tumors.

Knee Examination Proforma

1. **Gait, foot progression angle**
2. **Attitude**
3. **Inspection:**
   - **General findings:** Overlying skin, swelling, scar, and sinus
   - **Specific findings of the inspection:**
     a. **From front:** Deformity (varus/valgus), muscle wasting (thigh and calf), position of patella, limb length discrepancy, supra/parapatellar swelling, pelvis position, and ankle-foot
     b. **From side:** *Sagittal plane deformity*: Flexion/recurvatum deformity, and spine
     c. **From back:** Popliteal fossa, muscle wasting of calf, spine, pelvis, and ankle-foot
4. **Palpation:**
   - The local rise in temperature
   - *Tenderness*: Soft tissue and bony landmarks
   - Joint line tenderness, patellar tap, crepitus, synovial hypertrophy, retropatellar tenderness, and popliteal fossa
   - Confirmation of palpatory characteristics of swelling, scar, sinus, ulcer, and deformities
5. **Movements:** Active and passive
   - Flexion–extension, extensor lag, flexion deformity, and recurvatum
   - Crepitus
6. **Measurements:**
   - Limb length and thigh-calf circumference
   - Q-angle, intercondylar and intermalleolar distance
7. **Neurovascular examination**
8. **Special tests:**
   a. **Anterior stability tests for ACL:** Anterior drawer test, Lachman test, Pivot shift test
   b. **Posterior stability test for PCL:** Sag sign, posterior drawer test, and quadriceps active test
   c. **Tests for the stability of posteromedial corner:** Valgus stress test in 0° extension and 30° flexion
   d. **Tests for the stability of posterolateral corner:** Varus stress test in 0° extension and 30° flexion
   e. **Meniscus test:** McMurray's, Apley's grinding, and Thessaly test
   f. **Patella stability:** Apprehension test
9. **Joint above (hip, spine) and below (ankle)**
10. **Lymph node examination**

(PCL: posterior cruciate ligament; ACL: anterior cruciate ligament)

Common Conditions Affecting Knee and their Salient Features

1. **Discoid meniscus (DM):**
   - A congenital disorder wherein the meniscus is malformed like a disc or a coin (*Typically, it is semilunar*)
   - Usually bilateral, presentation is at any age. However, it commonly presents in growing children with painless/painful thuds.
   - *Presents with:* "Thud" in the knee during knee movements, knee pain with activity or locking.
   - *Pathologically:* Large, disk-like meniscus covering the whole plateau (complete DM) or nearly 80% (incomplete).
   - *Clinically:* Thud/click present over the joint line, which is demonstrable with knee flexion and extension. The meniscal tear test may be positive.

2. **Knee instability due to ligament tears (ACL/PCL/MCL/LCL/combination):**
   - *Affects:* Mostly, young patients
   - *Presents with:* Instability while running/jumping/pivoting sports/climbing stairs, etc. There may be associated pain and or locking. PCL instability is typically observed while descending stairs or ramp, or while lifting heavy weight overhead (professional weight-lifters or manual workers).
   - History of twisting injury/road traffic accident (RTA); usually, history of inability to stand and walk after the injury and immediate-early swelling. The patient resumes weight-bearing after symptoms subside. Chronically, recurrent instability is the primary symptom ± pain. Note that lone MCL and LCL tears may not present with instability.
   - *Pathologically:* Complete tear of the ligament. Usually, complete tears of MCL and LCL occur in combination with ACL/PCL/both.
   - *Clinically:* Appropriate tests are positive depending upon the type of ligament tear.
   - *Diagnosis:* X-ray of the knee- *Look for Segond fracture, which is the hallmark of an ACL tear.* MRI is diagnostic. In case of doubt, arthroscopy can confirm the tear of intra-articular ligaments such as ACL and PCL **(Figs. 8.31A and B)**.
   - *Treatment:* Rehabilitation. Surgical repair reconstruction (arthroscopic/open), if there is instability **(Fig. 8.31C)**. Multiligament injuries often require surgical reconstruction.

3. **Recurrent lateral dislocation patella:**
   - *Affects:* Adolescent and young adults. Females are affected more than males. These patients often have genu valgum (Increased Q-angle).
   - *Presents with:* Recurrent instability, occasional pain. Unlike ACL/PCL tear, which has a history of either significant trauma or a twisting injury, patellar dislocations often occur with a subtle or minimal twist during dancing, running, climbing stool, or stair.
   - *Pathologically:* Most common pathology is torn or stretched out MPFL. Others are trochlear dysplasia, patella alta, increased femoral anteversion, external tibial torsion, and increased ligament laxity.
   - *Clinically:* Apprehension sign +. Others signs elicited are increased- Q-angle, femoral anteversion, or external tibial torsion.
   - *Diagnosis:* X-ray—patella Alta; MRI—Torn MPFL, trochlear dysplasia or a loose body.
   - *Treatment:*
     1. **Conservative:** Usually reserved for 1st episode.
     2. **Surgery:** In patients with recurrent patella dislocation. Options—MPFL reconstruction is almost always required. Other bony procedures such as trochleoplasty may be required.

4. **Meniscal tear:**
   - *Affects:* Traumatic tears are common in young adults, while degenerative ones are seen in older population.
   - *Presents with:* Pain, especially on deep squats and cross-leg sitting, clicks, locking, and recurrent effusion.
   - *Pathologically:* Most common meniscal tears occur in the posterior third of the meniscus.

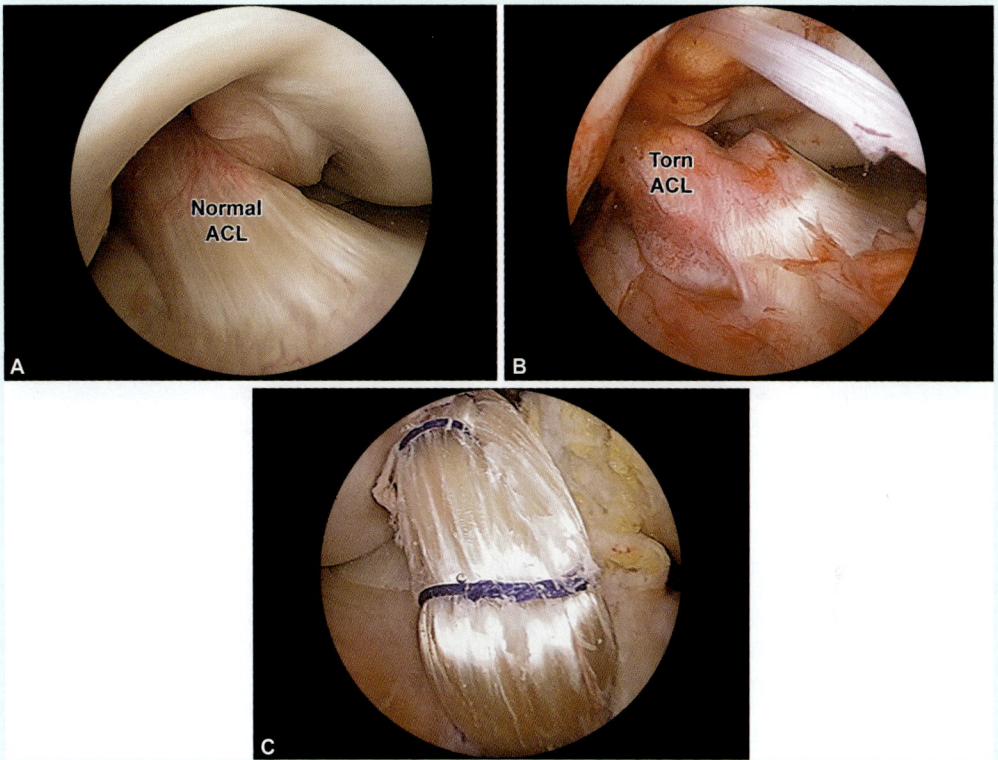

Figs. 8.31A to C: (A) Arthroscopic appearance of a normal ACL; (B) Arthroscopic appearance of a torn ACL; (C) Arthroscopic appearance of reconstructed ACL.

- ➢ **Clinically:** Quadriceps wasting, joint line tenderness, and painful deep flexion. McMurray and other meniscal tests may be positive.
- ➢ **Diagnosis:** MRI (Confirmatory)
- ➢ **Treatment:**
  - ♦ **Conservative:** It is especially adopted in degenerative tears with associated osteoarthritis.
  - ♦ **Surgery:** Tears >1 cm size, or which did not respond to the conservative treatment. Meniscal preservation (meniscal repair) and resection (partial meniscectomy) are two surgical options depending on the site and reparability of the tear.
5. **Primary osteoarthrosis of the knee (osteoarthritis):**
   - ➢ **Affects:** Adults >50–55 years of age; obesity is a significant risk factor.
   - ➢ **Presents with:** Mechanical pain, painful standing, walking, squatting, and sitting cross-legged.

Note: Patients with patellofemoral OA typically present with difficulty in stair climbing/descending and deep squats, whereas walking on a flat ground or standing is comfortable.

- ➢ **Pathologically:** Loss of articular cartilage in the joint due to wear and tear, osteophyte formation
  Clinically: Genu varum and flexion deformity
  - ♦ Joint-line tenderness, crepitus, and painfully restricted ROM
- ➢ **Diagnosis:** X-ray shows joint space reduction, subchondral sclerosis, and cyst, osteophytes, deformity. MRI is performed for detecting meniscal root tear, cartilage flaps. Arthroscopy, if performed, shows loss of cartilage and other pathologies (meniscal tear, cartilage loss) **(Figs. 8.32A and B)**.

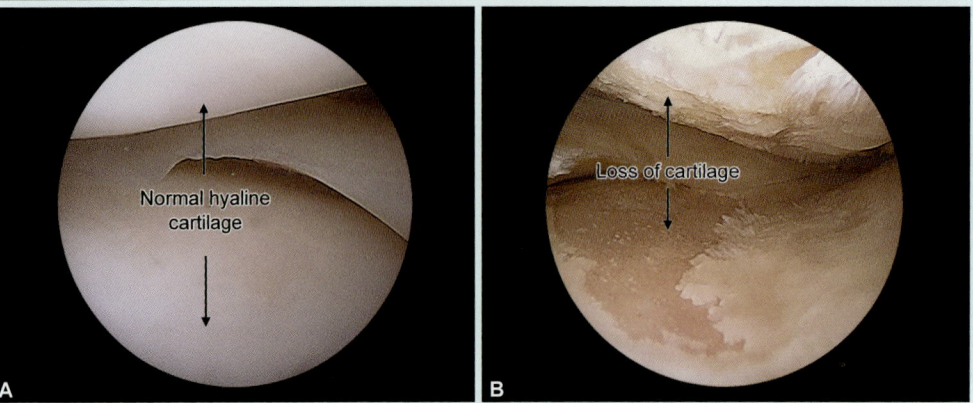

Figs. 8.32A and B: (A) Normal hyaline cartilage of knee joint; (B) Exposed subchondral bone due to cartilage loss in osteoarthritis.

- ➤ **Treatment:** Conservative options vary from nonsteroidal anti-inflammatory drugs (NSAIDs), physiotherapy, intra-articular steroid, platelet-rich plasma, or hyaluronic acid injection. Surgical options—arthroscopic debridement, high tibial osteotomy, and uni- or total knee replacement.

6. **Morrant Baker's cyst:**
   - ➤ **Affects:** Adults or older patients with coexisting arthritis or intra-articular pathology of the knee.
   - ➤ **Presents with:** Pain and swelling in the popliteal fossa, coexisting arthritis/synovitis of the knee, or any other pathology.
   - ➤ **Pathologically:** It is *not* a true cyst and is posteriorly located between the medial head of the gastrocnemius and capsular reflection of the semimembranosus (oblique popliteal ligament). There is an excess of synovial fluid formation whenever there is a chronic synovial irritation due to underlying intra-articular pathology. To accommodate excess joint synovial fluid with increased joint pressure, the knee synovium herniates posteriorly through the naturally occurring rent in the posterior capsule of the knee (through oblique popliteal ligament) with a unidirectional valve. The excess joint fluid keeps collecting in the cyst due to the unidirectional valve and forms Baker's cyst.

   > **Note:** A fact which we need to remember is that "Baker's cyst is almost always secondary to a primary intra-articular pathology in the knee, like OA or rheumatoid arthritis".

   - ➤ **Clinically:** Usually, the swelling is in the midline, slightly below the joint line. It becomes firm and prominent on an extended knee while soft and less prominent on the flexed knee (Foucher's sign). The knee may have clinical features of other pathology like OA/rheumatoid/chronic meniscal tear.
   - ➤ **Differential diagnosis:** *Semimembranosus bursa:* It is observed at the posteromedial aspect of the knee joint, slightly superior to the knee joint line.
   - ➤ **Investigation:** X-ray, ultrasonography (USG), and MRI (confirmatory)
   - ➤ **Treatment:** Always treat the intra-articular knee pathology; the Baker's cyst may subside. If Baker's cyst remains symptomatic even after conservative treatment of the primary condition, both primary condition and Baker's cyst can be managed arthroscopically.
   - ➤ **Complication:** Baker's cyst can rupture and mimic deep vein thrombosis of the calf.

7. **Chondromalacia patella:**
   - ➤ **Affects:** Young patients, especially females from the 2nd to the fourth decade. Often bilateral
   - ➤ **Etiology:** Typically idiopathic. However, other etiologies (trauma, infection, inflammation, etc.) must be ruled out.
   - ➤ **Presents with:** Knee pain, especially while keeping the knee bent for a long time (in the classroom, watching a movie- Theater sign), climbing stairs, squatting or sitting cross-legged.
   - ➤ **Pathologically:** Fraying and fibrillation of patellar cartilage

- **Clinically:** Clarke's test +, deep flexion painful, crepitus.
- **Diagnosis:** X-rays are normal. MRI may show cartilage changes; arthroscopy is diagnostic **(Figs. 8.33A and B)**.

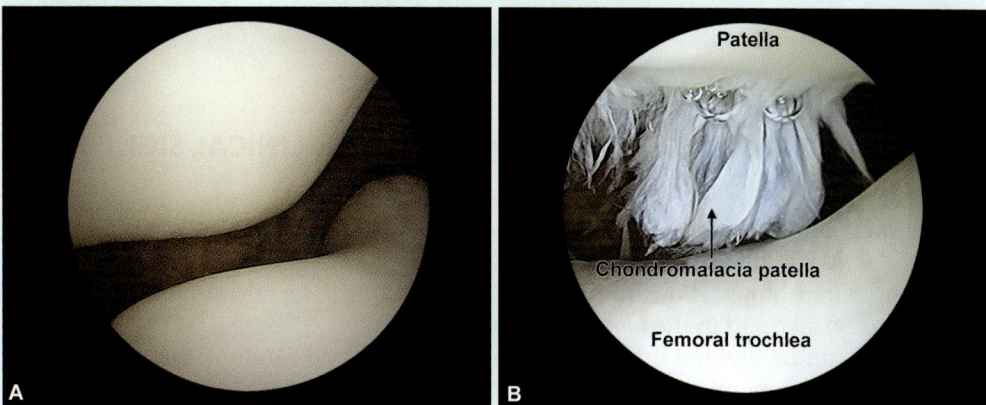

Figs. 8.33A and B: (A) Arthroscopic view of normal patella cartilage (from superolateral portal); (B) Arthroscopic view of cartilage fibrillation in chondromalacia.

- **Treatment:** Most patients are managed conservatively by activity modification, physiotherapy, and analgesics. Usually self-limiting by six months to a few years. Rarely, arthroscopic debridement of frayed cartilage is required.

8. **Osgood–Schlatter disease:**
   - **Affects:** Young adolescent kids who are active in sports, often bilateral.
   - **Presents with:** Anterior knee pain, especially while running, climbing stairs, and squatting
   - **Pathologically:** Avascular necrosis and fragmentation of tibial tuberosity (TT) apophysis
   - **Clinically:** Tenderness over the tibial tuberosity, prominent TT **(Fig. 8.34)**

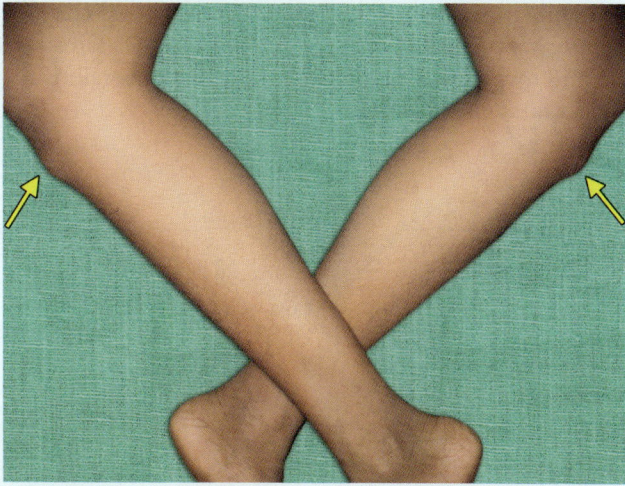

Fig. 8.34: Prominence of bilateral tibial tuberosity (yellow arrow) seen in Osgood–Schlatter disease.

CHAPTER 9

Clinical Evaluation of the Foot and Ankle Joint

SURGICAL ANATOMY OF FOOT-ANKLE AND ITS CLINICAL SIGNIFICANCE

1. **Osteology**
   - The *ankle joint* is formed between the lower end of the tibia, fibula, and talus, whereas the *subtalar joint* is formed between the calcaneum and talus.
   - Twenty-eight bones (Lower end of tibia and fibula, 7 tarsals, 5 metatarsal, and 14 phalanges) take part in the foot-ankle formation.
   - The foot can be divided into the hindfoot, midfoot, and forefoot. The bones of each component are mentioned in **Table 9.1**.

Table 9.1: Bones of the foot.

Hindfoot	Midfoot	Forefoot
Talus and calcaneum	Mid-tarsal (3 cuneiforms, navicular, cuboid)	All metatarsals and phalanx

2. **Major ligaments of ankle and foot**
   - The lower end of the tibia and fibula is supported by the anterior and posterior tibiofibular ligaments.
   - *Lateral ligaments of the ankle:* Three ligaments form the lateral ankle ligament complex: Anterior talofibular ligament (ATFL); calcaneofibular ligament (CFL); and posterior talofibular ligament (PTFL) ligament **(Fig. 9.1A)** *(Note: ATFL is the weakest of all three, and is most commonly injured in lateral ankle sprain)*. ATFL resists inversion of talus in plantar flexion and inversion; CFL prevents calcaneal inversion and talar tilt, and PTFL prevents posterior talar displacement.

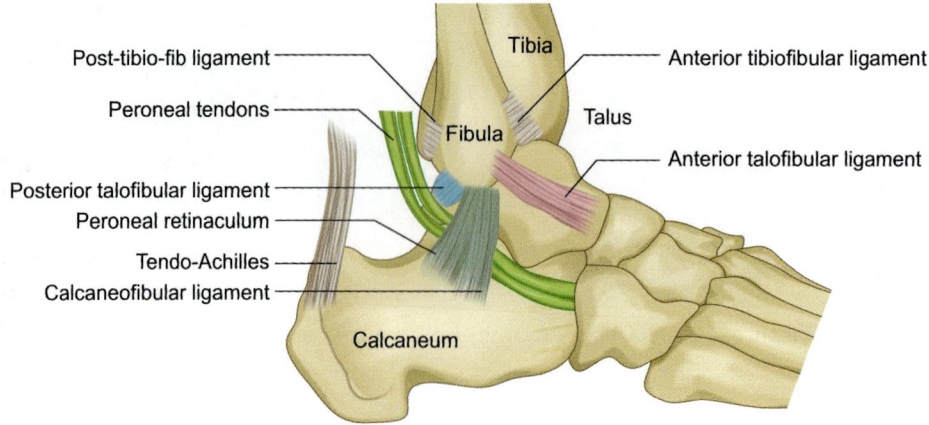

Fig. 9.1A: Lateral ankle ligament complex.

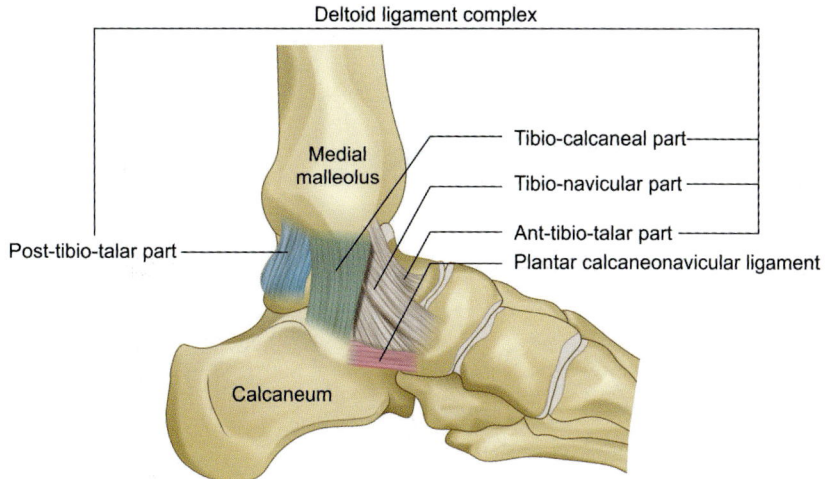

Fig. 9.1B: Medial ankle ligament complex.

- **Medial ligament of ankle:** Deltoid ligament supports the ankle on the medial side **(Fig. 9.1B)**. It has superficial and deep components. Superficial components are tibiocalcaneal, tibionavicular, and posterior superficial tibiotalar. Deep components are anterior tibiotalar and posterior deep tibiotalar.
- **Syndesmotic ligaments:** The tibiofibular syndesmosis has four ligaments: the anterior inferior tibiofibular ligament (AITFL), posterior inferior tibiofibular ligament (PITFL), inferior transverse ligament (ITL), and interosseous ligament (IOL).
- **Important ligaments of the foot:** Spring ligament (plantar calcaneo-navicular ligament), and short and long plantar ligaments.
- **Retinaculums of the foot:** There are three retinaculum of the foot, anterior, medial and lateral. The function of these retinaculum is to prevent bowstringing of the tendons, which pass under these retinaculum. Various structures passing under these retinaculum are mentioned in **Table 9.2**.

3. **Arches of the foot**
   - There are three arches in each foot: Medial longitudinal, lateral longitudinal, and transverse arch **(Fig. 9.2)**. Among all the arches, the medial longitudinal arch (MLA) is the most important as *loss of MLA results in flat foot*.
   - **How are the arches of the foot supported and maintained?** The arch of the foot is just like a structural arch. The integrity of foot and its arches are maintained by shape of interlocking bones, strength of various ligaments, plantar aponeurosis and various intrinsic and extrinsic muscles. Alteration in any of these structures could result in abnormal arch such as *pes planus* or *pes cavus*.
   - **Functions of the arch:** It distributes the weight between various tarsals and metatarsals, makes the foot flexible and easy to walk on uneven surfaces, helps propel the body in walking and running, and shock absorption.
4. The **primary function of the ankle and foot** is to transmit body weight during locomotion.
5. The **structures crossing the ankle under the extensor, medial and peroneal (lateral) retinaculum** are mentioned in **Table 9.2**.

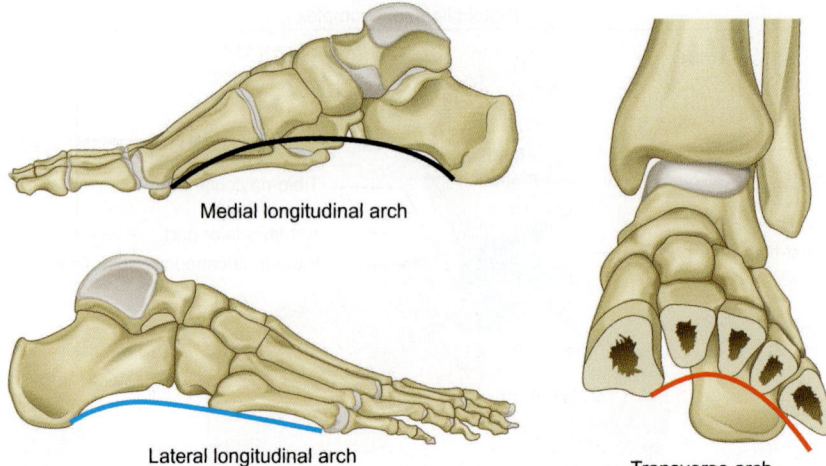

Fig. 9.2: Various arches of the foot. Curved black, blue and red lines represent medial, lateral and transverse arches, respectively.

TABLE 9.2: Structures crossing the ankle under various retinaculum.		
Anteriorly, under the extensor retinaculum	*Medially, under the medial retinaculum*	*Laterally, under the peroneal retinaculum*
Tibialis anterior, extensor hallucis longus (EHL), anterior tibial artery, deep peroneal nerve, extensor digitorum longus, and peroneus tertius (from medial to lateral)	Tibialis posterior, flexor digitorum longus (FDL), posterior tibial artery, posterior tibial nerve, flexor hallucis longus (FHL) (from anterior to posterior)	Peroneus longus and peroneus brevis

Types of joints in ankle and foot along with movements:
- *Ankle:* Hinge—Dorsi and plantar flexion
- *Subtalar:* Plane—Inversion and eversion
- *Intertarsal (Chopart Joint):* Gliding
- *Tarsometatarsal (Lisfranc joint):* Gliding
- *Metatarsophalangeal (MTP):* Condyloid—flexion, extension, some adduction and abduction.
- *Interphalangeal (IP) joint:* Hinge—flexion, extension

6. **Major extrinsic muscles of the foot-ankle**, their insertion, nerve supply, and action are mentioned in **Table 9.3**.

Before discussing the relevance of history taking and examination, it is important to know common conditions affecting the ankle-foot complex **(Box 9.1)**.

HISTORY AND ITS EVALUATION

Chief Complaints
- Pain and difficulty in walking
- Deformity
- Swelling
- Recurrent instability
- Tingling, numbness

CHAPTER 9 ♦ Clinical Evaluation of the Foot and Ankle Joint

TABLE 9.3: Major extrinsic muscles of foot-ankle.

Muscle	Insertion	Nerve supply	Principal action
Tibialis anterior	Medial cuneiform and first metatarsal bones	Deep peroneal nerve	Dorsiflexion of the ankle, inversion at subtalar joint
Extensor hallucis longus	The base of the distal phalanx (dorsal) of the great toe	Deep peroneal nerve	Dorsiflexion of the first interphalangeal joint
Extensor digitorum longus	Bases of the distal phalanges (dorsal) of the second, third, fourth, and fifth toes	Deep peroneal nerve	Dorsiflexion of distal interphalangeal (DIP) of lesser toes
Peroneus longus	Plantar side of the medial cuneiform and first metatarsal bone	Superficial peroneal nerve	Eversion, plantar flexion of the first metatarsal
Peroneus brevis	Tuberosity of the fifth metatarsal bone	Superficial peroneal nerve	Eversion
Tendo-Achilles	Calcaneal tuberosity on the calcaneus	Tibial nerve	Plantar flexion of the ankle
Tibialis posterior	Chiefly on navicular bone. However, it attaches to all the tarsals except for talus	Tibial nerve	Plantar flexion and inversion
Flexor digitorum longus	Bases of the distal phalanges (Plantar) of the second, third, fourth, and fifth toes	Tibial nerve	Plantar flexion at DIP joint of lesser toes
Flexor hallucis longus	The base of the distal phalanx (Plantar) of the great toe	Tibial nerve	Plantar flexion of the great toe IP joint

---

BOX 9.1: Common conditions affecting foot and ankle.

- **Congenital:** CTEV (clubfoot), flatfoot
- **Traumatic:** Ankle sprain, fractures, dislocation
- **Infections:** Post-traumatic osteomyelitis, tubercular synovitis, and arthritis
- **Inflammatory:** Rheumatoid feet with deformities of foot and toes
- **Metabolic:** Gout, pseudogout
- **Degenerative:** Plantar fasciitis, retrocalcaneal bursitis, tibialis posterior tendinitis
- **Neurological:** Charcot's feet, Morton's neuroma, Tarsal tunnel syndrome
- **Neoplastic:** Aneurysmal bone cyst, unicameral bone cyst

Note: Two questions remain the key to initiate the evaluation of the history of present illness. One, when were you apparently all right, and two, how did it start?

History of Present Illness

Pain and Difficulty in Walking

- One must enquire about the onset, location, duration, character, progression, and aggravating-relieving factors of the pain.
- A constant pain, especially at night, is a red-flag symptom and is suggestive of inflammation, infection, or tumor pathology.
  - ❏ The remission and exacerbation of the pain suggest a metabolic (gout/pseudogout) or inflammatory (RA) condition.

- Location/site of the pain can often give a clue to the diagnosis as pain arises from the underlying structures. For example, pain under the heel, which begins after placing the foot on the ground and decreases after walking for a few steps, is classic for plantar fasciitis. Pain at the back of the heel could arise from tendo-Achilles tendinitis/retrocalcaneal bursitis.
- Association of pain with change in the footwear or type of footwear must be asked for. A *tight shoe* could result in retrocalcaneal bursitis, Morton's neuroma, corns, and calluses. Prolonged wearing of *shoes with pointed and narrow toe box* (ballet shoes, stilettos) poses the risk of hallux valgus, while prolonged wearing of *stilettos* (high and pointed heel) can cause metatarsalgia and tendo-Achilles tendinitis.

Deformity

There are various common congenital and acquired deformities of the foot and ankle, such as congenital talipes equinovarus (CTEV), flatfoot (plano valgus), hallux valgus/varus, mallet, and hammer toes. One must ask about the onset (Congenital/acquired), progression of deformity, and painless or painful. Most deformities are painful, while deformities associated with Charcot's arthropathy is painless.

Swelling

Swelling could be unilateral or bilateral and localized or generalized. *Unilateral swelling* is usually due to local causes (trauma, tumor, infection, post-traumatic edema, varicose vein), whereas *bilateral swelling* indicates a systemic pathology (inflammatory arthritis, cardiac failure/renal failure/hypoalbuminemia). Swelling related to Charcot's arthropathy could be uni- or bi-lateral. *Intermittent swelling and redness* with pain at first MTP indicates gouty arthritis. Isolated proud swelling at the back of the heel is suggestive of Haglund's bump/retrocalcaneal bursitis, whereas swelling along the posteromedial aspect of the ankle may indicate tibialis posterior tendinitis.

Recurrent Instability

Recurrent giving away sensation/feeling of the ankle is due to the chronic ligament injury, which occurs after an ankle sprain.

Tingling and Numbness

The tingling and numbness in the ankle-foot could be due to local, proximal, or systemic cause. Systemic cause such as diabetes mellitus results in tingling and numbness in both legs and feet.
- *Local cause:* Tarsal tunnel syndrome (compression of tibial nerve under flexor retinaculum), Morton's neuroma.
- *Proximal cause:* Lumbar intervertebral disc prolapse.

Constitutional Symptoms

Symptoms such as fever, malaise, loss of weight and appetite may indicate an underlying infective, inflammatory or tumor disorder.

Effect on Activities of Daily Living (ADL)/Professional Activities

It is important to understand how the current complaints have affected the ADLs and professional activities, which may help plan the treatment.

Past History

Relevant history should be elicited. Diabetics are prone to foot ulcers and Charcot's arthropathy. Hypothyroid patients may present with ankle swelling. Past history of gout may explain bunion. A history of peripheral vascular disease may explain foot ulcers.

Personal History

History of smoking, alcohol intake, sleep, bowel-bladder, and type of shoe wear must be asked for.

Treatment History

A detail of treatment history can unfold the clues about the current diagnosis.

Family History

It may be positive in RA, hemophilia, and other congenital disorders.

Others: Allergies, Drug Intake, Menstrual History

At the end of history assessment, many common clinical ankle conditions can be reasonably well diagnosed based on age and key complaints. **Table 9.4** summarizes the important snippets for the clinical diagnosis of common ankle pathologies. However, all of them require confirmation with the specific examination.

TABLE 9.4: Foot and ankle clinical diagnostic snippets.

Symptoms and/or signs	Most likely pathology/diagnosis
A foot-ankle deformity since birth in which the ankle is in equinus and foot is inverted	*Congenital talipes equinus varus*
The deformity of the foot since birth in which the foot appears like rocker bottom chair-shaped	*Congenital vertical talus*
A young female presents with recurrent ankle instability with multiple episodes of slipping/giving away of the ankle while walking on uneven surfaces/running/descending stairs/while playing outdoor sports. Each episode was accompanied by pain and swelling around the ankle	*ATFL (Anterior talofibular ligament) and/CFL (Calcaneofibular ligament) tear*
A 47-year-old man presents with pain in the *undersurface of his heel* for two months. Pain is more in the morning as he keeps his foot on the ground, and the pain improves as he takes a few steps forward. The inferomedial calcaneal tuberosity is tender	*Plantar fasciitis*
A middle-aged male presents with chronic pain at the *back of the heel*. Pain increases after walking (*unlike plantar fasciitis*), and there is swelling at the back of both heels (right>left)	*Haglund's bump/retrocalcaneal bursitis*
A 55-year-old female presents with chronic pain and swelling on the inner aspect of the right ankle and proximal medial foot. Pain is more while standing, and the medial arch has collapsed compared to the left side. Swelling is present along the posteroinferomedial aspect of the ankle	*Tibialis posterior insufficiency/tendinosis* *Usually a problem in older women!*
A male patient presents with severe excruciating pain in the great toe with disturbed sleep. He said his pain-swelling phenomenon is episodic	*Hyperuricemia (Gout)* Always ask for reasons for hyperuricemia, such as non-vegetarian diet, excess alcohol intake, etc.

Contd...

Contd...

Symptoms and/or signs	Most likely pathology/Diagnosis
An adult male patient presents with forefoot pain between 3rd and 4th toes, with deep tenderness on the plantar aspect. Squeezing toes produced a click and tingling	**Morton's neuroma**
An elderly male with poorly controlled diabetes mellitus presented with diffuse swelling of the foot, minimal pain/no pain, loss of foot grip/feeling of midfoot instability/movement of foot bones while walking barefoot, following a recent trivial trauma. Clinician also notices the loss of the medial arch of the foot with the forefoot in abduction.	**Charcot's arthropathy**

EXAMINATION

General and Systemic Examination

General and systemic examinations should be performed in a standard fashion. Since many foot deformities and conditions are congenital, it is essential to examine the rest of the body to look for other abnormalities. Further, it is vital to examine the spine in patients with congenital abnormalities of the foot and ankle as the deformities in the foot and ankle could be due to neurological abnormalities of the spine. The radicular pain in the foot and leg is sometimes due to lumbar intervertebral disc prolapse, which may require spine assessment.

Examination of the Shoe/Footwear

Footwear inspection is quite relevant in assessing foot and ankle pathologies.

The shoe of a person with normal feet and arch would mildly wear on the *outer side of the heel and center of the sole* **(Fig. 9.3A)**. The shoe of the patient with cavus feet shows excess wear on the outer side of the heel and outer border of the shoe as they place more weight on the outer aspect of the foot **(Fig. 9.3B)**, whereas patients with flatfoot reveal excess wear on the inner side of the heel and medial border of the sole as they place more weight on the inner aspect of the foot **(Fig. 9.3C)**.

Local Examination

For the easy and systematic approach, the examination of the foot and ankle should be divided into five parts: ***forefoot*** (From the tip of toes to metatarsals), ***midfoot*** (cuneiforms, cuboid, and navicular), ***hindfoot*** (calcaneus and talus), ***ankle***, ***sole***, and ***skin***.

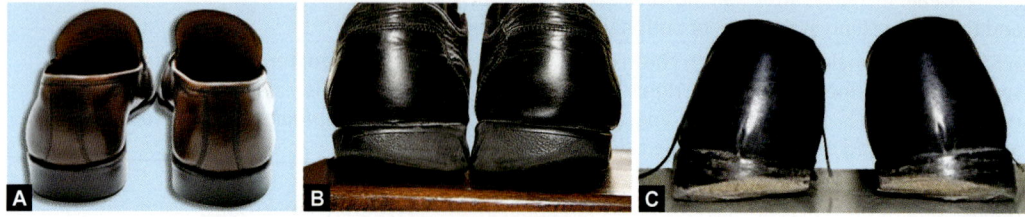

Figs. 9.3A to C: Shoe wear pattern in various type of feet. (A) Normal feet—mild wear on outer side of heel; (B) Oversupinator (cavus foot)—excess wear on lateral side of the heel; (C) Overpronator (flatfoot)—excess wear on medial side of the heel.

Gait

Assessment of type of gait is important. Further, check whether the patient is normally walking with the plantigrade foot with equal weight over the heel and forefoot (tripod) or they are walking on the heel (calcaneus), forefoot (equinus), or over the lateral border (CTEV).

Attitude

The attitude of the foot and ankle can be described in sitting or supine positions.

Inspection

It is crucial to examine the foot in ***standing*** (if possible) as the dynamic components of the foot, such as arches, are best observed in the standing position as various deformities such as heel varus/valgus often appear or increase during weight-bearing. Ask the patient to stand with both feet a few centimeters apart and look straight.

Now examine the ***forefoot, midfoot, hindfoot, ankle, calf, skin, sole, and size of the foot.*** If the patient cannot stand, then the examination can be performed in sitting or supine. The sole should be observed while sitting.

The general findings such as swelling, scar, and sinus should be described as per standard protocol. One must note any features of circulatory disturbance such as trophic changes in the nail, hair loss, varicosities, ulcers, and skin depigmentation around the ankle and foot. Specific findings of different regions are discussed below.

A. **Forefoot:** It reveals the *issues related to the toes, nails, and metatarsals.*
- Observe toes for any deformity such as hallux varus, valgus, mallet toe, hammer toes, or claw toes **(Figs. 9.4A and B)**. **Box 9.2** describes the common toe deformities.
- Nails must be examined for tropic changes (brittle, lusterless) or any disease characteristics such as Psoriasis.
- *Bunion*: Swelling over the 1st metatarsal head on the medial side.

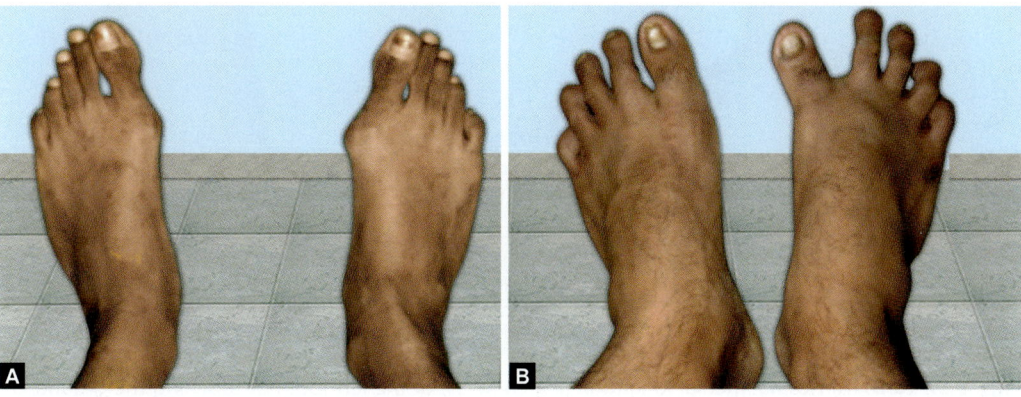

Figs. 9.4A and B: (A) Bilateral hallux valgus with bunion over 1st metatarsal; (B) Right great toe hallux varus.

> **BOX 9.2:** Common toe deformities.
>
> **Mallet toe:** DIP joint flexion deformity. Common in 2nd toe
> **Hammer toe:** PIP joint flexion, DIP extension, and MTP mild extension deformity. Common in 2nd toe
> **Claw toe:** PIP and DIP remain in flexion, whereas MTP in hyperextension
> **Hallux rigidus:** Limited dorsiflexion at first MTP joint

- *Bunionette (tailors bunion):* Swelling over the 5th metatarsal head on the lateral side.
- Look for forefoot deformity—abduction or adduction

B. **Midfoot:** The most important feature of the midfoot is the *arch of the foot, especially the medial longitudinal arch (MLA)*, which should always be assessed while the patient is standing. The normal MLA does not touch the ground, and the examiner can insinuate 1–1.5 cm of his index finger under the arch **(Figs. 9.5A and B)**.

The *exaggerated medial arch suggests "pes cavus,"* whereas the *attenuated arch suggests "pes planus" (flatfoot)* **(Figs. 9.5C and D)**. A **Heel raise test** can assess the flexibility of the arch. In this test, patient is asked to stand on his/her forefoot and elevate the heel. In a person with intact Tibialis anterior and Tendo-Achilles (TA) tendons, the medial arch accentuates and heel moves in inversion. However, there is no change in arch concavity in a person with rigid arch. Note that person cannot perform this test if the tibialis anterior or Tendo-Achilles are weak or ruptured (*watch video of Heel raise test*).

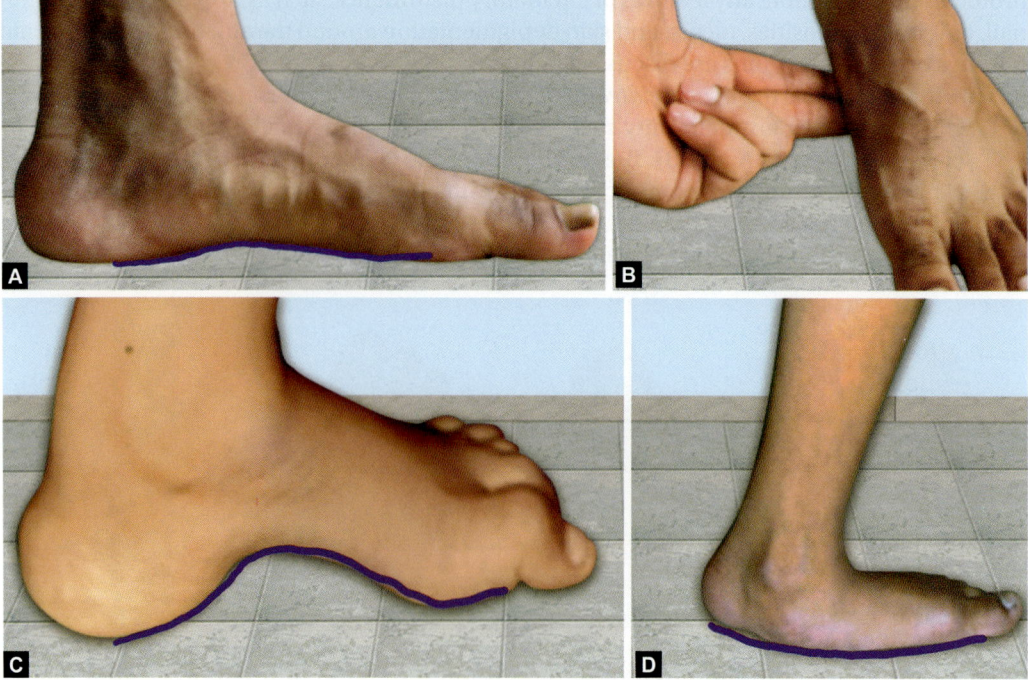

Figs. 9.5A to D: (A) Normal medial longitudinal arch (MLA) of the left foot not touching the ground; (B) Insinuation of a finger under the normal MLA; (C) Pes cavus (high arch) of the left foot; (D) Pes planus (flat arch) of the left foot.

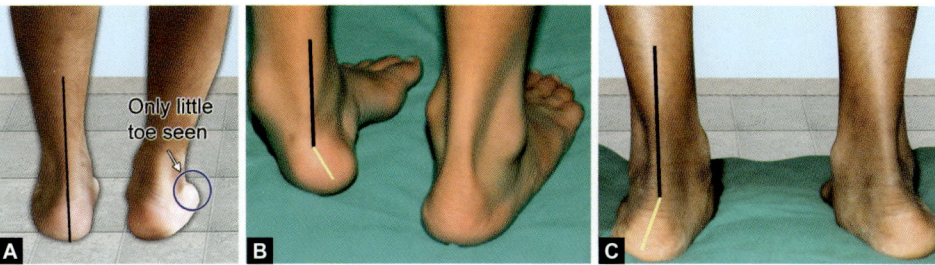

Figs. 9.6A to C: (A) Normal heel alignment with TA and calcaneum in the same line; only little toe is seen from behind; (B) Heel varus (left heel); (C) Bilateral heel valgus. The black line indicates the axis of TA, while the yellow line indicates the axis of the calcaneum.

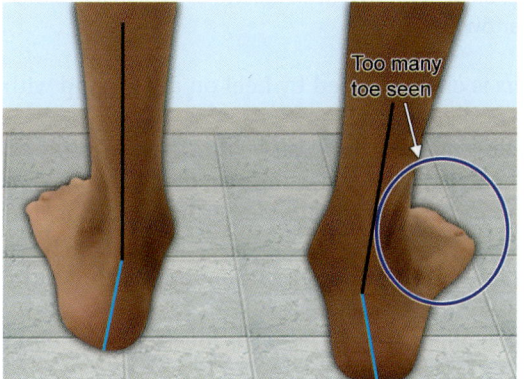

Fig. 9.7: 'Too many toes' sign in a patient with flatfoot, wherein more than two and half lateral toes are seen from behind. Also, note that the heel is in valgus with respect to TA in a patient with flatfoot. (Note the valgus angulation between black and blue line)

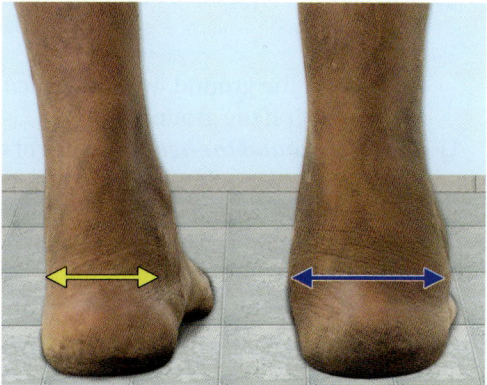

Fig. 9.8: Broad right heel due to malunited calcaneum fracture.

C. **Hindfoot and calf:** The hindfoot is examined from "behind and side", while asking the patient to stand with feet apart. Look for *heel alignment, back of the calcaneum, heel broadening, too-many-toe sign, tendo-Achilles (swelling, integrity), posteromedial-posterolateral aspect of ankle, and the calf.*
- **Hindfoot:** When observed from behind, normal hindfoot alignment is characterized by the axis of the tendo-Achilles (TA) axis and the calcaneum in the same line, and only the little toe is observed lateral to the silhouette of the leg **(Fig. 9.6A)**. In patients with **hindfoot varus or valgus deformity**, the axis of the calcaneum is in varus or valgus with respect to the axis of TA, respectively **(Figs. 9.6B and C)**. In a flatfoot, the heel moves in valgus, resulting in visualization of more than one toe lateral to the silhouette of the lower leg known as the *'too many toe sign'* **(Fig. 9.7)**. A **broadened heel** may suggest a malunited fracture of the calcaneum **(Fig. 9.8)**.
- **Equinus/Calcaneus deformity:** Hindfoot inspection from the side gives an idea of equinus/calcaneus deformity. *Equinus* is characterized by heel off the ground and

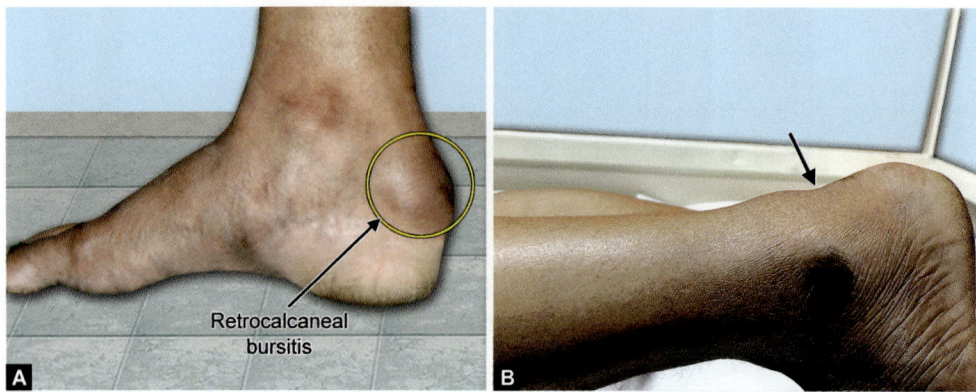

Figs. 9.9A and B: (A) Haglund's bump/retrocalcaneal bursitis; (B) Loss in Silhouette of TA due to rupture (black arrow).

forefoot on the ground, whereas *calcaneus* is characterized by heel on the ground with the forefoot off the ground.

- **Swelling around the heel:** Presence of swelling over the *back of the calcaneum may suggest* retrocalcaneal bursitis/Haglund bump **(Fig. 9.9A)**, while swelling over the *posteromedial and posterolateral aspect of the ankle is indicative of* tibialis posterior tendinitis and peroneal tendon tendinitis, respectively.
- Observe the **silhouette of TA** for any swelling (TA tendinitis) or apparent discontinuity (TA rupture) **(Fig. 9.9B)**. Note any calf muscles for wasting.

D. **Ankle:** Observe ankle for swelling, deformity, malleolar level (lateral is lower than medial), ulcers, and callosity.

E. **The skin over the foot (dorsum, medial, lateral, and posterior):** Look for swelling, varicosities, callosities, ulcers, scars, and sinus **(Figs. 9.10A and B)**. Also, observe for any foot muscle wasting.

F. **Sole:** Observe for normal concavity (loss or exaggeration), callosities, and ulcers.
- Typically, the sole is mildly concave. However, it is convex in Rocker bottom foot deformity (like a Rocker bottom chair) **(Fig. 9.10C)**. It is also convex due to collapsed arch in severe cases of Charcot's foot where the midfoot bones and joints are damaged **(Figs. 9.11A and B)**.

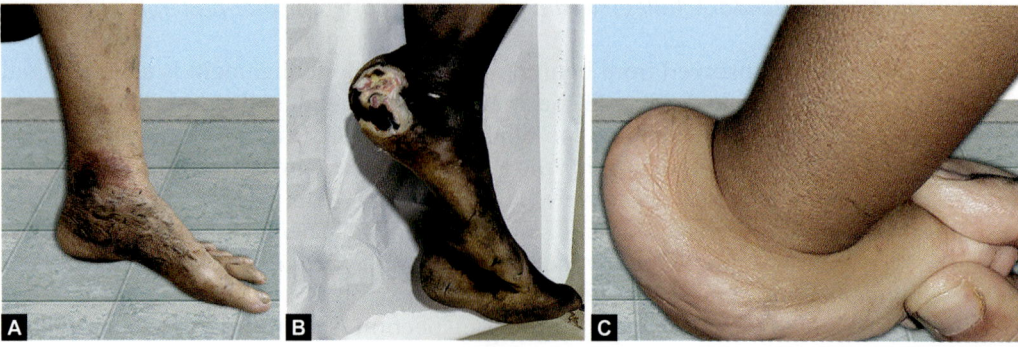

Figs. 9.10A to C: (A) Varicosities over the foot; (B) Non-healing ulcer over the heel; (C) Rocker bottom foot.

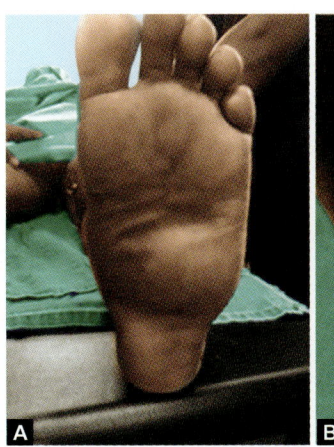
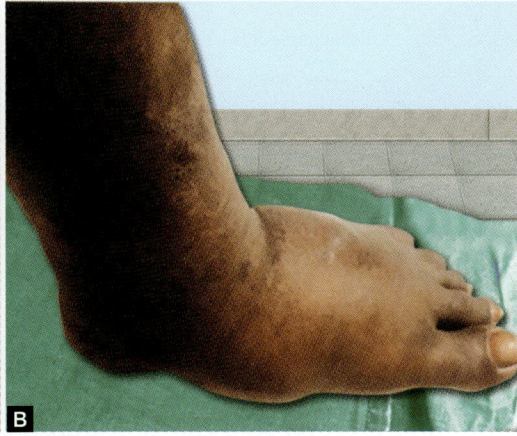

Figs. 9.11A and B: (A) Loss of foot concavity due to tarsal collapse; (B) Medial arch collapse in Charcot's foot.

G. **Borders and size of the foot:** Regarding *borders* of a normal foot, the medial border of the foot is longer than the lateral border. However, the lateral border is longer in the clubfoot, and the foot is smaller/bean-shaped in the clubfoot. The foot *size* can become smaller after a significant trauma/infection/tumor wherein a part of the bones is lost.

Palpation

The palpation of the foot-ankle must be done for assessment of a local rise in temperature, tenderness (soft tissue—bony landmarks and joint lines), intermalleolar relationship, and deformity. The bony landmarks are palpated for tenderness, irregularity and gap, while soft tissue landmarks are palpated for tenderness, thickening or defect.

1. **The local rise in temperature:** Entire foot and ankle.
2. **Tenderness:** The tenderness must be felt over anterior joint line and other important soft tissue-bony landmarks around the ankle joint.

The important landmarks around the ankle (anterior, medial, lateral, and posterior) to be palpated are mentioned below.

A. *Anterior:* Palpate the talus, lower third tibia, and syndesmosis **(Fig. 9.12)**. The syndesmosis is between the tibia and fibula, just above the ankle joint. Palpate the anterior ankle joint line, which lies 1 cm above the tip of the medial malleolus (MM). The joint line is felt and confirmed by gentle plantar and dorsiflexion of the ankle joint. A tender ankle joint line indicates intra-articular pathology.

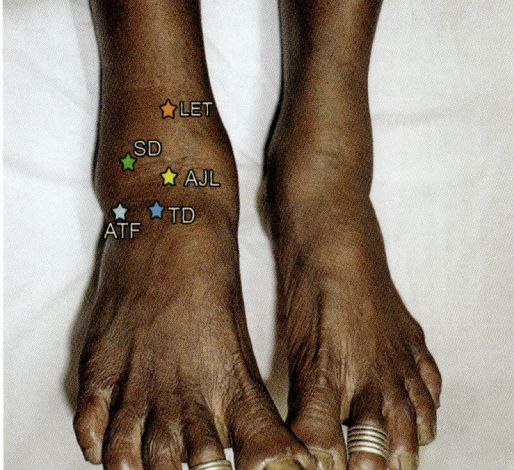

Fig. 9.12: Swelling over the right ankle can be noted. Major landmarks to be palpated on the anterior aspect of the ankle-anterior joint line (AJL), lower end tibia (LET), syndesmosis (SD), anterior talofibular (ATF) ligament, and talar dome (TD).

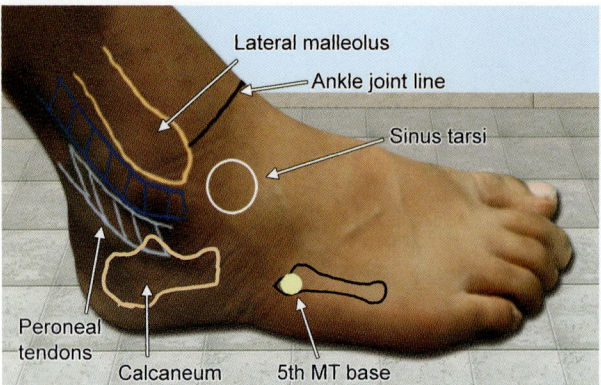

Fig. 9.13: Major landmarks for palpation around the ankle and foot lateral aspect. An anterior ankle joint line is illustrated for reference.

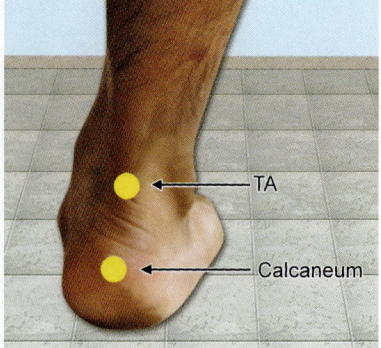

Fig. 9.14: Major landmarks for palpation of the posterior aspect of the ankle.

(TA: tendoachilles)

B. **Lateral:** Important lateral landmarks to be palpated are *Lateral malleolus, Peroneal tendons* (behind and below the lateral malleolus), *Calcaneum, and base of 5th metatarsal which are shown in* **Figure 9.13**.

C. **Posterior:** Posteriorly, there are two important landmarks to be palpated—*Tendoachilles (TA)* and *Calcaneum* **(Fig. 9.14)**. TA is tender in tendinitis and retrocalcaneal bursitis **(Fig. 9.9A)**, while a defect is palpable in TA rupture **(Fig. 9.15A)**. The Calcaneum is tender in infections, while a broad-irregular Calcaneum is felt in malunited fracture of Calcaneum.

D. **Medial:** Important landmarks to palpated medially are medial malleolus, medial tarsals, 1st metatarsal, Tibialis posterior tendon, and tibial nerve, which are shown in **Figure 9.15B**. *Tibialis posterior (TP)* is palpated behind MM and traced till the Navicular bone. TP is swollen and tender in TP tendinitis. A ruptured TP would result in a flatfoot. The *Tibial nerve* is palpated under the medial flexor retinaculum for any nerve entrapment/neuroma. Percuss the tibial nerve for Tinel's sign, which is positive in nerve entrapment (Tarsal tunnel syndrome).

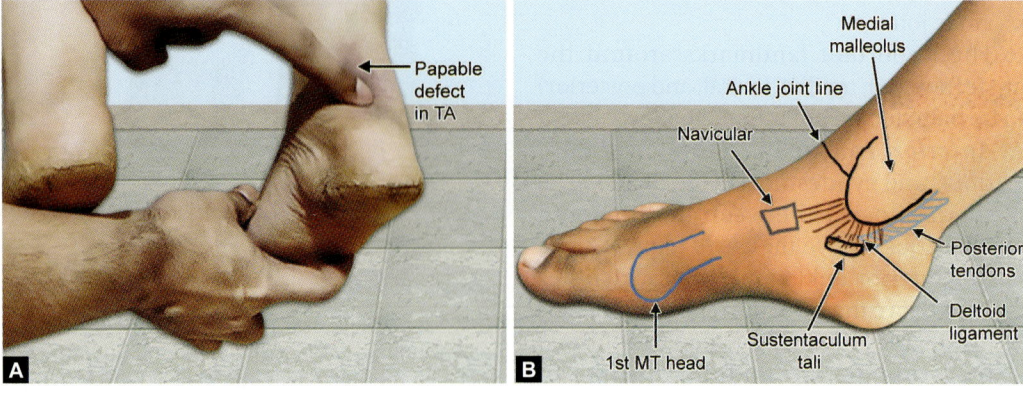

Figs. 9.15A and B: (A) Palpable gap after TA rupture; (B) Major landmarks for palpation of medial aspect of ankle and foot. Talus and medial cuneiform is not shown in the figure.

E. *Palpation of dorsum of foot:* Palpate cunieforms, cuboid, navicular, metatarsals, and dorsal tendons. There may be tenderness over 2nd metatarsal neck in stress fracture (March fracture). In Morton's neuroma, there is tenderness is felt between the 3rd and 4th metatarsals, and when the forefoot is squeezed together it results in a tingling sensation along with a click (*Mulder's click*)."

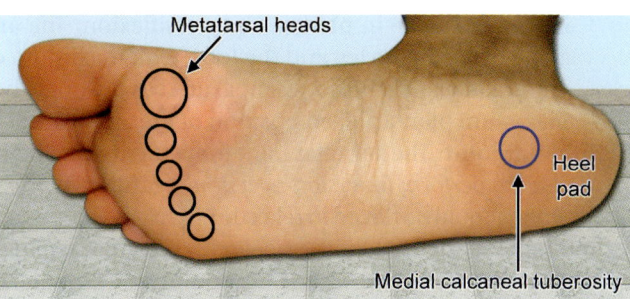

Fig. 9.16: Major landmarks for palpation of the sole.

G. *Sole:* Important landmarks to palpated on sole are heads of metatarsal and medial calcaneal tuberosity **(Fig. 9.16)**. Medial Calcaneum tuberosity is tender in plantar fasciitis.

Movements

Movements at the ankle, subtalar, midtarsal, and toe joints should be assessed.

1. **Ankle joint:** The typical movements at the ankle are "dorsiflexion and plantar flexion". The normal ankle ROM is mentioned in **Box 9.3**.

> **BOX 9.3:** Normal ankle and subtalar ROM.
> 1. Ankle dorsiflexion: 0–25°
> 2. Ankle plantar flexion: 0–50°
> 3. Subtalar inversion: 0–40°
> 4. Subtalar eversion: 0–20°

Always follow standard rules of movement assessment: Begin by assessing deformity, if any, and then observe active followed by passive ROM. Assess whether ROM is painless/painful, and crepitus during passive ROM (by keeping hand over the joint).

❑ Ankle dorsi- and plantar flexion is measured from the neutral position of the ankle, which is the position of the foot perpendicular to the leg **(Fig. 9.17A)**.

❑ *Method to assess passive ankle joint ROM:* The patient should be sitting or supine. The knee should be flexed to relax the tendo-Achilles as a tight TA in an extended knee would lead to less ankle dorsiflexion estimation **(Fig. 9.17A)**. The clinician holds the patient's heel with a cup of one hand, thumb, and index finger over the head of the talus and

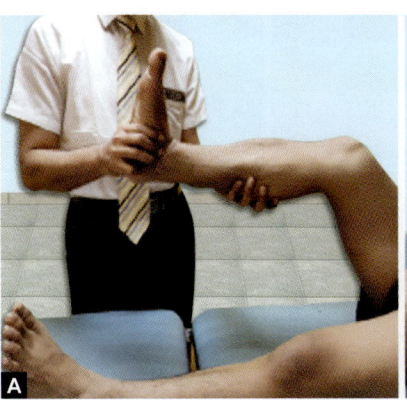 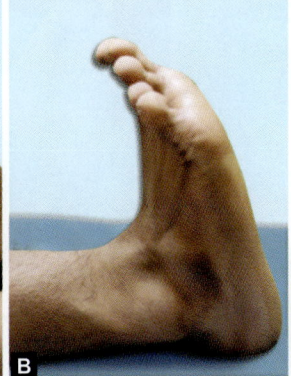 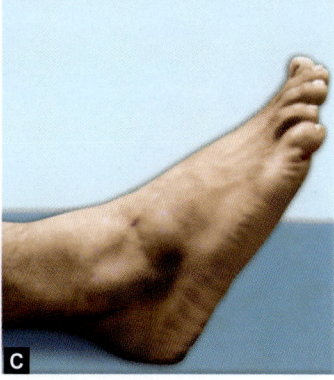

Figs. 9.17A to C: Assessment of the ankle ROM. (A) The neutral position of the ankle (with the knee flexed) followed by (B) Dorsiflexion; (C) Plantar flexion at the ankle joint.

moves the ankle in plantar and dorsiflexion. The ankle dorsiflexion is measured as the angle between the leg and the foot (with maximum dorsiflexed ankle) – 90° **(Fig. 9.17B)**. The ankle plantar flexion is measured as the angle between the leg and the foot (with the maximum plantarflexed position of the ankle) – 90° **(Fig. 9.17C)**.

2. **Subtalar joint:** The subtalar joint movements are "inversion and eversion."
   Method to perform inversion-eversion regardless of the patient's position (sitting or supine), the knee should be flexed to relax the TA. Next, the ankle is gradually moved in full dorsiflexion and holding the back of the heel with the palm while the thumb and index finger hold the head of the talus **(Fig. 9.18A)**. By completely dorsiflexing the ankle, the talus is locked into the ankle mortise as the broad anterior talar body comes inside the mortise (*Note: Talar body is trapezoidal where anterior half is wide and posterior half is narrow*). A dorsiflexed locked talus in the ankle mortise precludes any subtle rocking of the talus while performing eversion/inversion, which may contribute to false eversion/inversion. Then, the heel is inverted and everted to note the range of inversion-eversion **(Figs. 9.18B and C)**. Normal inversion is 40°, and eversion is 20°.

> **Note:** It is crucial to dorsiflex the ankle while measuring the inversion-eversion. Otherwise, the examiner may not agree to the findings. Conditions such as subtalar arthritis would render inversion-eversion ROM painful and decreased, whereas the tarsal coalition may have no/minimal subtalar movement.

3. **Movement at the toes:** Assess dorsi- and plantar flexion at the joints of the toes.

Measurement

1. **The foot size** should be measured from the back of the heel to the tip of the great toe (medial border) and the tip of the fifth toe (lateral border).

> The practical importance of foot size measurement is to assess the asymmetry of the foot. Also, it helps assess progress during the sequential 'cast' correction of the foot, especially in the case of CTEV. For example, in CTEV, the medial border is smaller than the lateral. The medial border becomes longer than the lateral with serial manipulation and cast application.

2. **Calf width** to quantify calf muscle wasting, if present.

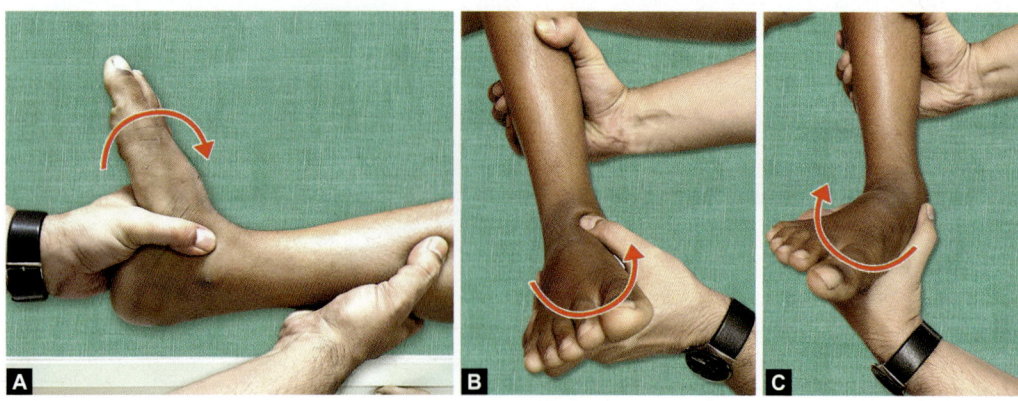

Figs. 9.18A to C: Assessment of the subtalar joint inversion-eversion. (A) Complete dorsiflexion at the ankle joint followed by (B) Inversion; and (C) Eversion.

Neurovascular Examination

A thorough vascular and neurological examination of the foot and ankle is a must. For vascular assessment; palpate both dorsalis pedis and posterior tibial artery.

The dorsalis pedis artery is felt just lateral to the EHL tendon over midtarsal region, while the posterior tibial artery is felt 1 cm below and behind the tip of the medial malleolus over the calcaneum.

The sensory and motor assessment of the foot and ankle are briefly described below.

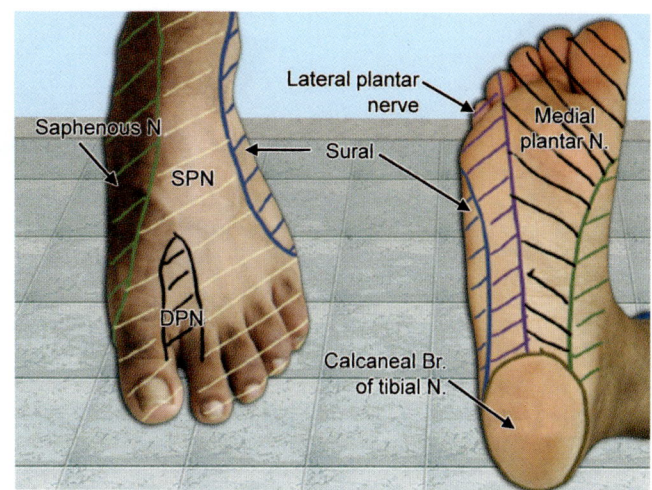

Fig. 9.19: Sensory innervation of the foot.
(SPN: superficial peroneal nerve; DPN: deep peroneal nerve; N: nerve; Br: branch).

Sensory assessment of the foot: The foot is innervated by sural, saphenous, superficial peroneal, deep peroneal, and tibial nerves **(Fig. 9.19)**.
- Medial border of the foot up to the ball of the great toe: ***Saphenous N.***
- Lateral border of the foot up to the ball of 5th toe: ***Sural N.***
- Entire dorsum of the foot except for 1st dorsal webspace: ***Superficial peroneal N.***
- 1st web space: ***Deep peroneal N.***
- Sole: ***Medial and lateral plantar nerves.***

Motor assessment: The clinician can assess the integrity of the nerve roots by the presence of various motor movements around the joint of the foot and ankle.
- *Dorsiflexion of the ankle:* L4
- *Plantar flexion of the ankle:* S1
- *Inversion:* L4, L5
- *Eversion:* L5, S1
- *Dorsiflexion of the great and smaller toes:* L5
- *Plantar flexion of the great and smaller toes:* S2

Special Tests

Various special tests are performed to assess ankle stability, medial arch flexibility, tendo-Achilles tendon integrity, and deep vein thrombosis.

Tests for Ankle Stability

The important ankle stability tests are mentioned below.
- **Anterior drawer test for anterior stability:** To test the integrity of the *ATF ligament*.
  Method: With the patient sitting on a couch and the knee flexed to 90°, the clinician holds the lower part of the leg from his left hand while the heel is held (cupped) from the right hand and the ankle is kept in 10° plantar flexion. Now, an anteriorly directed

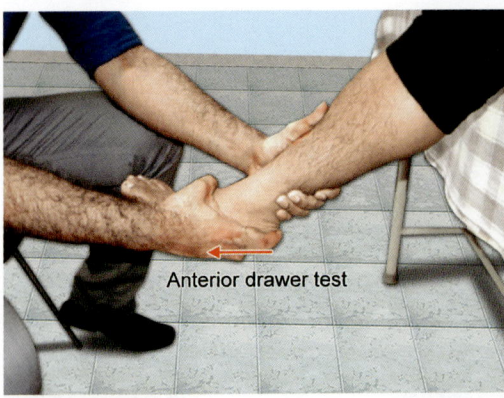

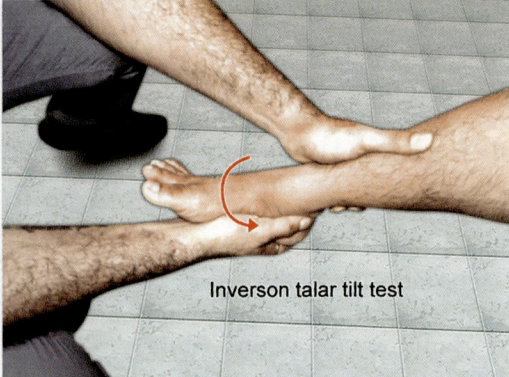

Fig. 9.20: Anterior drawer test. Red arrow indicates anterior pull.

Fig. 9.21: Inversion talar tilt test. Red arrow indicates inversion.

force is given (anterior drawer) to the heel **(Fig. 9.20)**. Always compare with the other side.
Interpretation: More than 8–10 mm anterior drawer or more than 3 mm compared with the contralateral side indicates insufficiency of the ATF ligament.

- **Inversion talar tilt test:** To test the integrity of the *calcaneofibular (CF) ligament*.
Method: With the patient sitting on a couch and the knee flexed to 90°, the clinician holds the lower part of the leg from his left hand while the heel is held (cupped) from the right hand and the ankle is kept in neutral flexion. Now, the ankle is inverted **(Fig. 9.21)**.
Interpretation: More than 5° tilt compared to the normal side with the soft mushy feel and or pain on the lateral side may indicate the insufficiency of the CF ligament.

Test for Flexibility of Medial Longitudinal Arch (MLA) for Flatfoot

- **Jack's test:** To assess whether the medial longitudinal arch of flatfoot is rigid/flexible type.
Method: While the patient is sitting, the clinician passively dorsiflexes the great toe of the index foot and observes for MLA exaggeration **(Figs. 9.22A and B)**.

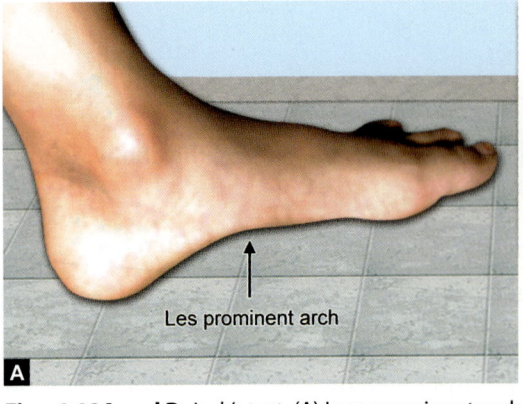

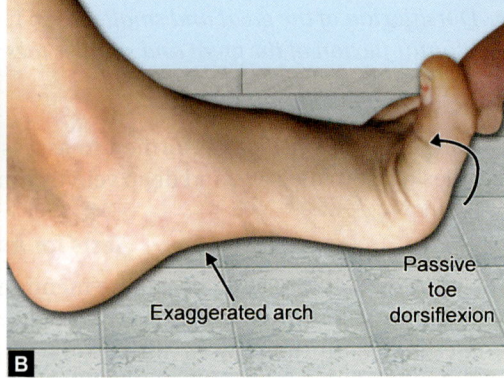

Figs. 9.22A and B: Jack's test. (A) Less prominent arch; (B) Exaggeration of the arch on passive dorsiflexing of the great toe indicates a flexible arch.

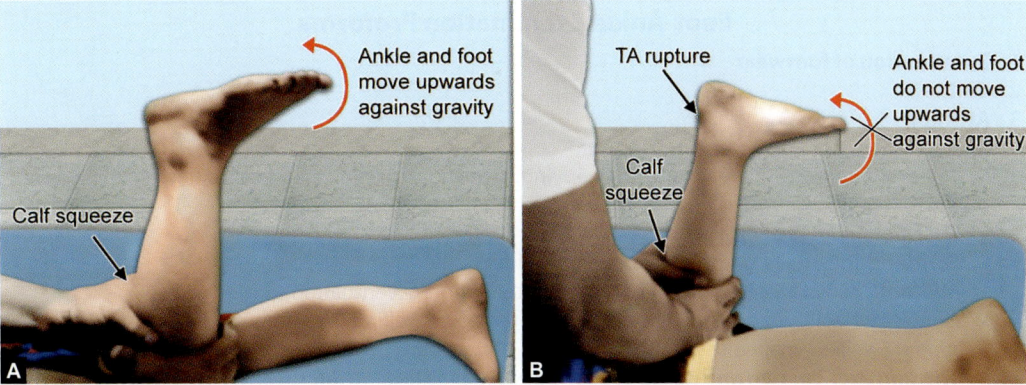

Figs. 9.23A and B: Thompson test (on squeezing calf). (A) Ankle plantar flexion against gravity in intact TA; (B) Absence of ankle plantar flexion in ruptured TA.

Interpretation: Exaggeration of MLA from its current flat position indicates a flexible type of flatfoot **(Fig. 9.22B)**, whereas no change in the arch (from flat position) indicates a rigid type of flatfoot *(often due to tarsal coalition)*.

Thompson–Simmond Test for the Integrity of Tendo-Achilles (TA) Tendon

Method: The patient should lie prone, and both the knees should be flexed 90° so that the foot faces upward. Now the calf is squeezed gently.

Interpretation: If the ankle moves in plantar flexion against gravity, it indicates intact TA. In contrast, if the ankle fails to move in plantar flexion, it indicates TA rupture **(Figs. 9.23A and B)**. *Note that patients with TA rupture cannot stand on the forefoot in a single-leg stance!*

Moses and Homan's Sign for Deep Vein Thrombosis (DVT)

Moses sign: The patient's calf is gently squeezed. A tender squeeze may suggest the presence of DVT. However, one must be careful during the Moses test, as a squeeze can theoretically dislodge a thrombus.

Homan's sign: The ankle is gently dorsiflexed. A painful dorsiflexion may suggest DVT of calf veins.

However, both signs have low sensitivity and specificity and must be interpreted along with risk factors, history and other signs such as subacute onset, swelling, and occasionally low-grade fever.

Examination of Other Joints Above

Standard knee, hip joint, and spine examination must be performed. Often spine affections such as spina bifida could result in ankle-foot deformities and hip dislocation.

Examination of Lymph Nodes

Inguinal and popliteal fossa lymph node examination is a must in all infective and tumor conditions.

Foot-Ankle Examination Proforma

1. **Examination of footwear**
2. **Gait**
3. **Attitude**
4. **Inspection:**
   - *General findings:* All areas for skin overlying, swelling, scar, sinus, and callosities. Examination of the footwear.
   - *Specifics findings of inspection*
   - *Forefoot:* Toes, nails, deformity, abduction/adduction
   - *Midfoot:* Medial longitudinal arch (normal/attenuation/accentuation)
   - *Hindfoot:* Heel (broadening, deformity), heel-rise test, swelling, TA silhouette, calf musculature
   - *Ankle:* Swelling, malleolus level, deformity
   - *The skin over dorsum and borders:* Skin creases, callosities
   - *Sole:* Shape, callosities, corns, skin, ulcers
   - *Size and borders of the foot*
5. **Palpation:**
   - A local rise in temperature
   - *Tenderness:* Bony landmark, soft tissues, joint line
   - Anterior, lateral, medial and posterior to ankle, squeeze test
   - Subtalar joint, midfoot and forefoot, sole, medial longitudinal arch
   - Normal intermalleolar relationship
   - Deformity
   - Confirmation of palpatory characteristics of swelling, scar, sinus
6. **Movements:** Active and passive
   - *Ankle:* Dorsiflexion and plantar flexion
   - *Subtalar joint:* Inversion, eversion
   - *Toes:* Flexion, extension
   - *Crepitus,* if any
7. **Measurements:** Size of foot, calf circumference
8. **Neurovascular examination**
9. **Special tests:**
   - *Test for ankle stability:* Anterior drawer for ATFL
   - *Medial longitudinal arch flexibility:* Jack test
   - *Tendo-Achilles integrity:* Thompson test
   - *DVT signs:* Moses' and Homan's signs
10. **Joint above:** Knee, hip and spine
11. **Lymph node examination**

Common Conditions Affecting Foot-Ankle and their Salient Features

1. **Clubfoot (CTEV):** It is the most common musculoskeletal birth defect.
   - **Affects:** Newborn child.
   - **Presents with:** Painless ankle-foot deformity, unilateral or bilateral.
   - **Pathology:** Soft-tissue contracture of the posterior and the medial side of the ankle and the foot. Medially rotated talar neck, calcaneal varus and medially rotated.
   - **Clinically:** Ankle equinus, hindfoot varus, cavus, forefoot adduction and inversion
     - Tight tendo-Achilles, small heel with varus
     - Prominent medial and posterior creases
     - Larger lateral border and smaller medial border of feet
     - Callosities over the lateral border of the foot in older children
     - Spine, hip, and knee are normal in idiopathic clubfeet.
   - **Diagnosis:** Clinical diagnosis. X-rays of the foot-ankle are done for the measurement of various angles.
   - **Treatment:** Serial manipulation (CAVE: Cavus, adduction, varus, equinus sequence) and cast application (Ponseti method), maintenance with an orthosis. Surgery in older children or failed conservative methods (Posteromedial soft-tissue release, osteotomy in children ≥5 years; JESS application/Ilizarov in older children, and triple arthrodesis in children >14 years.

2. **Congenital flatfoot/pes planus:**
   - **Affects:** Children and adults.
   - **Presents with:** Painless deformity.
   - **Pathology:** Medial longitudinal arch height is decreased (attenuated). Tarsal coalition is observed in rigid flatfoot. Calcaneonavicular and talocalcaneal coalitions are common.
   - **Clinically:** Presents at any age, unilateral or bilateral, flexible or rigid
     - Most of the cases are asymptomatic
     - *Too many toes sign* (seen from behind) in moderate-to-severe cases
     - *Rigid flatfoot may be due to tarsal coalition.* Jack's test is positive, while inversion-eversion is grossly limited due to the tarsal coalition.
   - **Diagnosis:** Primarily a clinical diagnosis. X-ray. CT scan help in diagnosing rigid flatfoot due to tarsal coalition.
   - **Treatment:** Usually, no treatment is required for the asymptomatic flexible flatfoot. Arch support orthosis and foot-ankle muscle stretching and strengthening are advised. Surgical intervention for severely symptomatic/rigid flatfoot is advised.

3. **Plantar fasciitis:**
   - **Affects:** Adults
   - **Presents with:** Heel pain when the patient takes a few steps and walks after a period of rest.
   - **Pathology:** Collagen degeneration associated with repetitive microtrauma to the plantar fascia.
   - **Clinically:** Tenderness is present over the medial calcaneal tuberosity at the plantar fascia attachment.
   - **Diagnosis:** Essentially a clinical diagnosis. Often, there may be a calcaneal spur. Furthermore, X-ray rules out other pathologies such as infection, tumor, and inflammation.
   - **Treatment:** Nonsteroidal anti-inflammatory drug (NSAID), soft heel shoe, rest, steroid injection. Rarely surgical release of the plantar fascia from medial calcaneal tuberosity may be performed.

4. **Retrocalcaneal bursitis (Hump-Bump/Haglund's deformity):**
    - ➤ *Affects:* Adult, common in repetitive trauma, sportsperson.
    - ➤ *Presents with:* Pain and prominent swelling at the back of the heel. In contrast to plantar fasciitis, the pain of retrocalcaneal bursitis usually does not subside while walking.
    - ➤ *Pathology:* Inflammation of the bursa, located between the Achilles tendon and the calcaneum.
    - ➤ *Clinically:*
        - ♦ Swelling over the posterior aspect of the calcaneum
        - ♦ Tenderness is present over the posterior aspect of the calcaneum over the TA insertion.
    - ➤ *Diagnosis:* Clinical diagnosis, X-ray, USG, MRI.
    - ➤ *Treatment:* NSAID, physical therapy (TA stretching), and shoe heel raise. Rarely, surgery may be required to excise the retrocalcaneal bursa, bony spur excision +/– TA repair.
5. **Tibialis posterior tendinitis/insufficiency:** It is the *most common cause of acquired flatfoot in adults*.
    - ➤ *Affects:* Mostly women, sixth decade onwards. Other risk factors are inflammatory arthritis (RA), diabetes, obesity, and steroid use.
    - ➤ *Presents with:* Painful/painless flatfoot deformity and swelling, on the medial side of the ankle along the tibialis posterior (TP) tendon.
    - ➤ *Pathology:* Progression of tendinitis to gradual insufficiency or tendon tear resulting in medial arch collapse.
    - ➤ *Clinically:*
        - ♦ Pes planus, swelling and tenderness along the course of TP tendon
        - ♦ Unable to perform a single-limb heel-rise.
    - ➤ *Diagnosis:* X-ray, MRI, USG.
    - ➤ *Treatment:* Orthosis (medial arch support), intrinsic foot muscle strengthening, and TA stretching. In severe cases, surgery may be required—tendon transfer (FHL), ligament repair, corrective osteotomy, and arthrodesis.
6. **Gouty arthritis:**
    - ➤ *Affects:* Adults, common in males. Commonly, small joints of the foot are affected.
    - ➤ *Presents with:* Episodic, sudden onset, severe pain with swelling of joints, especially 1st MTP joint **(Fig. 9.24)**.
    - ➤ *Clinically:*
        - ♦ Swelling, tenderness, and increased warmth at first MTP Joint.
        - ♦ Tophi in soft tissues (ear lobules)
    - ➤ *Diagnosis:* Clinical diagnosis, X-ray, uric acid level, renal function test.
    - ➤ *Treatment:* Acute episode is treated with NSAIDs, colchicine, or steroids. Chronic therapy involves treatment with uric acid lowering agents such as allopurinol or febuxostat. Also, treat the underlying cause, if any.

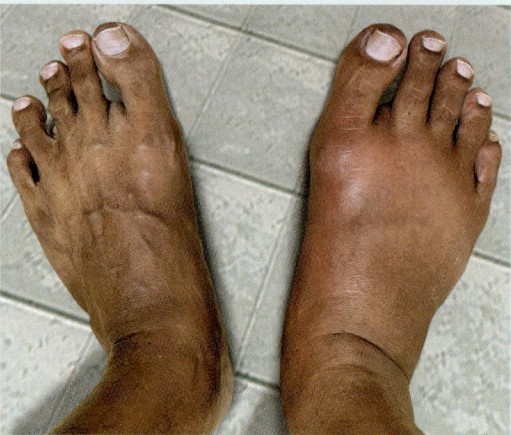

Fig. 9.24: Podagra of the right great toe.

7. **Ankle sprain:**
    - ➤ *Affects:* Mostly young patients. Lateral ankle sprain with injury to lateral ligaments is more common than medial side sprain.

- **Presents with:** History of twisting injury to the ankle (primary/recurrent), pain over the lateral aspect of the ankle, and recurrent instability of the ankle.
- **Pathology:** Tear of lateral ankle ligaments (most common—ATFL; followed by CFL and PTFL) due to inversion injury. Medial ankle sprain is relatively uncommon.
- **Clinically:** Tenderness anteroinferior/inferior/posterior to the tip of lateral malleolus depending upon the site of ligament injury (ATF/CF/PTF)
  - Painful plantar flexion and inversion, positive drawer tests, increased inversion.
- **Diagnosis:** X-ray, MRI (diagnostic).
- **Treatment:** Most cases are managed conservatively (RICE principle)—orthosis, below-knee cast, and rehabilitation. Surgical reconstruction of the ligament is performed in patients with recurrent instability.

8. **Morton's neuroma:** It is an interdigital neuroma commonly found between the 3rd and 4th metatarsal heads.
   - **Affects:** Present in adults, common with narrow shoe habit.
   - **Presents with:** Pain in the plantar aspect of the forefoot, worse with weight-bearing and wearing narrow toe-box shoes.
   - **Pathology:** Perineural fibrosis due to repetitive microtrauma.
   - **Clinically:** Tenderness over the 3rd interdigital space over the plantar aspect. Webspace squeeze test positive—Mulder's click may be positive.
   - **Diagnosis:** Clinical diagnosis, USG or MRI.
   - **Treatment:** Conservative treatment involves wider toebox shoe, avoiding heels, and local steroid injection. If still symptomatic—surgical excision.
   - **Differential diagnosis:** MTP synovitis, metatarsalgia, stress fracture, Freiberg disease

9. **Charcot's joint/neuropathic joint:**
   - **Affects:** Currently, diabetes is the most common cause of Charcot's arthropathy in the lower limb. Other causes are Hansen's disease, multiple sclerosis, syringomyelia, spinal cord injury, spina bifida, tabes dorsalis.
   - **Presents with:** Painless, progressive deformity and swelling of the foot and ankle.
   - **Pathology:** Two theories—neurovascular and neurotraumatic. *The neurovascular theory* states that autonomic dysfunction results in abnormally increased blood flow, causing osteopenia and bone resorption. *The neurotraumatic theory* implies that repetitive microtrauma to insensate joints results in progressive damage to the joints, which cannot adapt to the damages.
   - **Clinical presentation:** Painless, deformed foot and ankle. However, some patients do complain of mild pain.
     - Gross flatfoot or acquired Rocker bottom deformity
     - Swollen, warm, erythema: Clinical picture overlaps with cellulitis/osteomyelitis
     - Non-healing ulcers may be present over the foot, along with osteomyelitis
     - Exaggerated movement at the ankle and foot joints are observed
     - A neurological examination must be performed to assess sensorimotor deficit.
   - **Diagnosis:** X-ray is diagnostic—*dense bones, deformity, debris, dislocation of joints, destruction (gross) of the joints*. MRI helps in differentiating between infection and Charcot's arthropathy.
   - **Treatment:** Most cases require conservative treatment in the form of total non-contact orthosis, footwear modification, underlying disease control, protection of the foot against trauma, and gabapentinoids. Resistant cases with severe deformity, non-healing ulcers/severe infections may require amputation.

CHAPTER 10

Clinical Evaluation of the Spine

SURGICAL ANATOMY OF SPINE-SPINAL CORD AND ITS CLINICAL SIGNIFICANCE

1. **Brief osteology of the spine:**
   - *There are 33 vertebrae:* 7 cervical, 12 thoracic, 5 lumbar, 5 sacral, and 4 coccygeal vertebrae constitute the spinal column. A vertebra has body, pedicle, lamina, transverse process, and spinous process.
   - *Characteristics of the cervical vertebra:* C1–C6 cervical vertebrae have transverse foramen (foramen transversarium), which gives passage to the vertebral artery and vein, and a bunch of sympathetic plexus.
   - *Characteristics of the thoracic vertebra:* It has costal facets for rib articulation.
   - *Characteristics of the lumbar vertebra:* Lumbar vertebral bodies have the mammillary process and pars interarticularis (thick and strong tricortical bone at the junction of pedicle, lamina, superior and inferior articular processes).

2. **The spinal cord (anatomy, tracts, and blood supply), autonomic nervous system (ANS), and nerve roots:**
   - *Spinal cord:* The spinal cord starts from the foramen magnum as a continuation of the medulla oblongata and ends at the lower end of the L1 vertebra or the upper end of the L2 vertebra. The terminal end of the spinal cord is bulbous, which is known as *conus medullaris* **(Fig. 10.1)**. Conus medullaris gives rise to the lumbar and sacral roots, which continue to descend in dural coverings from the lower end of the spinal cord. These descending lumbosacral and coccygeal nerve roots (consisting of L2-L5, S1-S5, and one coccygeal root) collectively looklike a horse's tail, hence known as cauda equine **(Fig. 10.1)**. Spinal cord has 31 *transverse spinal segments* or *myelomeres*. Each spinal segment gives rise to a pair of nerve roots (ventral and dorsal). These roots combine to form a spinal nerve. It is important to note that spinal segment and vertebral levels do not match **(Fig. 10.2A)** as the vertebral column grows faster than the spinal cord. The general rule is that upper cervical vertebral levels match the spinal segment. For lower spinal segment

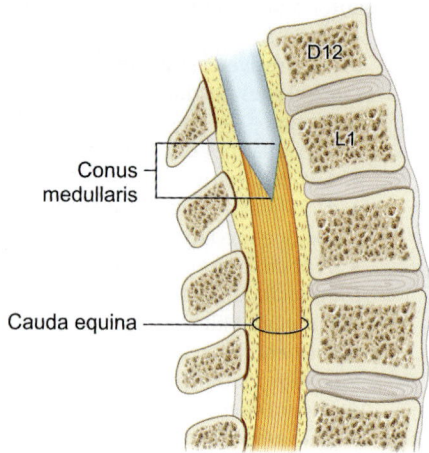

Fig. 10.1: Illustrated sagittal section of lumbosacral spine showing conus medullaris and cauda equina.

location, add one-two-three to the lower cervical, upper thoracic, and lower thoracic vertebra, respectively. There are several important sensory and motor tracts that cross the spinal cord **(Fig. 10.2B)** are briefly described below.

Major sensory tracts in the spinal cord:
i. *Posterior (Dorsal) column tract* carries sensations of touch, proprioception (position sense), tactile localization, two-point discrimination, stereognosis, and vibration. It is important to note that in the posterior column, the homunculus orientation of cervical to sacral sensory fibers is from lateral to medial, respectively **(Fig. 10.2B)**.

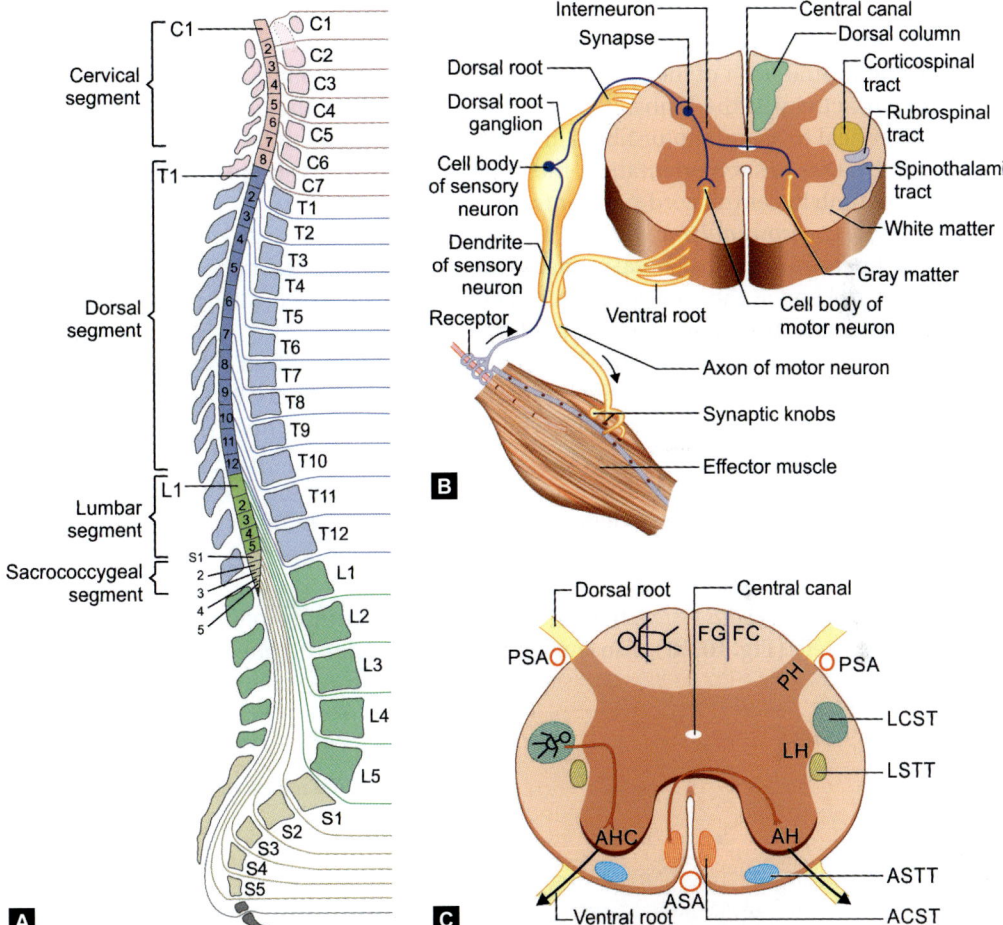

Figs. 10.2A to C: (A) Illustrated sagittal section of the spinal cord showing the myelomeres or spinal segments; (B) Spinal cord section showing major tracts with sensorimotor innervation; (C) Spinal cord cross-section showing various important sensorimotor tracts; dorsal column tract homunculus has sacral fibers most medial and cervical lateral, whereas CST homunculus has cervical fibers most medial and sacral ones lateral.

Note: Homunculus is a representation of small human being.

(FG: fasciculus gracilis; FC: fasciculus cuneatus; PSA: posterior spinal artery; LCST: lateral corticospinal tract; ACST: anterior corticospinal tract; LSTT: lateral spinothalamic tract; ASTT: anterior spinothalamic tract; PH: posterior horn; AH: anterior horn; LH: lateral horn; AHC: anterior horn cell; ASA: anterior spinal artery).

ii. *Lateral spinothalamic tract* carries pain and temperature
iii. *Anterior spinothalamic tract* carries touch and pressure.

Motor tract in the spinal cord: The corticospinal tract (CST) or pyramidal tract is the major motor tract, which is responsible for the voluntary motor activity of the body. Most CST fibers originate from the primary motor area of the brain (precentral gyrus and Brodmann area 4) and prefrontal area. After descending through the brainstem, almost 80% of CST fibers cross at the level of the medulla oblongata and form lateral CST, whereas the remaining 20% of uncrossed fibers form anterior CST.

i. *Lateral corticospinal tract (LCST):* LCST is the "principal-crossed motor tract" at the level of medulla oblongata containing 80% fibers from the opposite primary motor cortex of the brain, whose fibers synapse (end) with ipsilateral anterior horn cells (AHC) located in the ventral horn of the spinal cord. LCST is the main pathway to control voluntary motor activity in the limbs. It is important to note that the homunculus orientation of cervical to sacral motor fibers in LCST is from medial to lateral, respectively **(Fig. 10.2B)**. Due to such orientation, the upper limb weakness is more profound than the lower limb in central cord syndrome.

ii. *Anterior corticospinal tract (ACST):* It is an "uncrossed voluntary motor tract" containing 20% fibers from the ipsilateral primary motor cortex of the brain whose fibers eventually cross and end at the anterior horn cell of the opposite side. ACST primarily assists in axial muscle (trunk, neck, and shoulder) motor control.

Blood supply of the spinal cord: The spinal cord is supplied by a single anterior spinal artery (ASA) and two postero-lateral spinal arteries (PSA) **(Fig. 10.3)**. Single ASA supplies anterior two-thirds of the spinal cord, whereas two PSA supply posterior one-third of the spinal cord **(Fig. 10.3)**.

❑ **Autonomic nervous system:** There are two components of the ANS—sympathetic and parasympathetic. Both components of ANS start from the brain or spinal cord and end at ganglions as preganglionic neurons. After synapsing in the ganglion, postganglionic fibers end at the effector organ.

The sympathetic nervous system neurons originate from the thoracolumbar region's (T1-L2) lateral horn cells **(Fig. 10.2B)**, also known as *"thoracolumbar outflow."* These preganglionic

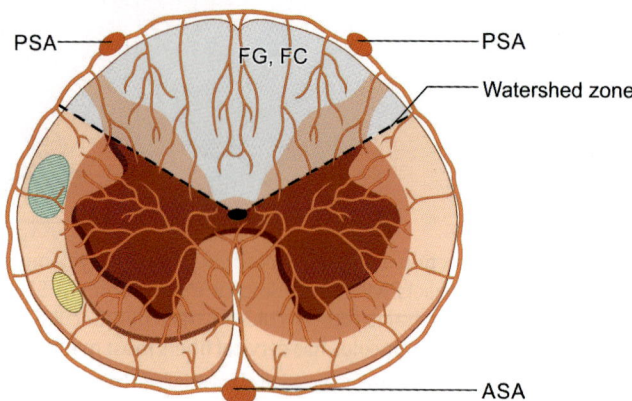

Fig. 10.3: Arterial supply of the spinal cord.
(ASA and PSA: anterior and posterior spinal artery; FG: fasciculus gracilis; FC: fasciculus cuneatus).

neurons synapse with postganglionic neurons and supply the heart, vessels (arterioles), and various other visceral organs. Therefore, *spinal cord injury at the cervical level disrupts sympathetic supply, causing hypotension.*

The parasympathetic nervous system of the body is via Vagus nerve and sacral roots (S2-S4) of the spinal cord known as *"craniosacral outflow."* Post-ganglionic neurons of PNS innervate effector organs (heart, lung, digestive system, urinary system, eye, and oral cavity).

3. **Urinary bladder (UB) and its innervation:** The supraspinal control centers of UB are located in the paracentral lobule (medial surface of the brain) and pontine nucleus **(Fig. 10.4A)**. Locally, UB is innervated by *somatic* (S2, 3, 4 via pudendal nerve), *sympathetic* (T10-L2) nervous system via hypogastric nerves, and *parasympathetic* (sacral outflow via pudendal nerve) nervous system via pelvic nerves **(Fig. 10.4A)**. The function of various components of the nervous system innervating the UB is mentioned in **Table 10.1**.

TABLE 10.1: Function of various components of nervous system innervating the urinary bladder.

Nervous system	Root value	Supplies	Function
Sympathetic *(via hypogastric nerve)*	D10-L2	Detrusor, IUS	• Detrusor—inhibition/relaxation: UB relaxed • IUS—stimulation/contraction
Parasympathetic *(via pelvic nerve)*	S2, 3, and 4	Detrusor, IUS	• Detrusor—stimulation/contraction: UB contracts • IUS—inhibition/relaxation
Somatic *(via pudendal nerve)*	S2, 3, and 4	EUS	EUS—contraction/relaxation depending upon cortical response
Sensory *(via hypogastric, pelvic and pudendal nerve)*			Sensations to the cortex

(EUS: external urethral sphincter; IUS: internal urethral sphincter; UB: urinary bladder)

4. **Intervertebral disc (IVD), spinal ligaments, and facet joints:**
   - *Intervertebral disc:* IVD consists of inner soft central-hydrated gelatinous "nucleus pulposus", outer fibrous "annulus fibrosus", and superior and inferior vertebral cartilaginous end plates **(Figs. 10.4B and C)**. The disc is innervated by the sinuvertebral nerve (Nerve of Luschka). IVD is stabilized by longitudinal ligaments and end plates.
   - *Ligaments:* Anterior longitudinal ligament, posterior longitudinal ligament, ligamentum flavum, inter- and supraspinous ligaments stabilize the spine **(Fig. 10.4C)**.
   - *Facet joints:* A facet joint is a plane synovial joint surrounded by a capsule and innervated by two small nerves. Facet joints are between the cervical, thoracic, and lumbar vertebra permit and constrain movements between the vertebrae **(Fig. 10.4C)**. They also share weight transfer along with IVD. Variable facetal orientation is partly responsible for different movements in different regions of the spine.
5. **The curvature of the spine, mobility, and function:**
   - *The normal sagittal curvature of the spine:* There is lordosis in the cervical spine, kyphosis in the thoracic spine, lordosis of the lumbar spine, and kyphosis in the sacrum **(Fig. 10.4D)**.
   - The *mobility of the spine* occurs at the IVD and facet joints. The cervical spine and lumbar spines are the most mobile, whereas the thoracic spine is the least mobile as it is encircled

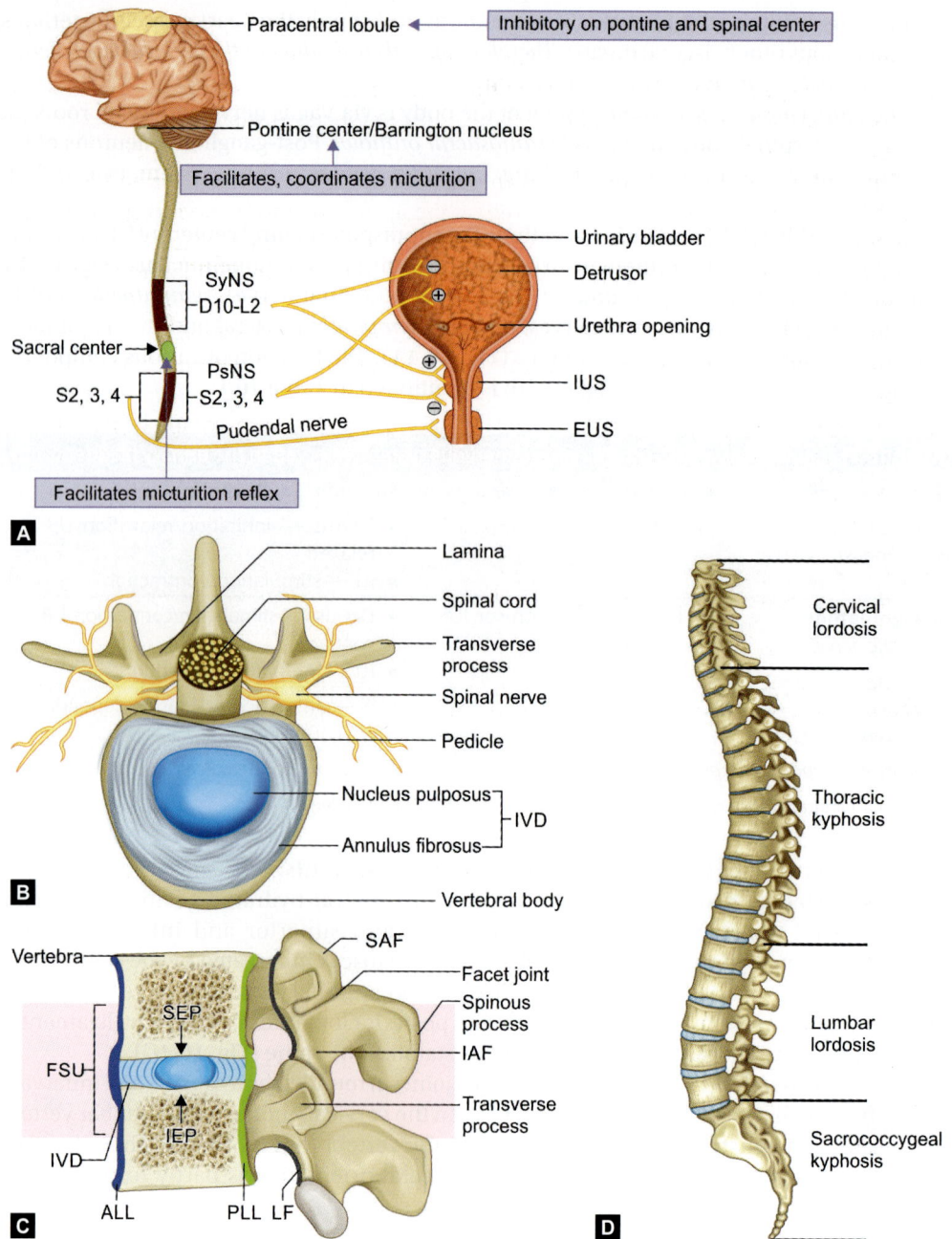

Figs. 10.4A to D: (A) Urinary bladder innervation; (B) Axial view of intervertebral disc and vertebra with nerve roots exiting from the spinal cord; (C) Functional spinal unit (pink- shaded area); (D) Normal spinal curvature in sagittal plane.

(EUS: external urethral sphincter; IUS: internal urethral sphincter; IVD: intervertebral disc; FSU: functional spinal unit; SEP: superior end plate; IEP: inferior end plate; ALL and PLL: anterior and Posterior longitudinal ligament; LF: ligamentum flavum; SAF and IAF: superior and inferior articular facet; SyNS: sympathetic nervous system; PsNS: parasympathetic nervous system).

by the rib cage. Degenerative spine and disc diseases are more common in more mobile regions, such as lower cervical and lumbar regions.
- ❏ *Functions of the spine:* Spine protects the spinal cord, provides attachment to various muscles and ligaments, maintains erect posture, and renders mobility.

6. **Movement at the spine:**
   - ❏ *Cervical spine:* While movements in cervical spine occur in all three planes, the predominance of movements is different at the upper and lower cervical spine. Flexion-extension (YES movement) at an atlanto-occipital junction, lateral rotation (NO movement) at the atlantoaxial joint, whereas lateral flexion in addition to all the above movements occurs at the lower cervical spine levels.
   - ❏ *Dorsal spine:* Predominant movement in the dorsal spine is *"rotations"*.
   - ❏ *Lumbar spine:* Predominantly, flexion-extension and lateral flexion occur in the lumbar spine.

Before we proceed with assessing the chief complaints and history assessment, it is essential to recollect the common conditions affecting the spine **(Box 10.1)**, which help in probing the various complaints of the patient.

> **BOX 10.1:** Common clinical conditions affecting the spine.
> - *Congenital:*, Spina bifida, scoliosis, kyphosis, Sprengel's/Klippel–Feil deformity, cervical rib
> - *Infection:* Tuberculosis (Pott's spine), brucellosis, and pyogenic
> - *Degenerative:* Intervertebral disc prolapse, spondylosis, lumbar canal stenosis, and myelopathy (cervical/thoracic)
> - *Inflammatory:* Ankylosing spondylitis and other seronegative spondyloarthropathies
> - *Metabolic:* Osteoporosis, osteomalacia, ochronosis
> - *Traumatic:* Fractures, dislocation, traumatic disc prolapse
> - *Tumors:* Multiple myeloma, secondaries, and osteoblastoma
> - *Others:* Thoracic outlet syndrome, fibromyalgia

HISTORY AND ITS EVALUATION

A detailed history plays a vital role in the diagnosis of the exact etiopathology of spine disease.

Before we evaluate the common symptoms of spine disorders, it is vital to understand the influence of age on various spine disorders **(Table 10.2)**.

TABLE 10.2: Age and common conditions affecting spine.

Age	Common conditions
Congenital	Spina bifida, scoliosis, muscular dystrophies
All Ages	Infective etiologies (Iatrogenic/secondary spine infections too are common in the adult and aging population following surgical interventions)
20–50 years	IVDP, ankylosing spondylitis
40–60 years	Degenerative conditions such as spondylosis (cervical/lumbar), lumbar spondylolysis, spondylolisthesis, and lumbar canal stenosis
>50 years	Spinal metastasis

Chief Complaints and History of Present Illness

The common symptoms of diseases affecting the spine are mentioned in the **Box 10.2**. Further, one must ask about the *onset of the complaints*, whether they were traumatic in onset or insidious, and then elaborate on all complaints sequentially.

> **BOX 10.2:** Common complaints in patients with spine pathology.
>
> Pain, neurological deficits, difficulty/restriction in movements, difficulty in walking, deformity, and dizziness are common symptoms in a patient with a spine pathology.

Pain

It is the most common symptom reported in spine disorders. To determine underlying etiology, one must probe into onset, duration, timing, site, nature, radiation, aggravating and relieving factors, morning stiffness, and claudication distance.

- **Onset of pain:** The pain could be sudden or insidious onset. Acute intervertebral disc prolapse, trauma, or sprain can present with sudden onset pain, whereas infective, inflammatory origin pain is insidious in onset.
- **Timing of pain:** One must always differentiate between mechanical pain (pain with activity) or pain at rest or night pain, as the reason for both is usually different.
    - *Pain at rest or night pain:* It may indicate infective, inflammatory, or malignant pathology.
    - *Mechanical pain (with activity)* is typically observed in degenerative conditions such as spondylitis, facetal arthropathy, IVDP, and osteoporosis.
- **Site of pain:** The region of pain such as cervical, thoracic, and lumbar gives an idea of the anatomical site of involvement.
    - **Nature of pain:** It could be dull aching or moderate-severe throbbing type. Dull aching pain is usually due to degenerative conditions (Disc disease, spondylosis), whereas throbbing type indicates localized infection, tumor, acute disc prolapse, acute trauma, or acute sprains.
- **Radiation of pain:** The radiating pain always suggests a nerve root involvement.
    - ***The area of radiation*** should be asked for (scapular region, upper limb, anterior aspect of the thigh, posterior aspect of the thigh, calf, or foot) as that will give a clue to the root involvement.
- **Aggravating factors:**
    - *An increase in pain during forward bending*, lifting weight in forward flexion position, coughing, sneezing, or turning in the bed is quite typical of lumbar IVDP.
    - *Pain during bending backward is* observed in lumbar canal stenosis, spondylolysis, spondylolisthesis, and facet arthropathy.
- **Relieving factors:**
    - Pain is often relieved at rest due to degenerative conditions such as spondylosis, canal stenosis, or spondylolisthesis. In contrast, inflammatory back pain due to seronegative spondyloarthropathy (AS) improves with activity (or worsens with rest).
    - Forward bending relieves pain in lumbar canal stenosis as canal diameter increases in forward flexion.

Associated stiffness in the back, *especially lumbar spine and SI joint area, in the morning and at rest:* It is commonly observed in AS and other inflammatory spondyloarthropathies.

TABLE 10.3: Clinical differences between neurogenic and vascular claudication.

	Neurogenic claudication	Vascular claudication
Common cause	Lumbar canal stenosis	Thromboangiitis obliterans, atherosclerosis of lower limb arteries
Pain characteristics		
Appears or increases	During standing, walking down-hill or downstairs, and descending the ramp	After walking for some distance. Uphill/downhill/ramp ascend-descend, pain will increase
Ramp/stair climbing	Decreases	Increases
Cycling	No effect or may decrease if the person is bending forward	Increases
Pain relieves	Bending forward, climbing upstairs, or ramp ascend	• No effect on bending forward • Increases while going upstairs/ramp
Claudication distance	Variable	Fixed
Associated back pain	Possible	Rare
Distal pulse	Normal	Feeble/absent
Sensory symptoms	Common	Rare
Trophic changes in limb	None	Likely

Walking/Claudication Distance

In patients with lumbar canal stenosis (LCS), the walking distance may decrease due to *neurogenic claudication*. Since walking distance is also decreased in vascular claudication, one must make all attempts to differentiate between the two types of claudication **(Table 10.3)**. Also, note that the two conditions can co-exist.

Neurological Symptoms

Motor weakness or sensory symptoms (tingling and numbness) in the limb indicate involvement of the spinal cord or nerve root or both. Bladder and bowel involvement (inability to pass or inability to control) indicates the involvement of the cauda equina/spinal cord while sexual dysfunction may indicate conus medullaris or cauda equina syndrome.

Restriction of Motion, Difficulty in Walking

The patient may complain of restricted motion due to pain, stiffness, or deformity caused by the underlying disease. Elderly patients suffering from chronic cervical spondylosis/disc disease may complain of imbalance while walking, clumsiness in the hands, and wasting of intrinsic hand muscles due to underlying cervical myelopathy.

Deformity

Deformity of the spine is a common presentation in *congenital* (torticollis and scoliosis), *idiopathic* (Scheuermann's disease, scoliosis), *post-traumatic, infective* (TB), *inflammatory* (AS), or *metabolic* (osteoporosis) disorders of the spine. Scheuermann's disease is seen in adolescence with gradually increasing thoracic kyphosis.

Swelling

Swelling over the spine and paraspinal (PS) region may be one of the presenting symptoms. Typically, it could be congenital (spina bifida aperta) or acquired (cold abscess). A cold abscess can track along neurovascular/muscular planes distal to the abscess and the clinician should be mindful of every single one of the said probability. Multiple swelling elsewhere in the body could indicate neurofibromatosis, which is often associated with scoliosis.

Dizziness

Dizziness or occasional blackouts are noted in cervical spondylosis due to osteophytes encroaching the vertebral artery foramen resulting in vertebrobasilar insufficiency.

Constitutional Symptoms

One must always ask for constitutional symptoms, such as history of fever, weight loss, and loss of appetite. It could be present in infection (TB, pyogenic) or tumors.

Red Flags of the Spine

One must always ask for symptoms such as severe unrelenting pain for weeks–months, night or rest pain, neurological deficits (sensorimotor deficit, bladder and bowel involvement, and sexual dysfunction) with/without recent worsening, increasing deformity, ongoing treatment for any infective or malignant condition, or any constitutional symptoms such as fever, weight loss, or loss of appetite. These red-flag symptoms may suggest an underlying infection, tumor, or an inflammatory disease process, therefore, require urgent attention.

Other Conditions

- Pregnancy, genitourinary, or gynecological pathologies (pelvic inflammatory diseases) could result in back pain or mimic back pain without any organic pathology in the spine.
- Prostate symptoms must be asked in men as prostate malignancy can metastasize to the spine and give rise to back pain with/without neurological deficit.

Occupational History

Desk-bound professionals, heavy manual laborers, heavy-weight lifters, or drivers are more prone to low back pain.

Past History

Similar complaints in the past must be probed, as remissions and exacerbations are common in IVDP, spondylosis, or other degenerative conditions. Any history of TB (of any region) is essential if there is current suspicion of Pott's spine.

Personal History

History regarding sleep, appetite, smoking, and alcohol intake must be noted.

Treatment History

The treatment history should be asked in detail, e.g., any prolonged drug intake in TB gives a diagnostic clue; a long-term steroid intake could result in osteoporosis.

TABLE 10.4: Clinical diagnostic snippets of the spine.

Symptoms and/signs	Most likely pathology/diagnosis
A 48-year-old man presents with chronic neck pain, which aggravates on activity (working on the computer, long hours in the office, watching TV or mobile) with radiation to the trapezius, scapula, or over the shoulder	*Cervical spondylosis, Cervical IVDP*
A 28-year-old male presented with progressive stiffness and low back pain. The back stiffness is worse in the morning, after prolonged sitting and improves after activity	*Ankylosing spondylitis or a seronegative spondyloarthropathy*
An older woman complained of generalized back pain, which exacerbates with activity and relieves on rest. Relatives also told the clinician that her posture had been progressively stooping. The clinician also noticed that there is an exaggeration of her entire dorsal spine kyphosis	*Osteoporotic vertebral body fractures, senile kyphosis.* If there are systemic features (loss of appetite and weight, anemia), keep multiple myeloma in mind!
A middle-aged male with aching pain in the back and stiffness of the spine associated with evening rise of temperature, weight loss, and history of pulmonary Koch's in the past	*Tuberculosis of the spine*
A 60-year-old man complained that he has been experiencing bilateral lower limb pain (right>left), tingling, numbness, and paraesthesia while walking for several months. Progressively over the last few months, his 'walking distance' has decreased. The lower limb pain aggravates when he walks down the ramp/stairs and is relieved with forward bending of the spine and sitting for few minutes. It is also associated with off and on chronic mechanical lower backache, which aggravates on activity and relieves at rest	*Lumbar spinal canal stenosis* Note: Always rule out vascular causes of claudication such as thromboangiitis obliterans
A 35-year-old man presents with intermittent lower back pain associated with pain radiating to the right lower limb and paresthesia and weakness for 6 weeks. Low back pain was sudden in onset while lifting weights in the gym, and the pain is worse while sitting, bending forward, coughing, and sneezing	*Prolapsed lumbar intervertebral disc with nerve root compression*

Family History

Patients with AS or other seronegative spondyloarthropathies might have a positive family history. Patients with suspected tuberculosis can have a history of contact in family or neighborhood.

Menstrual History

Post-menopausal women are prone to osteoporosis, which can cause back pain and osteoporotic fractures.

At the end of history assessment, many common clinical conditions of spine can be reasonably well diagnosed based upon a combination of age and key complaints. **Table 10.4** summarizes the important snippets for the clinical diagnosis of common spine pathologies. However, all of them require confirmation with the examination.

EXAMINATION

General and Systemic Examination

The general and systemic examination must be performed in the standard fashion. Several examples of how a general examination could give a clue about the current diagnosis are mentioned here:

- Congenital scoliosis could be associated with neurofibromatosis and café-au-lait spots, which need to be looked for during the general examination. Infective (tuberculosis) or tumors (secondaries, multiple myeloma) of spine can have constitutional features such as fever, pallor, or cachexia. Eye may have signs of iridocyclitis in patients with seronegative spondyloarthropathy.

Local Examination

Gait

If a person is ambulant, gait should be assessed before examining the spine.

> **Note:** Assessment of gait and examination of the patient in standing/sitting position should be avoided in patients with suspicion of an impending neurological deficit or an unstable spine (loading of the spine under physiological load might deteriorate the current neurological or structural status).

Attitude

The attitude can be commented upon while the patient is examined in supine.

Inspection

After appropriate consent, privacy, and chaperone, the spine examination should be performed. The patient is stripped, except for undergarments exposing the spine, upper, and lower limbs.

The clinician must inspect the patient from the front, side, and back. A hard bed should be used while examining the patient in supine position.

During the inspection of the spine—observe *alignment in the spine (front, side, behind), level of the shoulder and pelvis, neck and scapula, paraspinal spasm, skin over the back and elsewhere, swelling, deformities in the upper and lower limb, limb length, and scar-sinus.*

1. **Alignment of the spine:** The assessment of the spine alignment should start with the inspection of the head, neck, shoulder, pelvis, and natal cleft and should be done from the front, side, and back.

   a. *Alignment from the front and other findings:*
   Typically, the *head and neck* are aligned to the chest and lower spine. However, in torticollis, the neck is tilted to one side, with the chin rotated to the opposite side **(Fig. 10.5)**.

   b. *Alignment from the side and other findings:*
   - Ask the patient to stand upright and look for *natural lordosis of the cervical and lumbar spine and thoracic kyphosis.* Observe any deviation (exaggeration or attenuation) from the standard curves in cervical, thoracic and lumbar regions.
   - Thoracic kyphosis is exaggerated in many conditions (Osteoporosis, TB). The kyphosis could be localized (knuckle/angular) or *generalized* (round-back deformity) **(Box 10.3 and Fig. 10.6)**. *Note that a fixed/structural kyphosis is also known as gibbus.*

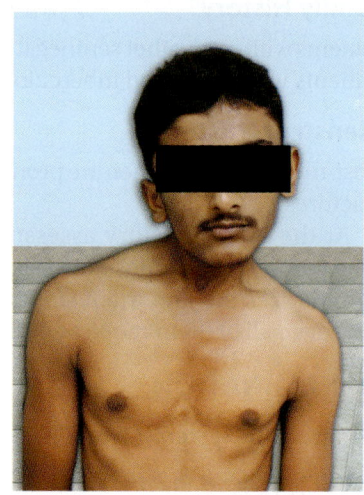

Fig. 10.5: Torticollis of right side.

> **BOX 10.3:** Nomenclature of kyphotic deformities of dorsal spine and its etiology.
> - *Collapse of a **single** vertebra*—"knuckle" deformity
> - *Collapse of **two to three** vertebrae*—"angular" deformity **(Fig. 10.6A)**
> - *Collapse of **four or more** vertebrae*—"round-back" deformity **(Fig. 10.6B)**. The round-back deformity is also known as Dowager's hump. 1–3 vertebral collapses are common in infections, trauma, and localized tumor, whereas round-back deformity (≥4 vertebral collapses) is observed in ankylosing spondylitis, Scheuermann's disease, multiple vertebral collapse due to osteoporosis/ secondaries and Paget's disease

- *Observe for exaggerated or attenuated lumbar lordosis:* Exaggerated lumbar lordosis is primarily compensatory, which is present in flexion deformity of the hip whereas attenuated (loss) lumbar lordosis is observed in surgical fusion of spine and ankylosing spondylitis.
c. **Alignment from behind:** Typically, both shoulders and pelvis are at the same level in a normal person, while the *head, neck, spine, and natal cleft are in one straight line* and the linear alignment of the head-spine-natal cleft is confirmed by drawing an imaginary plumb line from occiput to natal cleft **(Fig. 10.7A)**. Coronal malalignment results in scoliosis, which is defined as lateral bending and rotation of the spine **(Fig. 10.7B)**. Scoliosis is either *structural or functional*.

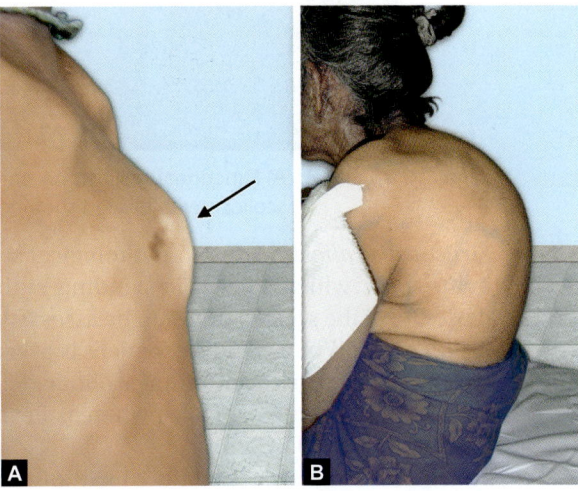

Figs. 10.6A and B: (A) Angular kyphosis; (B) Round-back kyphosis.

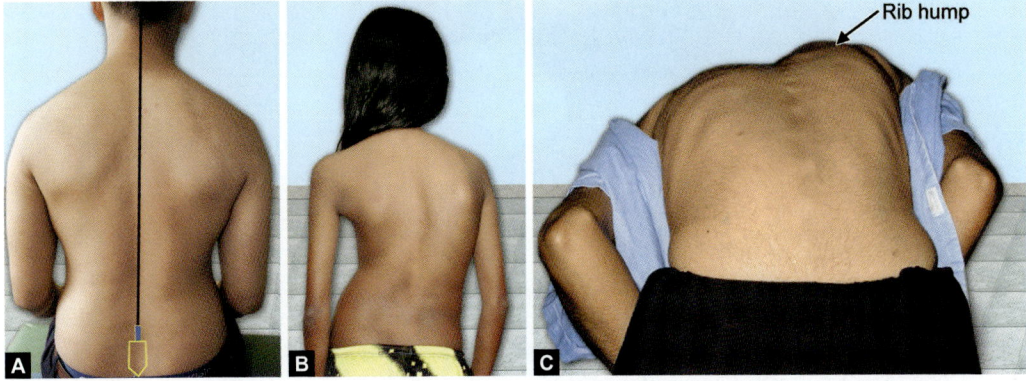

Figs. 10.7A to C: (A) Plumb line in a coronally normally aligned spine; (B) Scoliosis of dorsolumbar spine; (C) Adam's forward bending test showing persistent structural scoliosis with rib hump.

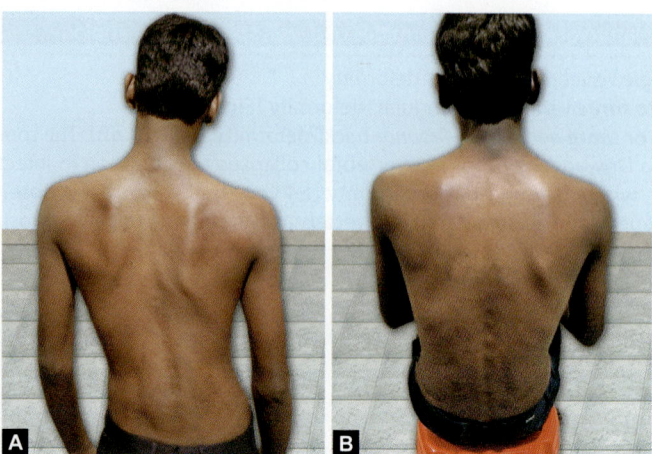

Figs. 10.8A and B: (A) Functional scoliosis on standing; (B) Obliteration of functional scoliosis with leveled shoulder, while sitting.

- *Structural scoliosis* is due to pathological structural changes (congenital/acquired) in the spine, which persists in standing, sitting, bending forward, or lying down. The flexibility of the spinal curve can be assessed by Adam's test:
- *Adam's test:* While standing, patient is asked to bend forward and attempt to touch toes by finger. A rigid structural scoliotic deformity persists on bending forward and a rib hump becomes obvious, whereas flexible structural scoliotic deformity might attenuate **(Fig. 10.7C)**.
- *Functional scoliosis* is functional without any structural changes in the spine. It is present in standing, whereas it disappears on sitting or bending forward **(Figs. 10.8A and B)**. Commonly, functional scoliosis is due to limb length discrepancy (LLD) or acute paraspinal (PS) muscle spasms.

2. **Neck and scapula:** Look for webbing of the neck and levels of two scapulae. Short-webbed neck is observed in Klippel–Feil syndrome **(Fig. 10.9A)**. The scapular levels are assessed by

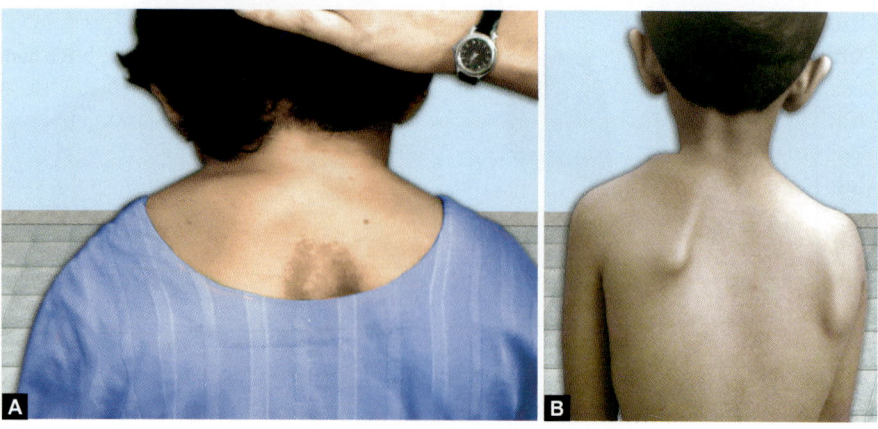

Figs. 10.9A and B: (A) Short, webbed neck in Klippel–Feil syndrome; (B) High riding scapula (left) in Sprengel shoulder.

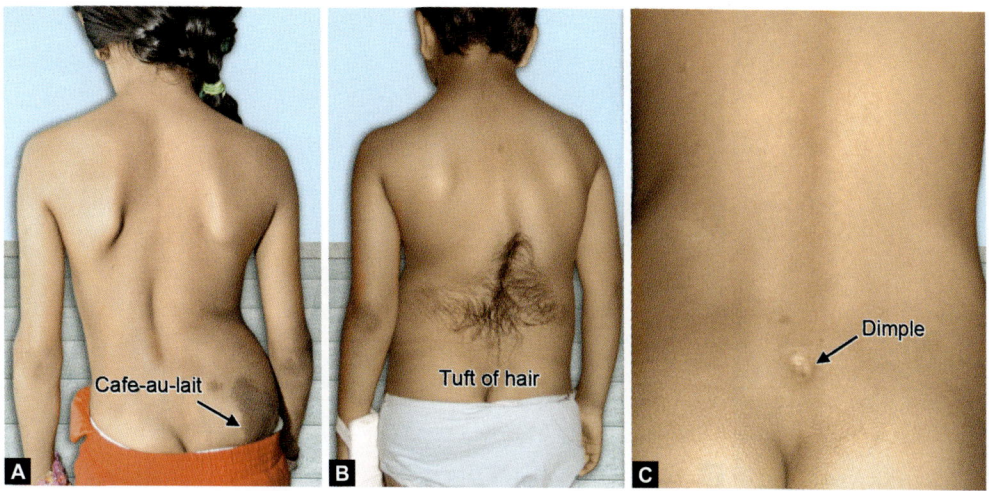

Figs. 10.10A to C: (A) Cafe-au-lait spots; (B) Tuft of hair over lumbar spine; (C) Dimple over the lumbosacral junction.

observing the levels of superior and inferior angles of the two scapulae. High-riding scapula is present in the Sprengel shoulder **(Fig. 10.9B)**.
3. **Paraspinal spasm:** One must note any paraspinal (PS) spasm indicated by a deepened midline furrow.
4. **The skin of the back and elsewhere:** Various cutaneous markers on the skin, such as *café-au-lait spots, axillary freckling, tuft of hair, dimple*, or *hemangioma* could provide a clue to an underlying diagnosis **(Figs. 10.10A to C)**. Café-au-lait spots are present in neurofibromatosis associated with scoliosis, whereas tuft of hair, dimple, or hemangioma is associated with spina bifida occulta.

> **Note:** CAFÉ-AU-LAIT SPOTS are considered significant only if they are more than 5 in number with each spot measuring 10–15 mm in size.

5. **Swelling:** Swelling in spine could present as *cold abscess*, which is observed in TB spine. Cold abscess could be present in the neck triangles, supra- or infraclavicular fossa, axilla, intercostal spaces, paraspinal region, abdomen, inguinal region, as well as Petit triangle depending upon the level of Pott's spine **(Fig. 10.11A)**. Swelling is also observed in *spina bifida aperta as* meningocele and meningomyelocele **(Fig. 10.11B)**.
6. **The deformity and muscle wasting in the upper and lower limb:** Any ipsilateral/bilateral wasting and deformity of upper limbs could be secondary to cervical spinal cord/roots involvement, especially cervical myelopathy.
7. Presence of any **scar, sinus, bedsore** should be described in standard fashion.

Palpation

One must palpate the spine to assess *local temperature, tenderness, alignment, step between two spinous process, PS spasm, deformity, swelling, important bony and soft tissue landmarks*, and other palpatory characteristics of swelling, scars, and sinuses.
1. **The local rise in temperature:** It should be checked all over the spine and PS regions.

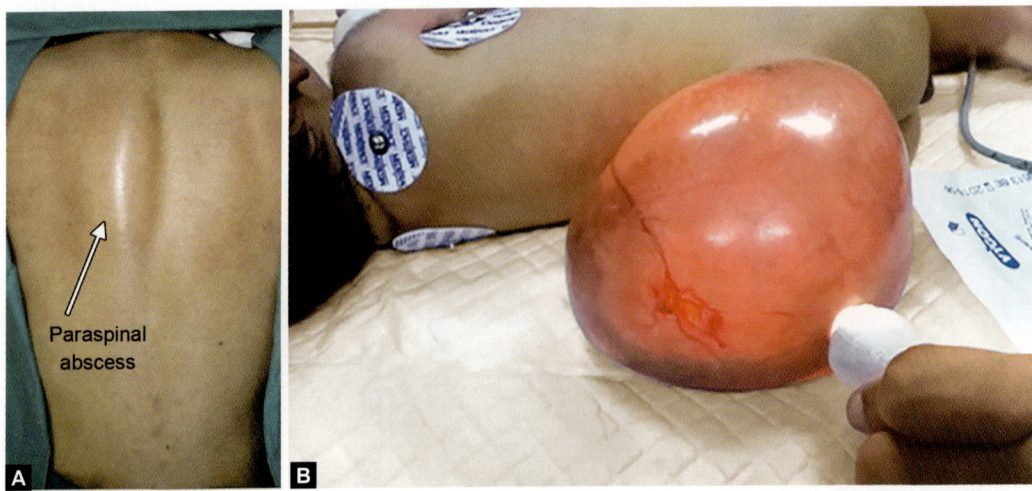

Figs. 10.11A and B: (A) Paraspinal abscess; (B) Meningocele over the lumbosacral spine (torch showing trans-illumination).

2. **Spine alignment and tenderness:** It should be elicited sequentially over the entire spine from the cervical to the sacral region **(Fig. 10.12A)**. The clinician should run his thumb from cervical to sacral spine and feel the *'linearity' of the spinous processes.* Any coronal alteration from this linearity may indicate underlying scoliosis. Any tenderness over the spinous process may help in localizing the level or site of the lesion **(Fig. 10.12A)**. The level of the vertebra is confirmed based upon specific bony landmarks **(Fig. 10.12B)**.
3. **Palpate step-off between two spinous processes:** While running the thumb from cervical to sacral region, the clinician must feel for any step between the two spinous processes, which is commonly observed in the spondylolisthesis or traumatic dislocations.
4. **Paraspinal spasm:** Paraspinal (PS) spasm is common in acute back pain, infections, and trauma. PS spasm is assessed by palpating PS muscle with pulp of the thumb or fingers **(Figs. 10.12C and D)**. Typically, PS muscles are soft on palpation but feel firm if there is a PS spasm.
5. **Palpatory characteristics of swelling, scars, and sinuses:** It should be done in standard fashion.

Movement of Various Regions of Spine: Cervical, Dorsal, and Lumbar

The methodology of ROM assessment at various regions of the spine is discussed below.

Cervical Spine Movement

The movement in the cervical spine occurs in *all three planes: flexion-extension, lateral flexion, and rotations.* The degree of movements are assessed with respect to vertical axis. Apart from movements, Occiput-wall distance assessment helps flexibility of spine in extension.
- **Extension:** 0–50°. Ask the patient to look towards the roof **(Fig. 10.13A)**.
- **Flexion:** 0–80°. Ask the patient to touch the chin on the chest without bending the dorsal spine **(Fig. 10.13B)**. Chin-manubrium distance can be measured for documentation purposes.

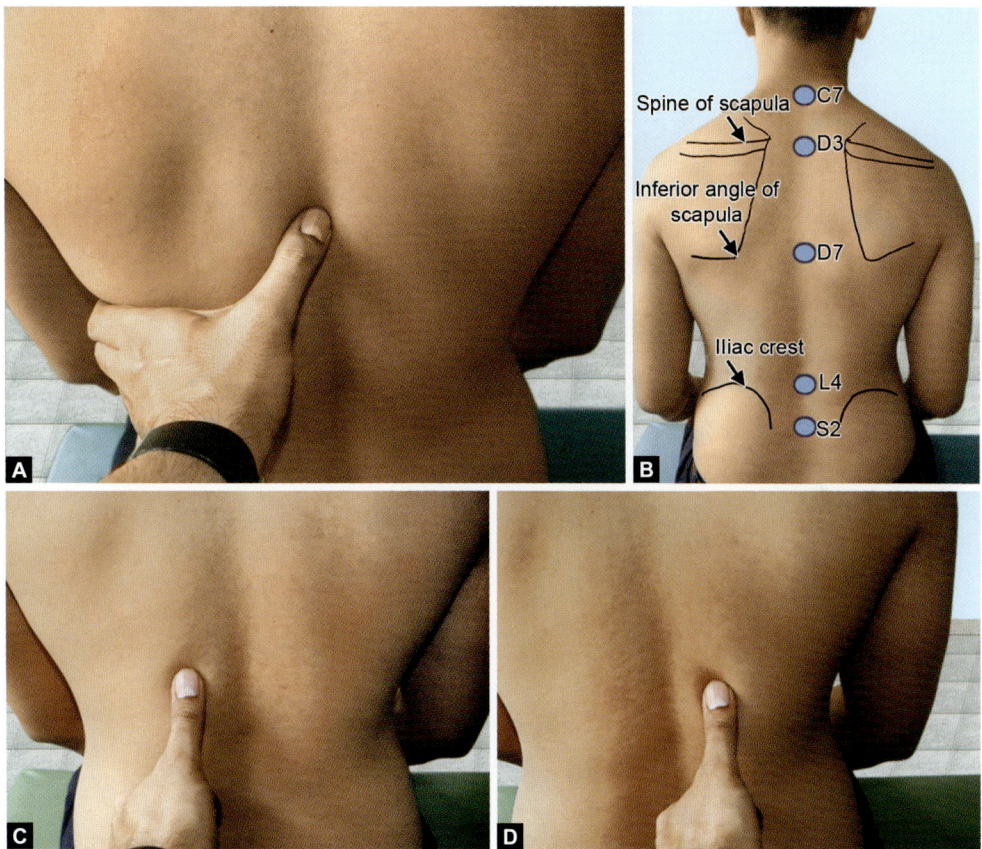

Figs. 10.12A to D: (A) Direct palpation of the spinous process; (B) Bony landmarks corresponding to the respective vertebral levels; C7 spinous process is the most prominent spinous process of the cervical spine, D3 vertebra spinous process at the level of spine of the scapula, D7 spinous process at the level of the inferior angle of the scapula, L4 vertebra spinous process at the level of the iliac crest, and S2 vertebra at the level of the PSIS dimple; (C and D) Assessment of the paraspinal spasm by placing thumb pulp of over the paraspinal muscles.

- **Lateral flexion:** 0–45° to either side. Ask the patient to tilt the head laterally and attempt to touch the shoulder with their ear without shrugging the shoulder **(Fig. 10.13C)**.
- **Rotation:** 0–80° to either side. Ask the patient to look on either side without turning the trunk **(Fig. 10.13D)**

Occiput-wall distance test (Flesche test): This method is typically used in measuring decreased "overall" spinal extension in AS, especially cervical spine extension.

Typically, when a normal person stands erect against a wall with heels, buttocks, back, and shoulder touching the wall, the occiput must touch the wall **(Fig. 10.14A)**. However, in patients with advanced AS wherein the upper dorsal and cervical spine are stiff, the occiput fails to touch the wall indicating loss of extension in the cervicodorsal spine **(Fig. 10.14B)**.

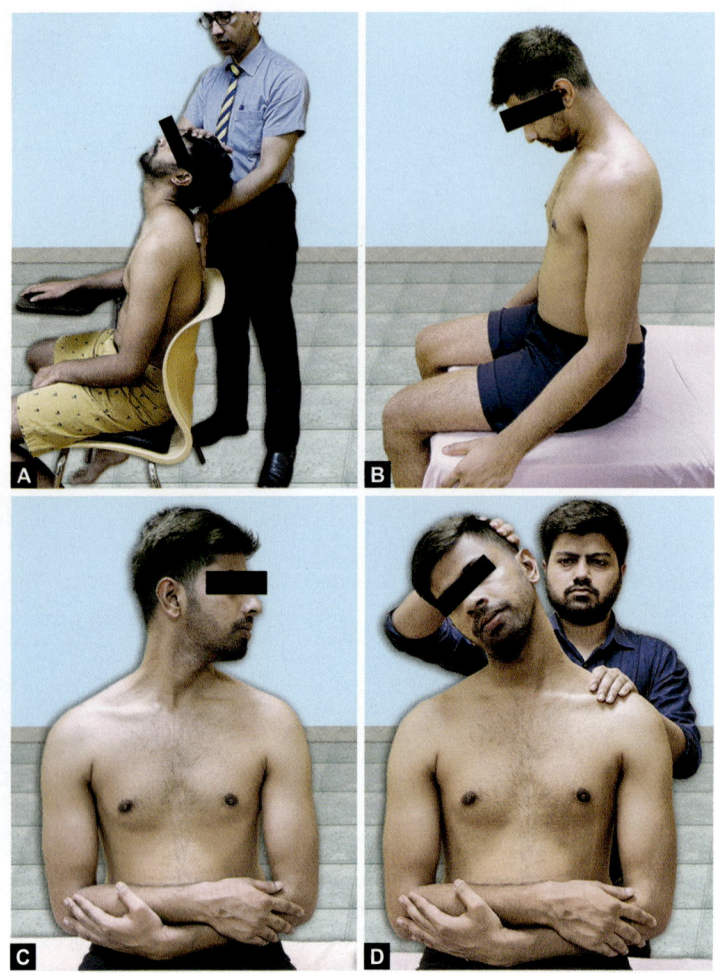

Figs. 10.13A to D: Assessment of cervical spine movements. (A) Cervical spine extension; (B) Cervical spine flexion; (C) Cervical spine lateral rotation (without rotating the trunk); (D) Cervical spine right lateral flexion.

Dorsal Spine Movement

The predominant movement in the dorsal spine is *lateral rotation* (0–50°).
Method: It is essential to note that dorsal–spine rotation assessment should be avoided while the patient is standing as there will be a 'rotational' contribution from the pelvis-hip complex resulting in an exaggerated assessment of dorsal–spine rotations. Therefore, to avoid such a fallacy, it is crucial to block movements from the pelvis-hip complex by asking the patient to sit on the couch or stool chair, which fixes the pelvis-hip complex. Now, the patient keeps their hands on the opposite shoulder by crossing the chest. Then, patient is asked to the trunk on either side, one by one **(Figs. 10.15A and B)**, and measure the angle between the static pelvis and mobile shoulder.

Lumbar Spine Movement

Typically, forward *flexion (0–60°)*, extension *(0–25°)*, and lateral flexion *(0–30°)* are assessed in the lumbar spine. The method to assess various ROMs is discussed below.

- **Lumbar spine flexion:** It is assessed by forward bending and modified Schober's method.
    - *Forward bending method:* Ask the patient to bend forward and try touching the toes/floor *"without bending the knee"* **(Fig. 10.16A)**. The patient's lumbar spine flexion movements must be noted as the ability to touch the ground or "how many cm away from the ground."
    - *Modified Schober's method to assess lumbar spine flexibility:* Flexion of the lumbar spine can also be measured by modified Schober's method. *Typically, this method is used in patients with AS to assess restriction in lumbar spine mobility.*

    Method: In an erect patient, three points are marked over the midline of the spine, a total of 15 cm apart. The first mark is over the midline at the level of the dimple of the PSIS, the second mark is 10 cm above the PSIS, and the third one is 5 cm below the PSIS mark **(Fig. 10.16B)**. Now, ask the patient to bend forward as much as possible and measure the distance between the highest and lowest mark **(Fig. 10.16C)**.
    Interpretation: In a normal person, the average distance between the highest and lowest mark during forward flexion should increase by 6–9 cm. *A <5 cm increase in the distance between the highest and lowest mark indicates decreased lumbar spine flexion.*

- **Lumbar spine extension:**
    Method: While the patient stands erect, the clinician stabilizes the pelvis with one hand (to avoid posterior pelvis tilt), and the other hand is kept over the shoulder. Now, the patient is

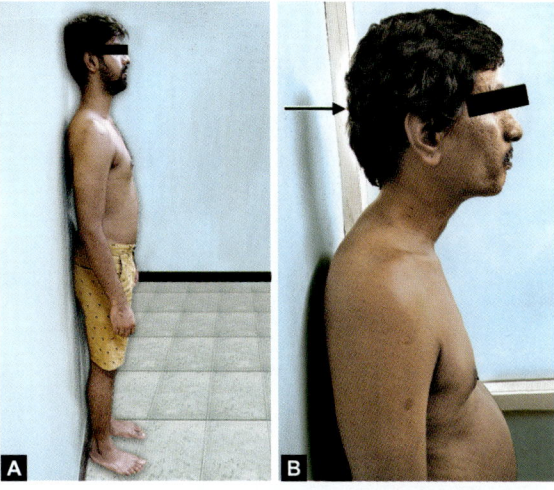

Figs. 10.14A and B: (A) Typically, head, dorsal spine, buttock, and heel touch the wall; (B) Increased occiput wall distance (black arrow) is observed in an AS patient.

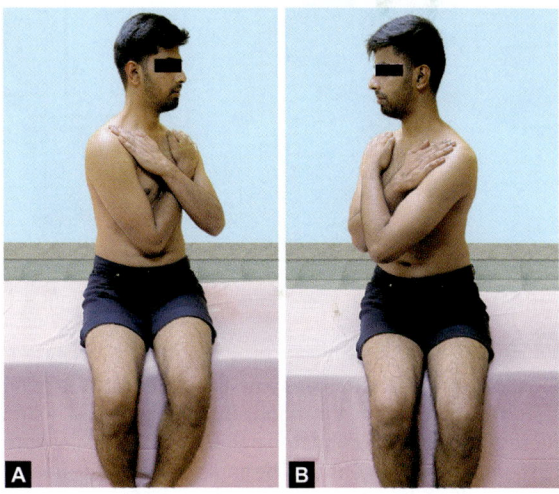

Figs. 10.15A and B: (A) Left lateral rotation of dorsal spine; (B) Right lateral rotation of the dorsal spine.
Note: Pelvis is fixed while the patient is sitting on the couch.

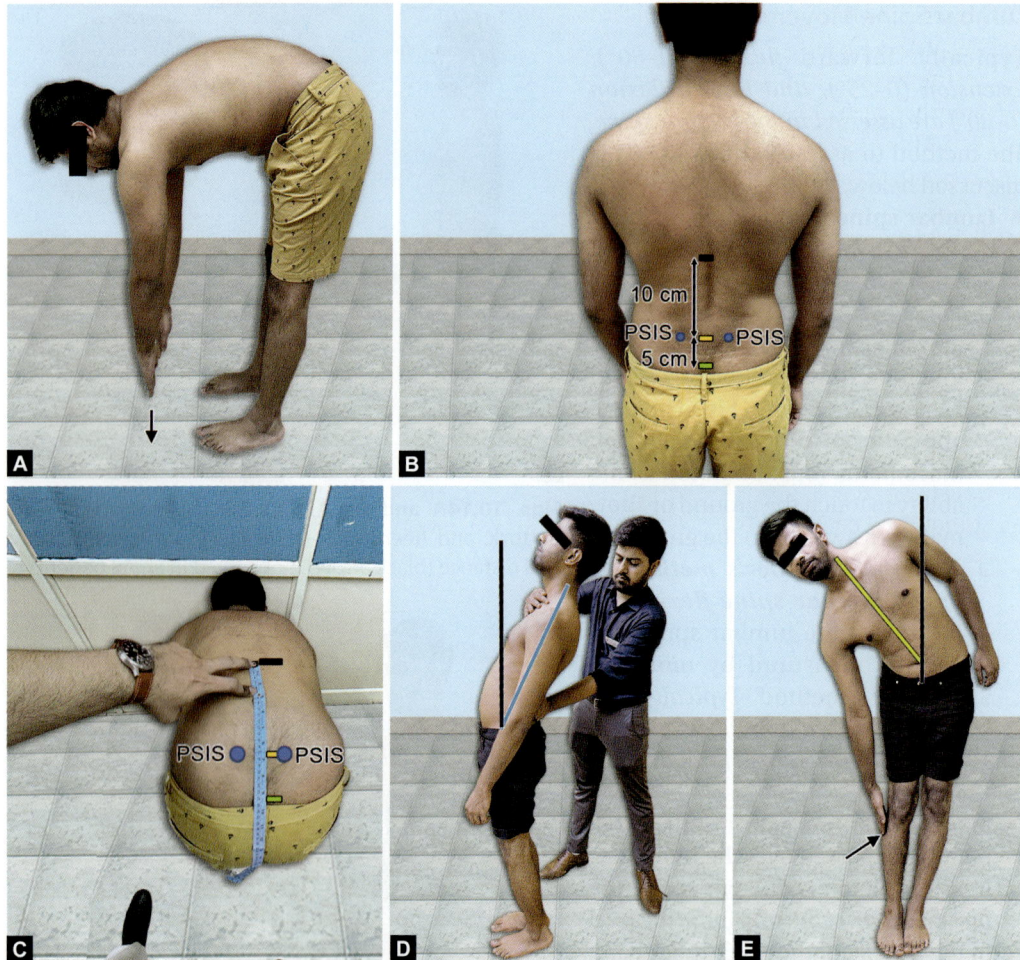

Figs. 10.16A to E: Lumbar spine movement assessment. (A) Lumbar spine forward flexion (black arrow shows distance from the floor); (B) Schober's test—standing erect with black, yellow, and green lines representing three designated points and blue circle represents PSIS; (C) Schober's test—forward bending; (D) Lumbar spine extension. The angle between the imaginary vertical black line and blue lumbar spine line indicates the extension measure; (E) Lateral flexion of the lumbar spine. The angle between the yellow line representing the dorsolumbar spine and midline black vertical line is a measure of lateral flexion. The black arrow indicates that finger can reach fibular head

(PSIS: posterior superior iliac spine).

asked to bend backward, and extension of the spine with respect to central vertical axis of the body is noted **(Fig. 10.16D)**. The average range of spine extension is 30°. The extension of the spine is decreased or not possible in AS.

- **Lateral flexion of the lumbar spine:**
  Method: The lateral flexion of the lumbar spine can be examined by asking the patient to bend on either side. The angle between the imaginary vertical midline axis and

the straight line joining T1 and S1 vertebra is measured as lateral flexion of the spine **(Fig. 10.16E)**.

The assessment of movement in the lumbar spine is quite helpful in diagnosing an underlying condition as specific movements are painful and restricted in certain diseases **(Box 10.4)**.

> **BOX 10.4:** Diagnostic clues with painful/limited movements of the lumbar spine.
>
> - *Painful forward flexion:* Noted in lumbar intervertebral disc prolapse
> - *Painful extension:* Noted *in lumbar canal stenosis, spondylolysis, spondylolisthesis, and* facet joint arthritis
> - *Painful rotation: Facet joint arthritis*
> - **Both flexion and extension of lumbar spine** are decreased in ankylosing spondylitis

Measurement

1. The linear measurement of the spine has less value in clinical diagnostics.
2. **Chest expansion:** The average chest expansion in an adult measured at the level of nipples is about 4–5 cm. Expansion <2.5 cm could be abnormal. It is decreased in AS.

Special Tests for Cervical Spine IVDP, Thoracic Outlet Syndrome, Lumbar Spine IVDP, and Sacroiliitis

Special Tests for Cervical IVDP or Spondylosis with Root Compression

1. **Spurling test:** It is performed when the patient complains of radicular pain in the upper limb due to nerve root compression ascribed to cervical IVDP/spondylosis.
   Method: The patient is asked to sit on a couch or chair. The clinician stands behind the patient, interlocks fingers of both hands, and keeps the volar aspect of his/her hand on the patient's head. Then, the clinician extends the neck completely, lateral flexes the neck to 30°, and gives mild downward axial pressure over the skull **(Fig. 10.17)**.

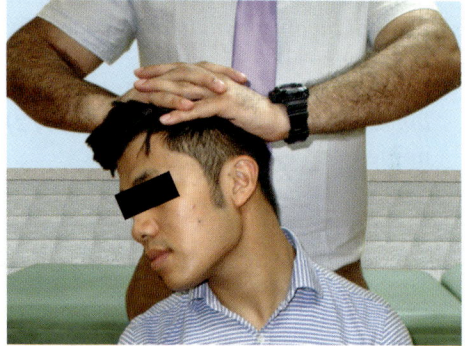

Fig. 10.17: Spurling test (neck in lateral flexion and extension).

   Interpretation: A radiating pain in the upper limb along the nerve root's dermatome during the maneuver indicates a positive Spurling test signifying root compression.

Special Tests for Thoracic Outlet Syndrome due to Cervical Rib or Scalenus Anterior/Medius Abnormality

> **Of note:** The ulnar side radicular pain pattern of TOS (medial arm, forearm and hand) due to pressure on C8, T1 trunk contrasts with the radial side radicular pain over the arm, forearm, thumb of cervical spine IVDP and cervical spondylosis, as the latter two primarily affect C5, C6, and C7 roots.

TOS can have vascular and neurological components. Various tests for TOS are *Adson's, and Roos tests, which assess vascular and neurological components of TOS.*

1. **Adson's test:** Provocative test for the *vascular component of TOS*.
   Method: The patient sits upright on a stool chair. The clinician holds the patient's wrist with one hand, gently *abducts the arm by 30°, extends, and externally rotates the shoulder* completely. The other hand of clinician holds the patient's neck and gently extends and rotates toward the affected side while asking the patient to take a deep breath and hold his breath. Now, the clinician palpates the radial pulse of the affected side **(Fig. 10.18A)**.
   Interpretation: If the pulse becomes feeble/disappears, Adson's test is considered to be positive. Always compare with the contralateral side.
2. **Roos test (elevated arm test):** Provocative test for the *neurological and vascular components of TOS*.
   Method: Patient is asked to sit on a stool chair and 90° abduct and externally rotate the shoulder with arm and forearms in the frontal plane of the body with the elbow flexed. Now, the patient is asked to repeatedly and slowly clench and open the fist for 3 minutes **(Fig. 10.18B)**. The appearance of neurological and vascular symptoms and the disappearance of the radial pulse are highly suggestive of TOS.

Special Tests for Lumbosacral Nerve Root Compression

Many clinical tests are described to assess lumbosacral nerve root compression, typically by a prolapsed IVD. For lower lumbar (L4, 5) and sacral (S1, 2) roots compression, straight leg raising test (SLRT), Lasegue, and well-leg raising tests are performed. For *higher lumbar root (L2, 3) compression, a* femoral nerve stretch test is performed.

If the pain radiates over the back of the thigh, leg, and foot, it indicates lower lumbar and sacral root involvement, whereas the pain over the front of the thigh suggests upper lumbar root involvement.

1. **Straight leg raising test:** It is performed to confirm the compression/irritation of the *lower lumbar (L4-5)* and *sacral (S1, 2)* nerve roots by placing tensile stresses at the sciatic nerve.

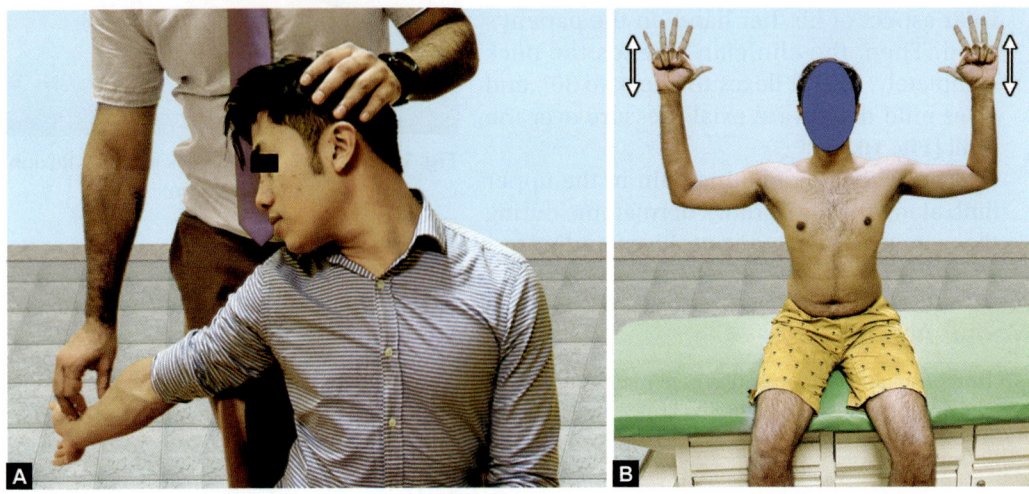

Figs. 10.18A and B: Tests for thoracic outlet syndrome. (A) Adson's test; (B) Roos test.

Prerequisite: There should be no fixed flexion deformity (FFD) at the knee, and the hip should be mobile.

Method: The patient lies supine on the couch without a pillow under his/her head. Ask the patient regarding the side (right or left) of the lower limb in which the pain is radiating, and start the SLRT from the normal lower limb, i.e., the limb with no radiation of the pain. In case of bilateral radiation of pain, the SLR test could be started from either side.

The clinician holds the distal tibia of the normal lower limb with one hand while keeping the other hand over the extended knee and gradually elevates the lower limb from the couch. While elevating the limb, the clinician watches the patient's face for discomfort due to radiating pain in the elevated limb. The clinician must stop elevating the limb when the patient complains of radiating pain in the limb and note the SLR angle between the couch and the elevated limb axis **(Fig. 10.19)**. A painful SLRT maneuver is called SLRT positive. Of note, *the clinician must confirm by asking the patient whether it is a pain that radiates up to the back of the thigh, leg, and foot or is it a mere tightness felt at the back of the thigh.*

Interpretation: In a normal person without any lower lumbar or sacral root compression, the limb can be easily elevated to 70–90°. In patients with positive SLRT, the limb cannot be raised >60°, and the patient would complain of radiating pain in the affected limb. *Note that the pain always radiates below the knee level in IVDP of the lumbar spine with compression of L4 root onwards.* In several patients with hamstring tightness, the patient reports no pain but mere tightness at the back of the thigh.

2. **Lasegue's or Bragard's test:** It is performed to confirm the lower lumbar (L4 onward) nerve root irritation/compression.

   Method: During SLRT, the clinician stops the limb elevation when the patient start experiencing pain radiating to the lower limb, followed by gradually lowering the limb until the radiating pain reduces completely. Next, the ankle is gently dorsiflexed. If dorsiflexion of the ankle reproduces pain along the posterior thigh, leg, or foot, the Lasegue's test is considered positive **(Fig. 10.20)**.

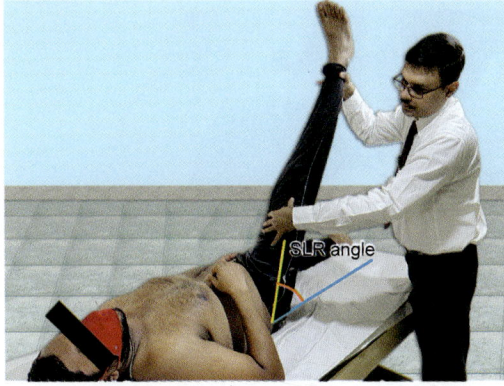

Fig. 10.19: Straight leg raising test.

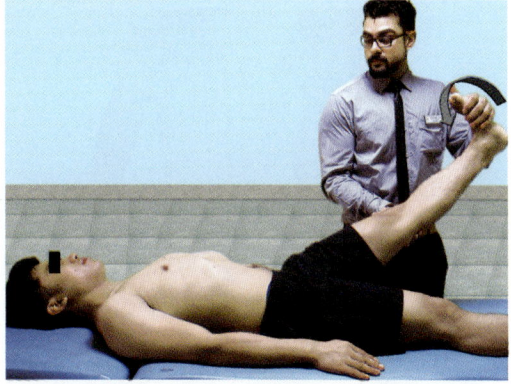

Fig. 10.20: Lasegue test (Gray curved arrow indicates ankle dorsiflexion).

3. **Well-leg raising test/crossed SLRT:** It has the highest specificity for IVDP (axillary type/medial disc prolapse) compared to SLRT, and Lasegue test.
   Method: It is similar to SLRT, but this test is characterized by elevation of "only normal limb." If the patient complains of radiating pain in the non-elevated/index limb while the normal leg is elevated, the well-leg test is positive. *A positive well-leg raising test is pathognomonic of lumbar IVDP.*
4. **Femoral nerve stretch/reverse Lasegue test:** It is performed for higher (L2, 3, and 4) lumbar nerve root irritation or compression (forming femoral nerve) where the patient complains of radiating pain in front of the thigh along with back pain.
   The front of the thigh radiating pain indicates L2–4 involvement.
   Method: The patient is made to lie prone on the couch. The clinician holds the ankle with one hand, flexes the knee, and starts gradually extending the hip while the other hand stabilizes the pelvis **(Fig. 10.21)**.
   Interpretation: A positive femoral nerve stretch test is indicated by tingling/pain in front of the thigh (femoral nerve distribution area).

Special Tests for Sacroiliac Joint

Sacroiliac (SI) joint involvement is frequent in seronegative spondyloarthropathy (ankylosing spondylitis) and infective conditions such as TB. *Figure-of-four and Gaenslen's tests* are performed to assess sacroiliac joint (SIJ). Direct palpatory tenderness over SIJ is also an important sign of SIJ involvement.

1. **Figure-of-four test:**
   Method: While the patient lies supine on the couch, the patient's knee is flexed to 90°, the hip is externally rotated, and the leg-ankle junction is placed over the lower end of the opposite thigh just above the knee. Subsequently, the clinician pushes the flexed knee downward with one hand, and another hand stabilizes the pelvis by keeping the hand over the opposite anterior–superior iliac spine (ASIS) **(Fig. 10.22)**.
   Interpretation: Pain over the ipsilateral SIJ during the maneuver is considered to be a positive figure-of-four test. A similar maneuver is repeated for the other side of the SIJ.

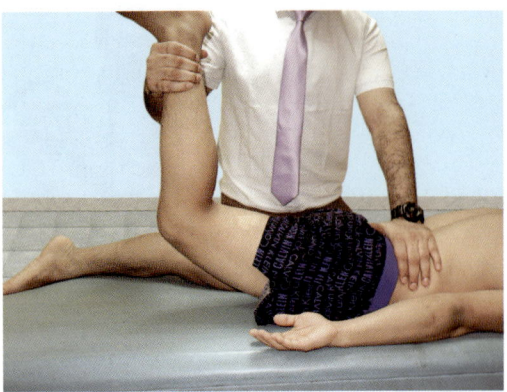

Fig. 10.21: Femoral nerve stretch test.

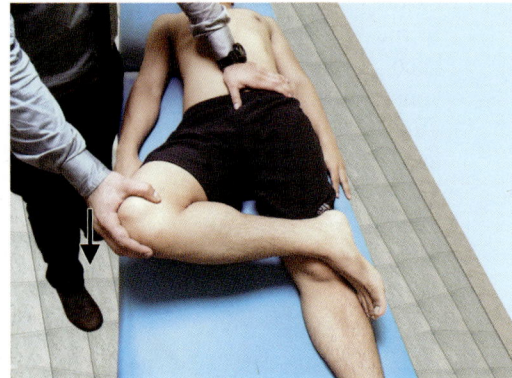

Fig. 10.22: Figure-of-four test. Black arrow indicates downward pressure over the knee.

2. **Gaenslen's test:**
   Method: The patient lies supine over the couch. One of the hips and knees are hyperflexed and the other hip is extended over the edge of the couch simultaneously **(Fig. 10.23)**. If this maneuver causes pain over SIJ on the flexed hip-knee side, the test is considered to be positive.

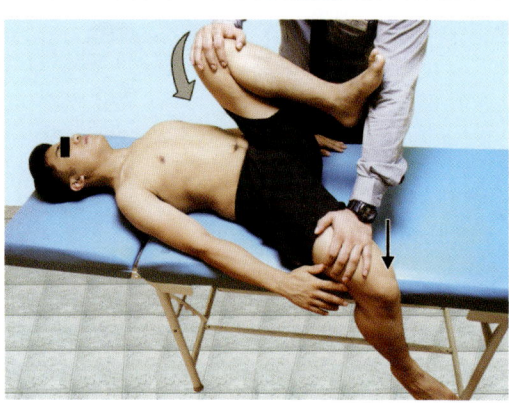

Fig. 10.23: Gaenslen's test. Black arrow indicates downward pressure on the thigh (for hip extension) and curved gray arrow indicates hyperflexion of the opposite hip.

Neurological Examination

Although spinal column/spinal cord pathology do not involve brain and cranial nerves, the neurological examination should be thorough, involving a quick assessment of the central nervous system. Nevertheless, this chapter does not intend to discuss a detailed and in-depth brain and cranial nerve examination.

A routine neurological evaluation of spinal cord injury must involve assessing *higher mental function, cranial nerves, gait, sensory-motor status, reflexes (superficial and deep), abnormal reflexes, bladder-bowel status, and skin condition.*

1. **Higher mental function:** A quick assessment of consciousness, alertness, orientation to time-place-person, memory, and speech gives valuable information about the overall health of the nervous system (brain).
2. **Cranial nerves:** Generally, cranial nerves are not involved in the spine or spinal cord pathology. However, a quick assessment of all (12) cranial nerves should be part of the neurological evaluation.
3. **Sensory examination:** *The principal objective of the sensory examination is to ascertain the "level of the lesion."* However, it is important to note that the principles of sensory examination are different in patients with "spinal cord and/or root level pathology" versus "peripheral nerve affection", as discussed below.
   i. In patients with spinal cord or nerve root involvement, the sensory assessment is according to the "dermatomal distribution of a nerve root" **(Fig. 10.24)**. In contrast, sensory assessment in a peripheral nerve affection is performed *"typically in the autonomous zone of a peripheral nerve".* For example, a patient with brachial plexus root level injury requires sequential assessment of sensation in all dermatomes from C5 to 8 and T1, whereas sensory assessment in the first dorsal webspace is sufficient in the radial nerve (C5–8, T1) injury.
   ii. In patients with spinal cord lesions, assessing at least one sensation from three important sensory tracts of the spinal cord (posterior column, anterior, and lateral spinothalamic tract) is essential. In contrast, quick assessment of a single sensation such as crude touch usually suffices in a peripheral nerve lesion.

A **dermatome** is an area of skin that is supplied by a single spinal nerve.

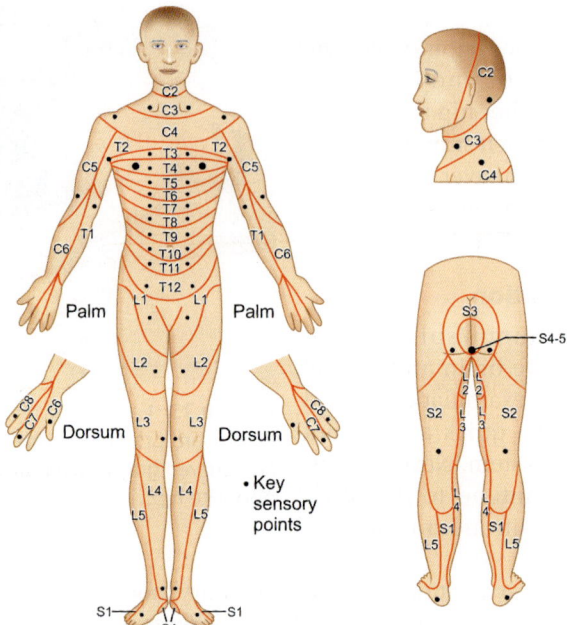

Fig. 10.24: Dermatomes of the body. Note that there is no C1 dermatome in the body.

The steps or methodology of sensory assessment are mentioned in **Box 10.5**, whereas the sensations tested in a patient with spinal cord affection are mentioned in **Table 10.5**.

BOX 10.5: Methodology of sensory examination in a spinal cord/nerve root affection.

- The clinician should explain the procedure and steps of sensory examination to the patient and ensure adequate privacy during the examination
- It is mandatory that the part to be tested should be exposed entirely (without any clothing) with adequate coverage of the private parts. *Note that the sensory examination should not be performed over the clothes*
- One should always compare the sensation of the affected part with the normal/contralateral side
- Once the steps and procedure of sensory examination are explained, the patient must keep his eyes closed during the sensory assessment
- The sensations must be tested dermatome-wise in the spinal cord or nerve root affection (cf. sensory assessment in autonomous zone is enough in peripheral nerve affection)
- While testing the touch, a constant stimulus is given simultaneously over the "same dermatome" bilaterally or over normal and affected parts of the body, and the patient is asked to differentiate between sensory perception over the normal and abnormal parts. Further probing may help in assessing whether there is hypoesthesia/anesthesia/hyperesthesia
- In case of doubt regarding the sensory perception findings, repeat the entire process of sensation testing after re-explaining the procedure to the patient
- In between, no sensory stimulus is given, and the patient is asked for sensory perception to check a malingerer

TABLE 10.5: Sensations carried by various spinal cord sensory tracts and their assessment.

Sensory tract	Sensations	How to test?
Anterior spinothalamic	• Crude/light touch • Pressure	• A light touch is tested with a wisp of cotton or a brush • Test pressure by applying firm pressure with a fingertip or blunt end of a pencil
Lateral spinothalamic	Pain	It is tested with a pin (not a hypodermic needle). Take care not to perforate/breach the skin
	Temperature	It is tested with test tubes containing cold and hot water
Posterior column	Fine touch	It can be tested using nylon monofilament (Semmes–Weinstein monofilament or von Frey hair) of variable diameter. The monofilament is placed perpendicularly over the skin for one second till it buckles, and ask the patient whether he/she felt it or not. If no response, use the next thicker diameter wire
	Stereognosis	Pick an common object (coin/key), place it in the patient's hand with eyes closed, and ask the patient to identify the object
	Proprioception and joint position sense	Move a joint through a small range of motion, and hold in a static position. Now, ask the patient to describe the 'held' position, or mimic the position on the other side
	Vibration	Tested with 128 Hz tuning fork over bony prominences such as malleoli, radial, and ulnar styloid process
	Two-point discrimination	It determines the ability to perceive two points applied to the skin simultaneously. It is tested with two points of blunt divider or compass esthesiometer, wherein two points of esthesiometer are applied to the skin simultaneously with the tip spread apart. The two tips are gradually brought closer together with each successive application until the stimuli are perceived as one. The smallest distance between the stimuli that is still perceived as two distinct points is measured
	Graphesthesia	The ability of the patient to identify a letter/number or design drawn on the body

4. **Motor examination:** The motor examination involves assessing the *bulk of the muscle, tone, power, coordination, and involuntary movements.*
   i. **Bulk:** The bulk or nutrition of the muscles may be reduced if there is muscle disuse after spinal cord/root affection. It can be assessed during the inspection and measured with tape.
   ii. **Tone:** Muscle tone is defined as 'the tension in the relaxed muscle' or 'the resistance felt by the clinician during repetitive passive movement of a joint when the muscles are at rest. Muscle tone (hypo- or hypertonia) alters after spinal cord or pan-plexus injuries.

Hypotonia is characteristic of lower motor neuron (LMN) lesions, whereas hypertonia (spasticity/rigidity) is present in upper motor neuron (UMN) lesions. To assess muscle tone, hold proximal and distal parts of the extremity and gently move a joint several times to feel the resistance offered to the passive movement. **Table 10.6** enumerates the differences between UMN and LMN lesions.

TABLE 10.6: Differences between an upper motor neuron (UMN) and lower motor neuron (LMN) lesion.

Characteristics	UMN	LMN
Wasting of muscle	Less	Pronounced
Tone	Hypertonia	Hypotonia
Superficial reflexes	±	–
Deep reflexes	Exaggerated	Absent
Babinski's	Present	Absent
Clonus	Present	Absent

iii. **Power:** Though in practice, combined power of any joint is acceptable. For example, ankle dorsiflexion power is grade 4. However, in detailed neurological assessment may require individual muscle power assessment also. Further, the muscle power must be graded between 0 and 5 according to the Medical Research Council (MRC) grade **(Box 10.6)**.

BOX 10.6: Medical Research Council (MRC) grading for muscle power.

- **Grade 0:** No power in the muscle
- **Grade 1:** Flicker in the muscle
- **Grade 2:** Movement present but with gravity eliminated
- **Grade 3:** Movement against gravity
- **Grade 4:** Movement against mild-moderate resistance
- **Grade 5:** Movement against full resistance

Of note- MRC grading does not involve plus (+) or minus (–); hence, clinicians should avoid concluding muscle power as 3+ or 2-, etc. The muscle power should be a whole number, such as 2/3/4, as per the test.

iv. **Coordination:** Finger-nose test, diadochokinesia (rapid pronation and supination of the forearm), heel shin test, tandem walking, and Romberg's test are performed for the coordination assessment.

All coordination tests must be determined with open eyes first, followed by closed eyes to differentiate between sensory and cerebellar ataxia. Sensory ataxia (posterior column lesions) improves with open eyes due to visual input correction from eyes, whereas cerebellar ataxia remains the same.

v. **Involuntary movements:** Many involuntary movements such as fasciculations, tremors (fine and pin rolling), chorea, athetosis, and hemiballismus are observed in different neurological disorders. However, almost all of these involuntary movements are common in disorders of the brain and not the spinal cord or nerve root.

5. **Reflexes:** A reflex is an involuntary, predictable, and specific response to a stimulus-dependent on an intact reflex arc. There are two types of reflexes—superficial and deep tendon reflexes (DTRs). One must elicit these reflexes in all cases of assessment of the spine and spinal cord.

   i. **Superficial reflex:** With receptors in the skin or mucous membrane, *superficial reflexes are polysynaptic reflexes with supraspinal brain control for execution.* Hence, completing the superficial reflexes requires anatomical continuity between the spinal cord and brain. Therefore, superficial reflexes are absent in complete spinal cord injury (complete transection), and the return of superficial reflex indicates incomplete cord injury (*a good prognostic sign!*).

Commonly evaluated superficial reflexes (with root values) in spinal cord injury/compression are abdominal (T7-T12), cremasteric (L1, L2), anal (S3, S4), and plantar (L5, S1). Other superficial reflexes assessed in brain or brainstem disorders are conjunctival, corneal, and gag reflexes.

ii. **Deep tendon reflex:** With receptors in the muscles, *the DTRs are executed at the local spinal level and do not require supraspinal control for execution (cf superficial reflexes).* Nevertheless, there is a supraspinal inhibitory control over the DTRs. Hence, the deep reflexes return after spinal cord injury, albeit exaggerated due to the absence of supraspinal inhibitory control. Occasionally, DTR could be hyporesponsive if the patient is apprehensive. In such a case, to distract the patient, the Jendrassik maneuver can be deployed to reinforce the DTR or else ask the patient to clench the teeth while the clinician performs DTR.

Various DTRs (with root values) to be assessed in the spinal cord or nerve injuries are biceps (C5, 6), supinator (C6), triceps (C7), knee (L2, L3, L4), and ankle (S1, S2). The jaw jerk can be assessed in brain disorders.

> **Note on Jendrassik Maneuver**
> In 1885, Erno Jendrassik reported that having the patient "hook together the flexed fingers of his right and left hands and pull them apart as strongly as possible" while the clinician taps on the tendon for deep tendon reflexes (DTR), enhances the DTRs of normal patients. Alternately, ask patient to clench teeth.

6. **Abnormal reflexes in UMN lesions:**
   i. **Babinski sign:** It is a sign observed in patients with UMN lesions.
   In a normal patient, stroking of the lateral side of the plantar aspect of the foot deviating toward the base of the great toe with a blunt-tipped object results in plantar flexion of the great and other toes.

   In patients with UMN lesions, the plantar response is an abnormal extensor type known as the Babinski sign, which involves dorsiflexion of the great toe in patients with or without fanning of all other toes and leg withdrawal.
   (Note that the Babinski sign is not reported as Babinski negative. It is either present or reported as plantar response).
   ii. **Clonus:** Clonus is a rhythmic, oscillating, stretch reflex. It is a sign of a UMN lesion. In patients with UMN lesions and hyperreflexia, one must look for "sustained" patellar and ankle clonus in lower limbs.

> **Of note:** Sustained clonus implies a minimum of 10 repetitions!

Method to elicit patellar clonus: In a supine patient with an extended knee, the clinician holds the patella and suddenly pushes it distally, and light pressure maintains the distal position. Each beat of the clonus is felt like a "repetitive jerky" proximal movement of the patella followed by relaxation to the distal end.

Method to elicit ankle clonus: With the patient supine, the clinician flexes the knee by keeping one hand in the popliteal fossa and holds the forefoot from the plantar side by other hand.

Now, the clinician suddenly dorsiflexes the ankle and maintains dorsal pressure. Each beat of the clonus is felt like a "repetitive jerky" dorsiflexion of the ankle followed by relaxation plantarwards.

7. **Bladder and bowel status:** The urinary bladder status should be assessed, which could be normal/automatic/atonic type of a bladder *(Read about types of the bladder under common conditions affecting the spine)*. Bowel status must be ascertained whether the patient has regular bowel movements, constipation, or incontinence.
8. **Skin condition:** One must check the skin for any bedsore/ulcer over the pressure points of various bony prominences such as occiput, scapula, sacrum, greater trochanter, fibula head, lateral malleolus, and heel.

Examination of the Abdomen and Pelvis

The abdomen and pelvis examination is essential in all cases of back pain as many intra-abdominal organ pathologies could result in back pain. The palpation of the iliac fossa and groin is necessary as TB of the lumbar spine could present as a psoas abscess that may descend in the iliac fossa or groin and present as a palpable mass. Another example, abdominopelvic malignancies (renal, ovarian, endometrial) could present as metastasis in the spine.

Lymph Nodes Examination

As per indications of the case (TB spine, lymphoma, malignancy, etc.)

Notes

Spine Examination Proforma

1. **Gait**
2. **Attitude**
3. **Inspection:**
   - **General findings:** All areas for overlying skin, swelling, scar, sinus, and ulcer
   - **Specific findings of the inspection:**
     a. **Alignment of spine and rest of body:**
        - *From front:* Head and neck alignment, neck tilt, shoulder level
        - *From the side:* Cervical lordosis, dorsal kyphosis, lumbar lordosis, (normal/exaggerated/attenuated)
        - *From the back:* Alignment of head, neck, spine, and natal cleft, scoliosis (functional/structural), list (if any)
     b. **Level of shoulder and pelvis**
     c. **Neck and scapula:** Hairline, webbing, scapula (level and shape)
     d. **The skin of the back and elsewhere**
     e. **Swelling**
     f. **Deformities in the upper and lower limb**
     g. **Muscle spasm and atrophy**
4. **Palpation:**
   - The local rise in temperature
   - *Spinous process:* Tenderness, step, deformity, and any absence of spinous process
   - *Paraspinal spasm*
   - *Other bony (scapula, PSIS, and iliac crest) and soft tissue landmarks*
   - *Deformities in upper and lower limb*
   - *Confirmation of palpatory characteristics of swelling, scar, and sinus*
5. **Movements:** Active and passive
   - *Cervical spine:* Flexion, extension, rotation, lateral flexion, and occiput wall distance
   - *Dorsal spine:* Rotation
   - *Lumbar spine:* Flexion (forward bend and modified Schober's test), extension, and lateral flexion
6. **Measurements:** Chest expansion, scoliosis inclination (if applicable), limb length (if relevant), arm span, and upper: lower segment ratio
7. **Special tests:**
   - *Test for cervical root compression in IVDP/spondylosis:* Spurling test
   - *Test for thoracic outlet syndrome:* Adson's test, Roos test
   - *Test for lumbar spine root compression in IVDP:* Straight leg raising test, Lasegue test, Well leg raising test and femoral nerve stretch test
   - *Sacroiliac joint test:* Figure-of-four test, Gaenslen's test
8. **Neurological examination:** Gait, higher mental function, cranial nerve examination, sensorimotor examination, superficial and deep reflexes, abnormal reflexes, bladder and bowel status assessment, and skin condition.
9. **Other areas and lymph nodes:** Examination of regions such as chest, abdomen, per-rectal, and lymph nodes of cervical and other areas is a must in suspected spine tuberculosis or malignancy.

(IVDP: intervertebral disc prolapse; PSIS: posterior superior iliac spine)

Common Conditions Affecting Spine and their Salient Features

1. **Thoracic outlet syndrome (TOS):** TOS describes a syndrome resulting from compression of the brachial plexus and/or subclavian vessels as they exit through the thoracic outlet.
   - **Pathology:** There are various causes of TOS. **Osseous causes:** Cervical rib, 1st rib exostosis, malunited clavicle fracture; **Soft tissue causes:** Hypertrophied scalenus muscle, fibrous bands, tumors; **Chronic overuse causes:** Repetitive shoulder use in extreme position (frequent overhead activities involving hyperabduction, hyperextension) in athletes involved in weight-lifting, rowing or swimming; overworking on a computer keyboard
   - **Clinically:** Features of TOS are either neurological (95%) or vascular (5%). Features are usually quite variable.
     - *Local features:* Neck pain radiation to occiput, rhomboid, trapezius. Occasionally, the cervical rib is obvious and palpable (**Fig. 10.25A**).
     - *Neurological features:* About 90% of cases show involvement of lower trunk resulting in pain, tingling, numbness, paraesthesia along the ulnar nerve with typical radiation toward the medial side of the arm and forearm.
     - *Vascular symptoms:* Venous congestion causing heaviness in the upper limb, swelling, and episodic cyanotic discoloration. Arterial obstruction causes Raynaud's-like features in hand (episodic coolness, cyanosis, erythema and worsening in cold temperature).
     - Various provocative tests (Adson's, Roos) may be positive.
   - **Diagnosis:** X-ray (**Fig. 10.25B**), CT scan, MRI, Doppler scan, and nerve conduction velocity (NCV)
   - **Treatment:** Conservative—shoulder shrugging and cervical isometric exercises, activity modification, analgesics, and gabapentinoids (Pregabalin). Surgical option is reserved for patients with severe neurovascular symptoms.

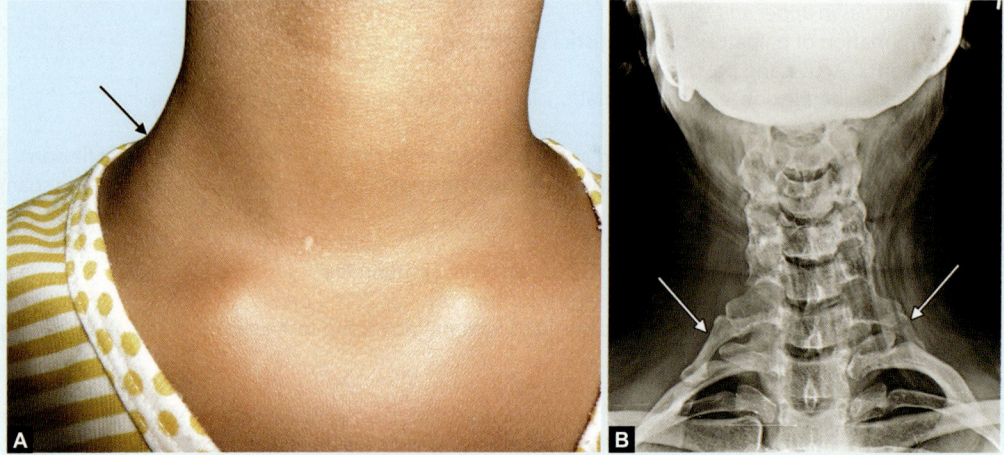

Figs. 10.25A and B: (A) Cervical rib (black arrow shows a prominent subcutaneous cervical rib); (B) Cervical spine anteroposterior X-ray showing cervical rib (white arrows).

2. **Tuberculosis of the spine:**
   - **Affects:** Mostly young adults, but can affect person of any age. TB spine commonly involves "thoracolumbar junction."
   - **Presents with:** Neck/back pain, especially at night, and stiffness. Low-grade fever, and weight loss.
   - **Pathology:** Musculoskeletal TB is always secondary to the primary elsewhere (occult/overt/past history). Commonly affects dorsolumbar junction (50%). *Paradiscal site* is most commonly involved.

- **Clinically:** Vertebral tenderness and/or kyphosis is present at the respective site of the vertebral involvement. Paraspinal spasm present. Movements of the spine are painfully restricted, and there may be clinically apparent cold abscess. The patient may present with a neurological deficit.
- **Diagnosis:** X-ray, MRI, and other investigations for TB. Always investigate for primary focus.
- **Treatment:** Anti-tubercular treatment (ATT), bracing, surgical decompression, and stabilization
- **Differential diagnosis:** Tumor, other infections of the spine such as pyogenic spondylodiscitis and brucella infection.

3. **Degenerative spondylosis (old term: spondylitis):**
   - **Affects:** Middle age and elderly.
   - **Region affected:** Lower cervical and lumbar (mobile spinal areas are commonly affected).
   - **Presents with:** Chronic mechanical pain (neck and low back) is the chief complaint. Sometimes, there can be radicular pain at the affected nerve root region.
   - **Pathology:** Degeneration in the IVD, instability, osteophytes, hypertrophy of facet joint capsule and synovium, and ligament(s) hypertrophy (posterior longitudinal, ligamentum flavum).
   - **Clinically:** Mechanical pain, painful restricted ROM.
   - **Diagnosis:** X-ray, MRI.
   - **Treatment:** Conservative treatment is the mainstay (analgesics, physiotherapy, gabapentinoids, muscle strengthening, and soft cervical collar).

4. **Intervertebral disc prolapse (IVDP) of the cervical/lumbar region:**
   - **Affects:** Mostly young adult.
   - **Presents with:** Acute or chronic neck/low back pain with/without radiation to the scapular region, upper limb or lower limbs. In lumbar IVDP, pain often increases while bending forward and lifting weights. The lumbar IVDP pain also increases on coughing, sneezing, and turning in the bed at night. Neurological examination is a must to correlate the level of disc prolapse.
   - **Pathology:** Typically, cervical and lumbar IVDP is common in the lower cervical spine (C4-5, C5-6, and C6-7) and lower lumbar (L3-4, L4-5, L5-S1) region. IVDP is characterized by rupture of annulus fibrosus followed by the protrusion, extrusion, and sequestration of the IVD **(Fig. 10.26)**. A prolapsed disc can compress the cord and nerve roots.
   - **Clinically:** Local pain which may radiate to the the limbs. Vertebral tenderness is present at the affected level along with a painful range of motion. In cervical region, *Spurling test could be positive*. In lumbar IVDP, List (postural scoliosis) could be present in acute cases. Other signs are *painful forward flexion, positive SLRT, and Lasegue tests. A positive crossed SLR is highly specific for an IVDP*.
   - **Diagnosis:** X-rays may show degenerative changes (osteophyte, decreased disc space). MRI is diagnostic.
   - **Treatment:** Mostly conservative—analgesics, muscle relaxants, gabapentinoids (Pregabalin), soft cervical collar, activity modification, and physiotherapy. Rarely, discectomy if worsening neurological deficit or unrelenting pain which is not responding to conservative treatment.

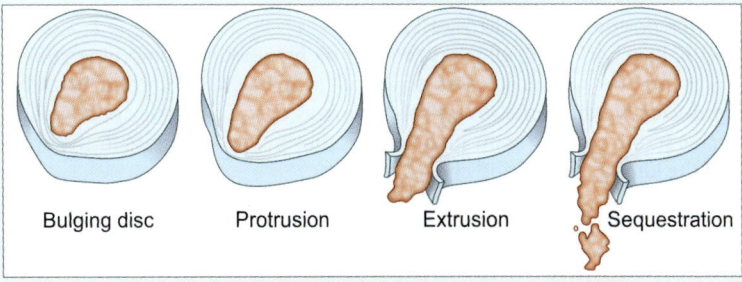

Fig. 10.26: Stages of disc herniation or prolapse.

5. **Spondylolysis and spondylolisthesis:**
   - ➤ *Affects:* Mostly middle age, elderly, and young athletes.
   - ➤ *Pathology:* Spondylolysis is characterized by a break in pars interarticularis, whereas spondylolisthesis is characterized by slipping an upper vertebra over the lower one.
   - ➤ *Clinically:* Both conditions present as low back pain with/without radiation to the limbs. Spondylolisthesis is characterized by a palpable step between two vertebral spinous process. Extension is painful.
   - ➤ *Diagnosis:* Spondylolysis can be diagnosed with lateral X-ray of spine **(Fig. 10.27A)**. Oblique view of the spine may show Scottish Terrier dog sign, while AP view shows Napolean hat sign. Spondylolisthesis would show slippage of the vertebra **(Fig. 10.27B)**.
   - ➤ *Treatment:* Conservative (as described in lumbar IVDP). Surgical—Decompression and stabilization

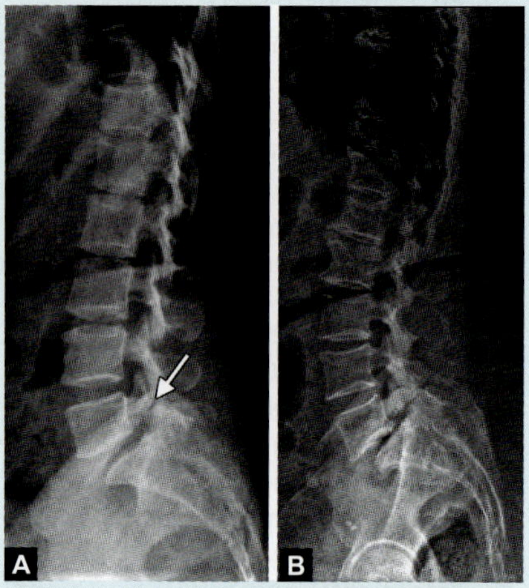

Figs. 10.27A and B: (A) Spondylolysis (White arrow indicates lysis in the pars interarticularis); (B) Spondylolisthesis L5 over S1.

6. **Lumbar canal stenosis (LCS):**
   - ➤ *Affects:* Typically affects older patients (>55–60 years)
   - ➤ *Presents with:* Radicular pain in lower limbs (uni- or bilateral) is the most common presentation, followed by *neurogenic claudication*. There may/may not be low back pain.
   - ➤ *Pathology:* Chronic degenerative lumbar spondylosis coupled with multilevel IVDP is the most common cause of LCS. Lumbar canal space available for lumbosacral nerve roots is stenosed due to multilevel disc prolapse, hypertrophied ligamentum flavum, osteophytes encroaching the canal, and hypertrophy of the facetal joint capsule.
   - ➤ *Clinically:* Extension of the spine is often painful. There may be some sensory deficits, but motor deficits are rare. Further, there are no specific clinical tests to confirm the diagnosis of lumbar canal stenosis, and it should be confirmed with history and imaging. *Always rule out vascular causes of claudication!*
   - ➤ *Diagnosis:* X-ray, MRI—diagnostic for LCS.
   - ➤ *Treatment:* Conservative—analgesics, physiotherapy, brace, gabapentinoids (Pregabalin), and epidural injections. If conservative options fail, laminectomy and decompression with/with stabilization can be performed.

7. **Ankylosing spondylitis:**
   - ➤ *Affects:* Young to middle age, predominantly men
   - ➤ *Genetics:* Often positive family history, HLA-B27+
   - ➤ *Presents with:* Low back pain, which is more at night, along with morning stiffness, is the most common presentation. Advanced cases may result in spinal deformity and hip arthritis.
   - ➤ *Pathology: Sacroiliitis* and *Enthesitis* are the hallmarks of seronegative spondyloarthropathy. Most cases are characterized by SI joint involvement, progressive stiffness in the spine, followed by ankylosis of the lumbar, dorsal, and cervical spine.

- **Clinically:** Tests for sacroiliitis are positive. Schober's test+, kyphotic deformity in the dorsal spine, decreased cervical spine ROM, increased occiput-wall distance, decreased chest expansion, and hip arthritis and ankylosis. Several patients also have eye (iridocyclitis) and cardiac (conduction defects) features.
- **Diagnosis:** X-ray (sacroiliitis, bamboo spine, and dagger spine), HLA-B27+. MRI shows sacroiliitis in early cases where X-rays are normal.
- **Treatment:** Conservative—nonsteroidal anti-inflammatory drugs (indomethacin), DMARDs (sulfasalazine, methotrexate) physiotherapy, and chest physiotherapy are the mainstay of treatment. Hip replacement and rarely spinal corrective osteotomy for severe dorsal kyphosis may be required.
- **Differential diagnosis:** Other seronegative spondyloarthropathies which can affect the spine are:
  - Psoriatic arthropathy (with skin and nail changes), Reiter's disease (urethral infection, conjunctivitis), and inflammatory bowel disease-related spondyloarthropathy

8. **Osteoporosis:** A disorder characterized by low bone mass.
   - **Affects:** Old age, postmenopausal. Women are more affected than men due to the loss of estrogen protective effect on bones.
   - **Presents with:** Mechanical low back pain. History of fracture in the spine, hip, or wrist.
   - **Pathology:** Decreased bone mineral density (BMD), especially in cancellous bones (spine, pelvis, end of long bones).
   - **Classification:** Type 1: Postmenopausal; Type 2: Senile
   - **Clinically:** Kyphosis, pathological fractures in the hip, spine, distal radius, or other cancellous bones.
   - **Diagnosis:** X-ray (Thinned cortices, loss of trabecular bone, fractures), BMD assessment by DEXA (dual-energy X-ray absorptiometry)—*Normal:* T score –1.5 to +1.5 SD, *osteopenia:* –1.5 to –2.5 SD, and *osteoporosis:* T-score less than –2.5 SD
   - **Treatment:** Conservative options: Bisphosphonates, calcitonin intranasal spray, parathormone injection, denosumab, calcium, vitamin D, anabolic steroid injection, healthy diet, exercise, and braces. *Surgical treatment:* Vertebroplasty and kyphoplasty.

9. **Osteomalacia:** A disorder of defective mineralization in a mature skeleton (Rickets in counterpart in children)
   - **Affects:** Women in the childbearing age group are commonly affected. Often after pregnancy/multipara
   - **Presents with:** Mechanical back pain, muscle pain, and fractures
   - **Etiology:** Usually due to vitamin D deficiency, malabsorption, renal osteodystrophy, drugs
   - **Pathology:** Defective mineralization of osteoid area in a mature skeleton
   - **Clinically:** Proximal muscle weakness, fractures, especially in the femoral neck, other long bones, ribs and vertebra, waddling gait due to proximal hip muscle weakness
   - **Diagnosis:** X-ray: *looser's zone* (medial femoral cortex, medial border of scapula, ribs, pubic rami), biconcave vertebral bodies (codfish), vertebral fractures. *Lab studies:* Low Ca, P, vitamin D3 while ALP and PTH are elevated.
   - **Treatment:** Large dose of vitamin D and calcium. Treat the underlying cause. Fracture fixation, if necessary.

10. **Central cord syndrome:**
    - A condition wherein the spinal cord tracts crossing the spinal segment adjacent to the central canal are affected **(Fig. 10.28)**. It is commonly observed in *syringomyelia* (dilation of the central canal) and *hyperextension injury in the stiff cervical spine* (spondylotic, ankylosing spondylosis) of the elderly. It presents with loss of pain and temperature sensation as nerve fibers carrying these sensations cross to the opposite side (adjacent to central canal) to enter contralateral lateral spinothalamic tract (LSTT), more power loss in upper limb than lower limb as cervical motor area [lateral corticospinal tract (LCST)] is more medial than lumbosacral to the central canal.

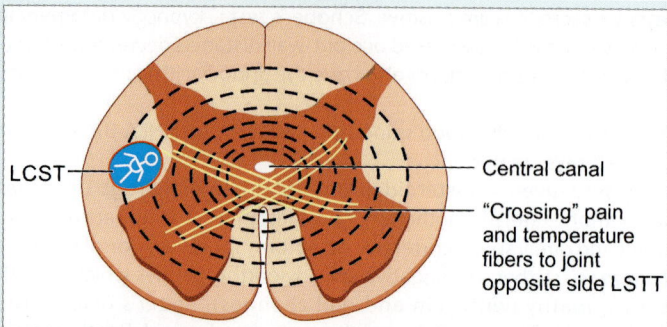

Fig. 10.28: Central cord syndrome. Circular hashed lines represent area gradually affected in central cord syndrome in a centrifugal fashion. Body representation (homunculus) in LCST (blue-circled area) is from cervical (medial) to sacral (lateral).

(LCST: lateral corticospinal tract; LSTT: lateral spinothalamic tract).

11. **Lateral cord syndrome/Brown–Sequard syndrome/hemisection of the spinal cord:**
    ➢ Classically described after a pointed knife injury/stab injury to the back.
    ➢ The spinal cord's hemisection results in loss of ipsilateral sensations carried by the posterior column and motor power, while loss of pain and temperature sensation of the opposite side below the level of the lesion **(Figs. 10.29A to C)**.

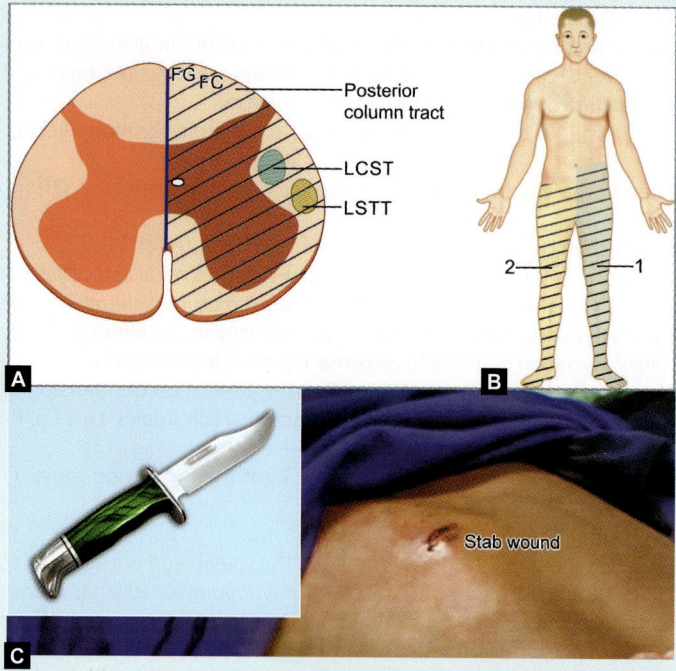

Figs. 10.29A to C: Lateral cord syndrome, its mechanism of injury and clinical presentation. (A) Continuous lines depict the area affected in lateral cord syndrome; (B) Green-shaded area (1) represents damage to the ipsilateral posterior column and corticospinal tracts, while yellow-shaded area (2) represents damage to opposite LST tract; (C) The typical mechanism of lateral cord syndrome by a stab injury to the back by a knife.

(LCST: lateral corticospinal tract; LSTT: lateral spinothalamic tract; FG: fasciculus gracilis; FC: fasciculus cuneatus).

12. **Posterior cord syndrome:** It is a syndrome due to posterior spinal artery blockage resulting in ischemia of the posterior one-third of the spinal cord followed by subsequent damage to the posterior column tract and later a part of the lateral corticospinal tract **(Fig. 10.30)**.

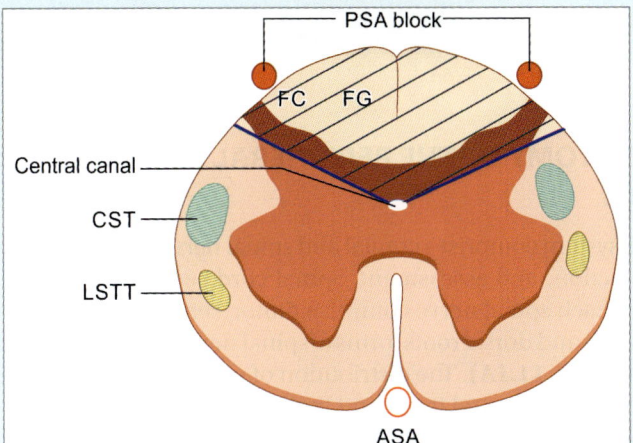

Fig. 10.30: Posterior cord syndrome. Continuous lines represent area affected in posterior cord syndrome.
(ASA: anterior spinal artery; CST: corticospinal tract; LSTT: lateral spinothalamic tract; PSA: posterior spinal arteries).

13. **Anterior cord syndrome:** It is a syndrome due to ASA blockage resulting in ischemia of the anterior two-thirds of the spinal cord followed by subsequent damage to the motor tracts and spinothalamic tracts. However, the posterior column is spared **(Fig. 10.31)**.

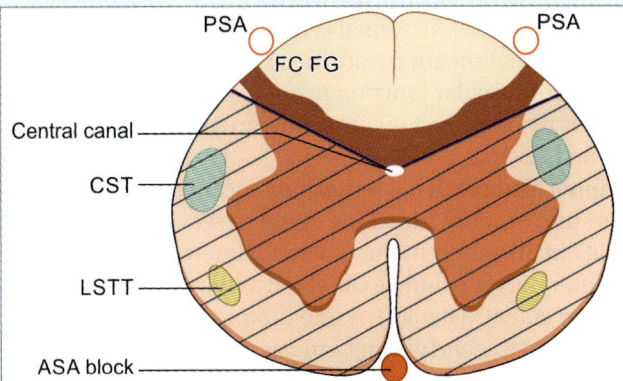

Fig. 10.31: Anterior cord syndrome. Continuous lines represent area affected in anterior cord syndrome.
(ASA: anterior spinal artery; CST: corticospinal tract; LSTT: lateral spinothalamic tract; PSA: posterior spinal arteries).

14. **Conus medullaris and cauda equina syndrome:**
    - **Conus medullaris syndrome (CMS):** Compression of conus medullaris is characterized by *acute low back pain, loss of sensation in the saddle area, and frequent sexual dysfunction.*
    - **Cauda equina syndrome (CES):** Compression of the cauda equina (L2-L5; S1-S5, and coccyx nerve roots) resulting in asymmetric severe radicular pain and sensorimotor involvement. Both conditions are orthopedic emergencies.

CHAPTER 11

Clinical Evaluation of the Peripheral Nerves

SURGICAL ANATOMY OF THE PERIPHERAL NERVE AND ITS CLINICAL SIGNIFICANCE

Peripheral nervous system comprises cranial and spinal nerve. This chapter will focus on spinal nerve anatomy, function, and assessment. Spinal cord segment gives rise to a spinal nerve (A total of 31 pairs). Each spinal nerve comprise motor, sensory, and autonomic components.

- The union of ventral and dorsal roots forms a 'spinal nerve', which further divides into ventral and dorsal ramus **(Fig. 11.1A)**. The distribution of ramus is mentioned below.
  - **Ventral ramus/root:** Ventral trunk and limb muscles
  - **Dorsal ramus/root:** Dorsal trunk-skin and muscles of the back

  Two or more ramus (dorsal/ventral) join to form a peripheral nerve, which could be mixed (sensory, motor, and autonomic fibers) or a pure sensory/motor nerve.

- A peripheral nerve fiber is surrounded by loose connective tissue known as **endoneurium/ neurilemmal sheath**. A group of many nerve fibers forms a **fascicle** surrounded by **perineurium**. Between multiple fascicles of nerve lies **mesoneurium**. Multiple fascicles form a nerve surrounded by **epineurium (Fig. 11.1B)**.

- **Basic unit of a peripheral nerve** is an axon **(Fig. 11.2)**. An axon has a cell body (lies in the anterior horn of the spinal cord), an axonal cylinder covered by a myelin sheath, and terminal dendrites. The neurilemmal sheath covers the axon and myelin sheath. The axonal cylinder terminates at the neuromuscular junction in a muscle fiber or a sensory organ.

  The axonal cylinder is responsible for ante- and retrograde conduction from the cell body to the axon terminal and reverse.

- **Function of a peripheral nerve:** It has *sensory, motor, and autonomic functions*. Any affection could compromise one or more functions of the nerve. Peripheral nerves could be purely sensory (superficial radial), purely motor (posterior interosseous) or mixed in function (Ulnar, Median). Mixed motor nerves could be classified as nerves with fine motor activity (Median, Ulnar) or gross motor activity (Radial). A fine motor nerve is the one that is involved in the fine skills of the hand and fingers (playing a musical instrument), whereas gross motor nerve is involved in gross functions such as dorsi- and palmar flexion of wrist. Autonomic functions of a peripheral nerve include control of smooth muscles, blood vessels, glands, and internal organs. The autonomic assessment of a peripheral nerve are out of scope of this chapter.

- **Classification of nerve injury:** The nerve injuries are classified in two ways: *Seddon's and Sunderland's*. Seddon's classification is more commonly used in clinical practice, classifying nerve injuries into three types: *neurapraxia, axonotmesis,* and *neurotmesis*. Neuropraxia is a focal block in the axonal cylinder without any structural/anatomical damage to the axon/endoneurium. Axonotmesis involves injury to the axonal cylinder, whereas neurilemmal sheath/endoneurium is intact. Neurotmesis is a complete severance of axon and neurilemmal sheath. An injury to a peripheral nerve results in **Wallerian degeneration** followed by **Wallerian regeneration**.

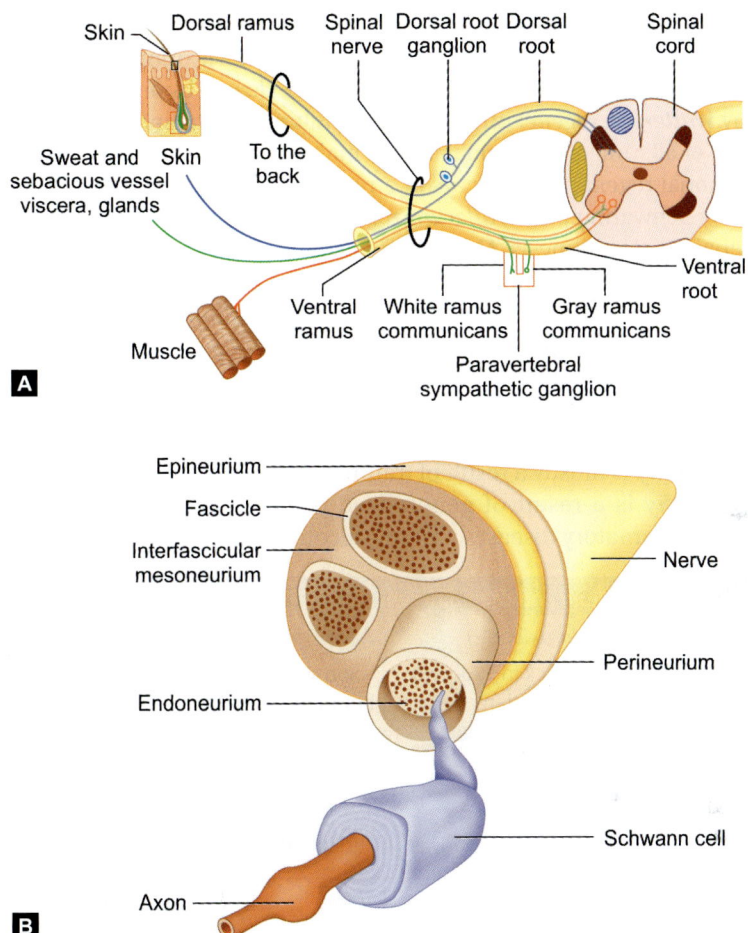

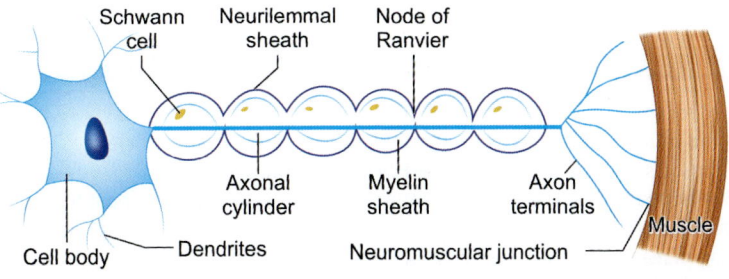

Figs. 11.1A and B: (A) Illustrative figure showing formation of the peripheral nervous system; (B) Structure of a nerve.

Fig. 11.2: Illustrative figure of an axon along with neuromuscular junction.

Structural nerve injuries (Axonotmesis, Neurotmesis) results in **Wallerian degeneration**. Wallerian degeneration is characterized by breaking down of myelin sheath and axonal cylinder till the proximal node of Ranvier. The debris are cleared by phagocytosis. Degeneration is followed by **Wallerian regeneration**, wherein multiple axonal sprouts arise out of proximal axon end. Out of all, one of the axonal sprout makes a connection with distal neurilemmal sheath. The axonal regeneration occurs at a rate of 1 mm/day, which gradually undergoes myelination by Schwann cells. *Wallerian regeneration*, it is observed in axonotmesis and 'surgically repaired' neurotmesis. No Wallerian changes are observed in neurapraxia as the nerve has no anatomical/structural Wallerian regeneration is associated with **Tinel's sign** and *Motor march*. Therefore, these two signs are present in Axontmesis and repaired neurotmesis, whereas it is absent in neuropraxia.

The differences among these three types of injuries are mentioned in **Table 11.1**.

- **Conditions affecting a peripheral nerve:** Nerve function could be affected by various diseases. The affection could be *mononeuropathy* or polyneuropathy **(Box 11.1)**.
    - **Mononeuropathy** is mostly a result of traumatic, compressive or infective causes
    - **Polyneuropathy** is a result of generalized causes, such as metabolic, endocrine, chemicals, inflammatory diseases, chronic alcoholism, and medications.

TABLE 11.1: Types of nerve injury and their differences.

	Neurapraxia	Axonotmesis	Neurotmesis
Definition	Focal block in axon, no anatomical damage to axon/endoneurium	Axon damaged, whereas neurilemmal sheath/endoneurium intact	Complete severance of axon and neurilemmal sheath
Severity	Mild	Moderate	Severe
Wallerian D, R	No	Yes	Yes. Progression of regeneration only if repaired
Tinel's sign	No	Yes	Only if repaired
Motor march	No	Yes	Only if repaired
NCV distal segment excitability	Maintained	Lost	Lost
EMG fibrillation	Absent	+ at 2–3 weeks	+ at 2–3 weeks
Recovery	4–6 weeks	6–18 months	None without repair
Prognosis	Excellent	Good	Fair-Poor

BOX 11.1: Common conditions affecting nerves (mono/polyneuropathy).

1. **Traumatic:** Mechanical, thermal, chemical, surgical (iatrogenic)
2. **Metabolic and endocrinal:** Diabetes, vitamin deficiency—B_1, B_6, B_{12} deficiency
3. **Infection:** Hansen's disease, Lyme's disease, HIV, Herpes simplex
4. **Compressive neuropathy:** Carpal/Tarsal tunnel syndrome—Idiopathic, post traumatic (Malunited or displaced fracture)
5. **Autoimmune diseases:** RA, SLE, sarcoidosis, Guillain–Barré syndrome
6. **Alcohol, chemicals:** Chronic alcoholism, lead toxicity, exposure to glue, solvents, insecticides
7. **Genetic:** Friedreich's ataxia, Charcot–Marie–Tooth disease, Fabry's disease
8. **Others:** Medication (anticonvulsant, anti-HIV), radiation

HISTORY AND ITS EVALUATION

Chief Complaints and History of Presenting Illness

The patients with nerve injury mostly come up with two categories of complaints. First, *complaint pertaining to etiology* such as trauma, infection, tumors, which has led to nerve affection, and second will be the complaint *about the effect* arising out of the nerve involvement such as motor weakness, sensory deficit, and autonomic disturbances.

Motor symptoms: Inability or weakness to use a specific part or move a joint.

Sensory symptoms include loss or blunting of sensation in a specific area; tingling, numbness, or radiation of pain or shock-like sensation in the limb.

Autonomic symptoms include altered sweating pattern in the extremity, and altered sensitivity to pain and temperature.

While asking about these symptoms, one must ask about the onset, duration, and progression of the complaints, as it is essential to understand that whether nerve affection is static, improving, or deteriorating, which helps in planning the future course of the treatment. Further, the clinician must always probe into *how the nerve involvement has affected the patient's activities of daily living (ADL)*. As far as the etiology of the nerve injury is concerned, the following undermentioned causes could be reasons for nerve affection. The details about the etiology must be probed.

1. **Trauma:** Traumatic injuries are one of the common causes of nerve injury. Many types of injuries could result in nerve palsy.
   a. A *closed traumatic injury* (fracture or dislocation) commonly causes neuropraxia or axonotmesis and rarely neurotmesis of a single/group of nerves. Since neuropraxia and axonotmesis has excellent to good prognosis, these injuries are given a trial of conservative management.
   b. *An open traumatic injury* (laceration, crush injury, and gunshot) usually causes neurotmesis unless proved otherwise. Hence, open wounds mandate exploration of the associated nerve injuries to check the continuity of the nerve.

> The site of injury may give a clue to the type and level of nerve injury, e.g., a sutured wound over the palmar aspect of the wrist may indicate injury to the underlying median or ulnar nerve, or a wound over the fibular neck risks the injury to the underlying common peroneal nerve.

   c. *A tight plaster cast* can injure a single nerve, especially if the edge of the plaster lies just above the nerve. For example, the upper edge of the below knee cast can compress the common peroneal nerve. A tight cast can also cause compartment syndrome, resulting in damage to the nerves traversing the compartment leading to variable motor and sensory damage.
   d. *A temporary pressure* over the nerve (Saturday night palsy) can cause transient palsy of the nerve (usually neuropraxia).
   e. *Delayed onset paralysis* after a fracture may indicate nerve entrapment in the callus or fibrous tissue. The nerve might also be affected due to the friction over a deformed bony fragment, such as tardy ulnar nerve palsy due to cubitus valgus.
   f. *Iatrogenic injury* wherein the patient complains that his movements and sensations were normal before the surgery to the index limb and were affected after the surgical intervention/other procedure. An unintentional injury to the nerve during the surgery could occur by pressure, prolonged traction or transection of the nerve.

g. *History of an injection* adjacent to the nerve. An injection injury could damage a nerve in two ways—first, by *chemical injury to the nerve* (due to preservatives in the injected medicine) and second, by *direct trauma to the nerve*. Such injection injuries often result in extensive inflammation and fibrosis of the nerve, causing a delayed or poor recovery.
2. **Infections of the nerve:** One of the common infective causes of nerve affection is *Hansen's disease*, especially in developing countries. Such patients give a history of hypopigmented or erythematous numb skin patches in other parts of the body. The patient may also have non-healing ulcers in the affected areas. Another infective cause of nerve affection is '*Poliomyelitis*', which is characterized by sudden onset of patchy paralysis in a limb without sensory loss. Such patients may give history of fever with diarrhea before paralysis. Other infective causes of nerve damage are *HIV, herpes zoster* (chickenpox and shingles)*, Cytomegalovirus, and Lyme's disease*.
3. A **tumor** in the vicinity of a nerve can compress, stretch, or infiltrate into the substance of the nerve, which could affect the functioning of the nerve.
4. **Metabolic conditions like diabetes** usually cause sensory affection, but motor palsy is a rare possibility. Chronic diabetic neuropathy can lead to Charcot's arthropathy, especially in the foot and ankle joints.
5. **Other causes:** *Autoimmune diseases, drugs, exposure to toxins, nutritional and vitamin deficiency, connective tissue disorders, hereditary diseases, chronic alcohol intake, chronic kidney or liver disease*. The list is exhaustive, but the clinician must probe into the etiology of the nerve affection as the management also involves treating the cause.

Constitutional Symptoms

Symptoms such as fever, malaise, loss of weight and appetite may indicate an underlying infective, inflammatory, or tumor disorder.

Effect on Activities of Daily Living (ADL)/Professional Activities

It is important to understand how current complaints have affected the ADLs and professional activities, which may help plan the treatment.

Past History

Patients with diabetes mellitus, thyroid disorder, RA or other collagen vascular diseases are also prone to mono/polyneuropathy. Hemophilia patients can present with compressive neuropathy.

Personal History

History of smoking, diet, alcohol intake, and occupation are important. Smoking and alcohol consumption can delay nerve recovery. Chronic alcohol intake is a risk factor for peripheral neuropathy (PN). Strict vegetarians could present with PN due to vitamin B_{12} and folate deficiency.

Patients in a particular occupation are more prone to nerve injury. For example, carpal tunnel syndrome is common in workers handling vibratory pneumatic tools (quarry workers, construction). Prolonged keyboard operators are prone to upper limb compressive neuropathies.

Treatment History

A detail of treatment history including drug intake can unfold the clues about the current diagnosis. Many drugs could result in PN, such as *chemotherapeutic agents* [Vinca alkaloids, Cisplatin, Bortezomib and thalidomide (used for multiple myeloma), paclitaxel and docetaxel (used for breast carcinoma)], *antimicrobials* (INH, ethambutol, linezolid), *cardiovascular* drugs (amiodarone), *immunosuppressive* (adalimumab, infliximab, and etanercept), *antiretroviral* drugs), and anticonvulsants (phenytoin, carbamazepine, phenobarbitone).

Family History

Hereditary neuropathies are a group of inherited disorders affecting the peripheral nervous system. The most common type is Charcot–Marie–Tooth disease (CMTD), one of the hereditary motor and sensory neuropathies. CMTD is characterized by progressive muscle weakness, muscular atrophy, and sensory disturbances with pes cavus, claw toes as major clinical features.

EXAMINATION

General and Systemic Examination

The etiology of the nerve affection could be systemic such as Hansen's disease (look for hypopigmented patches over skin), connective tissue disorders, chemical toxicity (lead poisoning features—blue line on gums, anemia), nutritional deficiency, or malignancy. Hence, a thorough head-to-toe general and systemic examinations in a standard fashion is recommended, especially in a systemic cause of neuropathy.

Local Examination

Rather than just the affected part, the entire limb up to the spine and trunk should be adequately exposed, including the normal side, for comparison. If the patient is ambulatory, *gait must be examined in patients with the involvement of nerves of the lower limb.*

Attitude

The attitude of the affected limb should be described in a standard fashion.

Inspection

The inspection involves assessing *deformity, muscle wasting, scars, condition of skin, and nail changes* in the involved extremity. Other findings, such as ulcers, sinuses can be described in the standard fashion.
1. **Deformity:** One must look for deformity in the affected part **(Figs. 11.3A and B)**. Box 11.2 mentions classic deformities observed after various nerve injuries.
2. **Wasting of muscles:** In chronic nerve injury, the affected muscles are wasted due to disuse **(Fig. 11.3C)**.

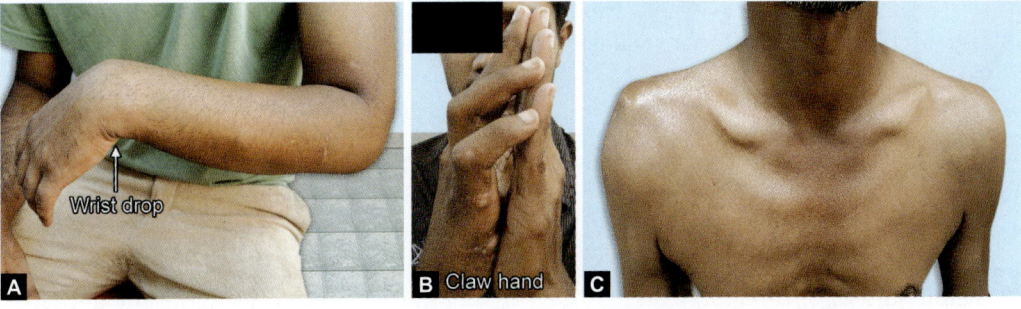

Figs. 11.3A to C: (A) Wrist drop (left); (B) Claw hand (right); (C) Wasting of right deltoid.

BOX 11.2: Typical feature in specific nerve palsy.

- **Policeman's tip hand:** Erb's paralysis
- **Scapula winging:** Long thoracic nerve (supplying serratus anterior) injury causes medial winging. Spinal accessory nerve (supplying trapezius) injury causes lateral winging
- **Wrist and finger drop:** Radial nerve palsy
- **Claw hand:** Ulnar (partial claw) or median-ulnar combined nerve palsy (total claw hand)
- **Pointing finger:** High median nerve palsy
- **Foot drop:** Sciatic/common peroneal nerve palsy

3. **Scars:** A traumatic or surgical wound or scar overlying the anatomical location of the nerve may explain the cause of nerve injury. For example, a scar over hypothenar eminence indicates injury to ulnar nerve, whereas scar due to a lymph node biopsy in the posterior triangle of the neck may suggest damage to the spinal accessory nerve causing trapezius palsy and consequent scapular winging **(Figs. 11.4A and B)**.
4. **Local and distal swelling:** A local swelling over the nerve could be due to a tumor or infective abscess (observed in Hansen's disease). The distal edema occurs due to poor muscle function resulting in poor venous and lymphatic drainage.
5. **Skin:** The skin of the involved area shows variable changes due to the dysfunctional sympathetic nervous system—Look for trophic change.
   - ❑ *In early stages of nerve injury:* Erythematous and glossy
   - ❑ *In late stages of nerve injury:* Dry and scaly.

   The skin may have *trophic ulcers* due to loss of sensation.
6. **Nail changes:** The nail changes are due to local sympathetic system dysfunction resulting in brittle and ridged nails with loss of shine.

Palpation

The palpation involves assessment in *temperature difference* over the skin compared to the normal side, *scar tenderness along course of nerve, nerve thickening, underlying bone, deformity, and assessment of swelling.*

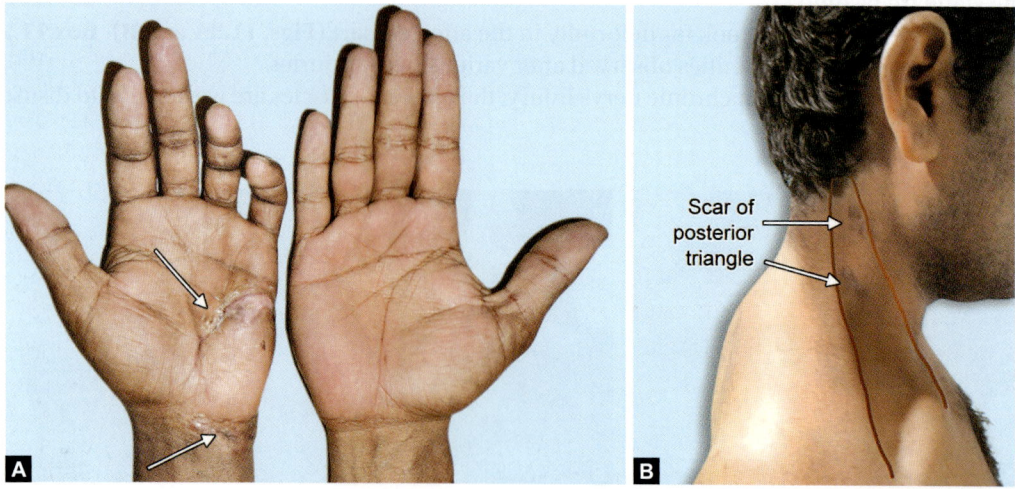

Figs. 11.4A and B: (A) Scars over the left wrist and hypothenar eminence (ulnar nerve site); (B) Scar in posterior triangle of the neck (spinal accessory nerve site).

1. **Temperature difference over the skin** compared to the normal side:
   - *Early-stage:* Increased (Warmer)
   - *Late-stage:* Decreased (Colder)
2. **Scar:** Scar must be palpated for tenderness, mobility, or fixity to the underlying structures.
3. **Palpation along the course of affected nerve:** There may be point tenderness along the nerve course, indicating neuroma formation, peripheral neuritis, or a nerve sheath abscess. Also, feel for the thickening of the nerve along the course, which may be present in Hansen's disease.

> **Note:** Peripheral nerves, which are prone to Hansen's disease—greater auricular nerve, superficial radial nerve, ulnar nerve, and common peroneal nerve.

4. Further, **palpate the underlying bone** for any bony irregularity due to any old fracture. Assess and describe the deformity, swelling or other characteristics of the local etiology responsible for nerve palsy.

Movements

Assess deformity, active and passive movements at all the affected and unaffected joints.
a. First, **check for any fixed deformity** in the affected joints due to chronic nerve injury.
b. **Assess active movement of the affected and uninvolved joints:** It helps assess overall power of the muscles crossing the joint. Furthermore, a detailed motor power assessment of individual muscles should be performed.
c. **Assess passive movement of the affected joints:** It gives an estimate of the stiffness at the joint.

Measurement

1. The **length of the limb** should be measured in a standard fashion.
2. **Wasting of muscles** indicates chronicity of disease and motor involvement.

Neurological Examination

Essentially, examination of the peripheral nerve (s), which is a part of the peripheral nervous system (PNS), is different from examination of the central nervous system (CNS) examination as the latter is more elaborate than the former. The CNS affection also involves examining the higher center (brain), cranial nerves, and superficial reflexes. Further, the pattern of sensory examination is different. Sometimes, what appears to be a PNS disorder could have a CNS component too. For example, a preganglionic brachial plexus injury due to root avulsion may have associated spinal cord involvement. Therefore, in all patients with PNS disorder, it is prudent to perform a quick survey of CNS, which involves assessing higher mental function, cranial nerves, and any evidence for UMN type of lesion (increased tone, clonus, extensor plantar reflex, and exaggerated deep tendon reflexes). Once it is clear from history and a quick CNS survey that the patient has only isolated PNS disorder, the neurological examination of the involved part can be divided into four parts:
1. Sensory examination
2. Motor examination
3. Autonomic examination
4. Clinical signs of nerve recovery: *Tinel's sign and motor march*
1. **Sensory examination:** *The principal objective of the sensory examination is to establish the level or site of the lesion.* There is a difference in sensory examinations of CNS and PNS disorder as discussed below.

❑ **CNS/UMN/nerve root level disorder:** The sensory examination is *"as per dermatomal distribution"* of nerve roots. In UMN disorders, one must check sensation in dermatomal fashion such as C5, C6, C7, etc. Further, though root level lesions (Brachial plexus, intervertebral disc prolapse) are LMN type of lesions, one must check sensation as per dermatome as these roots carry all types of sensations. Various dermatomes of the body are depicted in **Figures 11.5 and 11.6**.

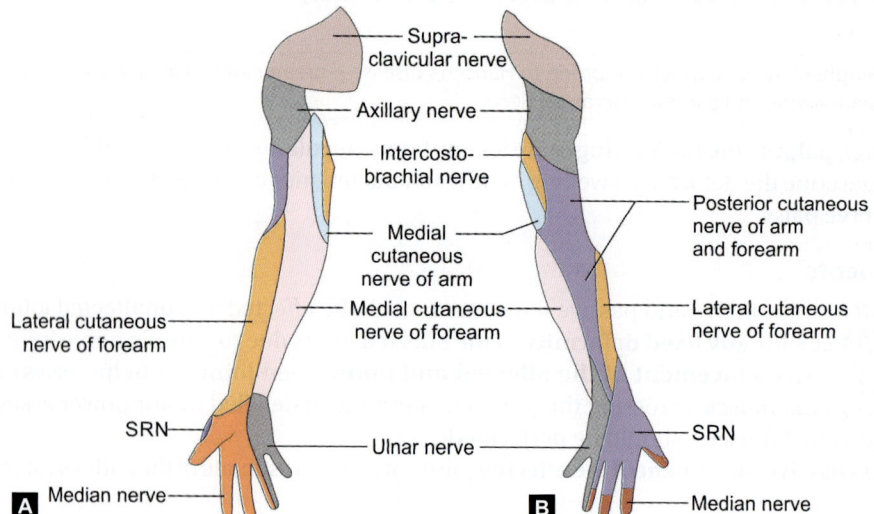

Figs. 11.5 A and B: (A—front; B—back) Sensory innervation of the upper limb. (SRN: superficial radial nerve).

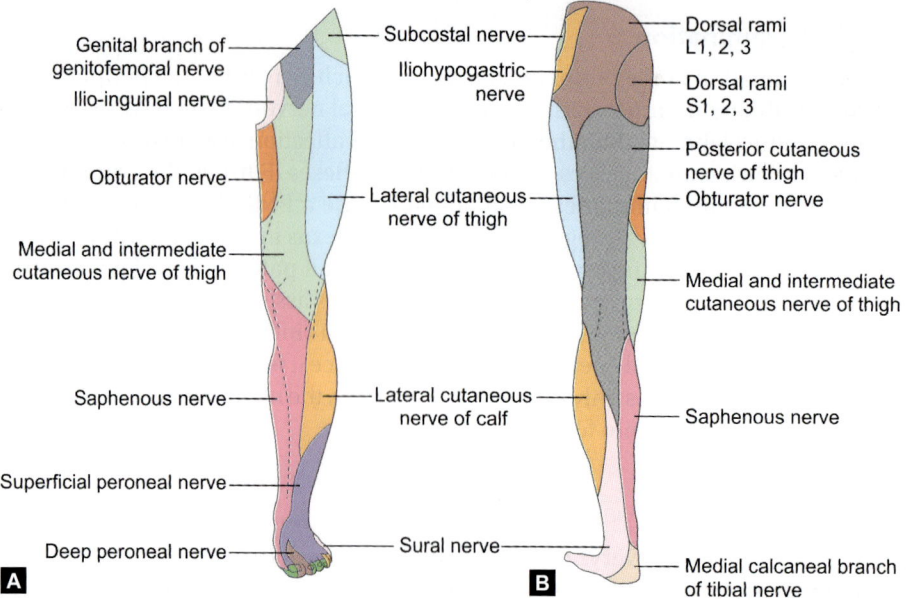

Figs. 11.6A and B: (A—front; B—back) Sensory innervation of the lower limb.

CHAPTER 11 ♦ Clinical Evaluation of the Peripheral Nerves

❑ **PNS/LMN disorder:** The sensory examination is "as per nerve" distribution, and not in a dermatomal fashion because a peripheral nerve is a mixture of many roots. Clinically, one could check the sensation in the 'autonomous zone' rather than the entire nerve area. The autonomous zones of various peripheral nerves are mentioned in **Box 11.3**.

The methodology of sensory examination is mentioned in **Box 11.4**. While 'which sensation' to be checked in CNS and PNS disorder is mentioned in **Box 11.5**.

BOX 11.3: Autonomous zone of major peripheral nerves.

- **Axillary nerve:** Upper lateral aspect of arm (also known as regimental badge sign)
- **Radial nerve:** Dorsum of first web space of the hand
- **Median nerve:** Volar digital pad of the index finger
- **Ulnar nerve:** Ulnar border of the little finger
- **Femoral nerve:** Anterior aspect of the thigh
- **Obturator nerve:** Mid-medial aspect of the thigh
- **Superficial peroneal nerve:** A central strip on dorsum of the foot
- **Deep peroneal nerve:** First interdigital space of dorsum of the foot
- **Saphenous nerve:** Medial border of the foot (ends just before the ball of the great toe)
- **Sural nerve:** Lateral border of the foot
- **Tibial nerve:** Plantar aspect of the foot

BOX 11.4: Method of performing the sensory examination.

- Obtain consent, ensure privacy, and chaperone. Explain to the patient about the examination. Note that sensory examination findings are often incorrectly elicited as the clinician fails to explain the due process of sensory examination to the patient.
- Remove the clothes and expose the part completely. The sensory examination should not be attempted over a part covered with clothing.
- The patient must keep his eyes closed during the sensory examination.
- Perform the sensory test (especially comparative sensations such as touch and temperature) on the normal and index side "simultaneously" and "repeatedly" and ask the patient whether they can feel the sensation, and "if any difference" in sensory perception between the two sides.
- It is also essential to do "negative testing" to ensure that patient has well understood the test and he/she is not malingering. Negative testing means that the part is not touched, but the patient is asked for the response.

BOX 11.5: Which sensation to test in PNS and CNS disorder?

- **In PNS:** A peripheral nerve carries all sensations from skin to the spinal cord. Hence in a peripheral nerve injury, *touch (light/crude) is commonly tested*, which gives a fair assessment of the sensory capability of a nerve.
- **In CNS/UMN type injury:** All the sensations carried by a peripheral nerve are distributed to the spinal cord's three major sensory tracts: posterior column, anterior, and lateral spinothalamic tract. Hence, in case of CNS/UMN, *at least one sensation from each tract* must be checked to confirm the integrity of all three sensory tracts.

> **What is autonomous zone?** An area that is exclusively innervated by *'a particular nerve'* without supply from collateral sprouting of adjacent nerves. Therefore, anesthesia in an autonomous zone indicates a complete lesion of that particular nerve. In contrast, with incomplete nerve lesion, sensation is retained in the autonomous zone.
>
> **What is dermatome?** It is an area of the skin that is innervated by a *'single nerve root'*.

2. **Motor examination:** The motor examination should be performed under the following heads:
   i. The ***bulk of the muscles*** can be observed during the inspection.
   ii. The ***tone of muscles:*** The clinician must gently move the joint several times to assess the tone in the muscles. LMN lesion causes hypotonia/flaccidity in muscles, whereas UMN lesion causes spasticity.
   iii. ***Power of muscles:*** It should be graded according to the MRC (medical research council) grades from 0 to 5, while the patient is asked to move a joint actively. *Grade 0*: No power; *Grade 1*: Slight flicker in muscle while attempting to move the joint; *Grade 2*: Movement of the joint with gravity eliminated; *Grade 3*: Movement of the joint against gravity; *Grade 4*: Movement of the joint against mild-moderate resistance; *Grade 5*: Movement of the joint against complete resistance.

   If the muscle is palpable due to its superficial location, it is essential to palpate the muscle contraction while assessing its power. Note that almost all figures in this chapter show that the clinician keeps his hand over the contracting muscle (if the muscle is palpable) while assessing the strength of the muscle. The methodology to assess the power of muscle is mentioned in **Box 11.6** below.

> **BOX 11.6:** Principles/method of motor power examination.
>
> - Always start power assessment from the "normal" side.
> - Ask the patient to move the joint actively to give a fair idea of any stiffness in the joint. Further, check passive ROM at the affected joint if active ROM is not a full range.
> - Always start with a grade 3 power assessment on the index side. If grade 3 is present, check grade 4 followed by grade 5.
> - If grade 3 is absent, then check grade 2 power followed by grade 1.
> - While assessing the muscle power, always palpate the muscle being tested as sometimes patients use trick movement to move a joint. In addition, the joint movement could be painful in acute injuries along with nerve involvement. In such cases, palpation of the muscle during an attempted joint movement gives an idea of its contractility and innervation.

   iv. ***Reflexes (superficial and deep tendon):*** Both superficial and deep tendon reflexes (DTR) must be assessed in the case of CNS/UMN lesion, whereas only appropriate/applicable DTR should be assessed in PNS/peripheral nerve lesion. The specific nerve injuries will affect following DTRs: *Musculocutaneous nerve*—Biceps reflex; *Radial nerve*—Triceps (proximal lesion), supinator reflex (distal lesion); *Femoral nerve*—Knee reflex; and *Tibial nerve*—Ankle reflex.
   v. ***Coordination and abnormal movements:*** It should be assessed in UMN lesion.
3. **Autonomic nervous system examination** involves examining vasomotor, sudomotor, and pilomotor function.
   The cutaneous ANS functions can be assessed as discussed below.
   i. **Vasomotor function:** A warm and pink limb indicates a limb with normal vasomotor function. A sympathetically dysfunctional limb appears cold and mottled.
   ii. **Sudomotor function:** It implies a function related to a normal sweating pattern over the limb. A sympathetically dysfunctional limb has altered/poor sweating (anhidrosis). It

can also be assessed with starch iodine and axon reflex test. However, it is not routinely performed in clinical practice.

4. **Clinical signs of nerve recovery:**
   i. ***Tinel's sign:*** It is a sign of peripheral nerve recovery. Since Tinel's sign is observed only in the case of a progressive Wallerian regeneration, it is present in axonotmesis and a surgically repaired nerve in neurotmesis due to progressive Wallerian regeneration. *It is absent in neuropraxia as there is no structural damage, and hence, no Wallerian changes.*
   Method: The part is exposed, and the procedure is well explained to the patient that while tapping the nerve, they may experience a tingling or shock-like sensation along the course and distribution of the nerve. Now, gentle tapping is performed with the index finger *along the course of the nerve from distal to proximal.*
   Interpretation and clinical significance: A *positive Tinel's sign* is indicated by the presence of a sudden shock/current-like sensation along the course and distribution of the nerve while the nerve is being tapped.

   ==A Tinel's sign is 'clinically significant' only if it progresses distally with every follow-up.==

   It implies that the tingling/shooting sensation must be elicited at a level distal to the previous one at every follow-up after a few weeks-months, considering that nerve regenerates at the rate of 1 mm/day. For example, a *Tinel's sign* elicited after three months (90 days) of the injury should be elicited approximately 90 mm (9 cm) distal to the original site of injury. *The point is that it must progress distally!*

   If Tinel's sign remains static, i.e., at every follow-up, the shock-like sensations are elicited at the same level with no distal progression; it indicates a neuroma formation as tapping a neuroma too produces a shock-like sensation. Thus, a static Tinel's sign indicates no recovery of the nerve and is a *poor prognostic sign.*

   ii. ***Motor march phenomena:*** It is another sign of nerve recovery where the muscle nearest to the site of injury recovers first, followed by other distal ones as the nerve reinnervates muscles from proximal to distal. For example, in a patient with a radial nerve injury in the spiral groove, the first muscle to recover would be brachioradialis followed by extensor carpi radialis longus and so on (recovery in proximal to distal order).

> **Note:** Tinel's sign and motor march phenomena happen during Wallerian regeneration, observed after axonotmesis or surgically repaired neurotmesis. Tinel's sign and motor march are not observed in neuropraxia, as there is no Wallerian degeneration or regeneration in neuropraxia.

Lymph Node Examination

Examination of the lymph node is important, especially in cases of infection.

Once the local examination of the affected extremity is over, a specific nerve examination should be performed. A total of 15 important nerves supply various muscles around the shoulder girdle, upper and lower limb; ***seven nerves around the shoulder girdle*** (dorsal scapular, spinal accessory, long thoracic, thoracodorsal, medial-lateral pectoral, suprascapular, and upper-lower Subscapular nerves), ***five nerves in the upper limb*** (axillary, musculocutaneous, radial, median and ulnar) and ***three nerves in the lower limb*** (Sciatic with divisions— common peroneal and tibial, femoral and obturator). **Flowcharts 11.1 and 11.2** illustrate the general schema of the nerves supplying the shoulder girdle and upper limb, respectively. This chapter will discuss all the nerves mentioned above except the suprascapular and subscapular (upper and lower) nerve, whose assessment has been discussed in Chapter 4 (Shoulder-rotator cuff).

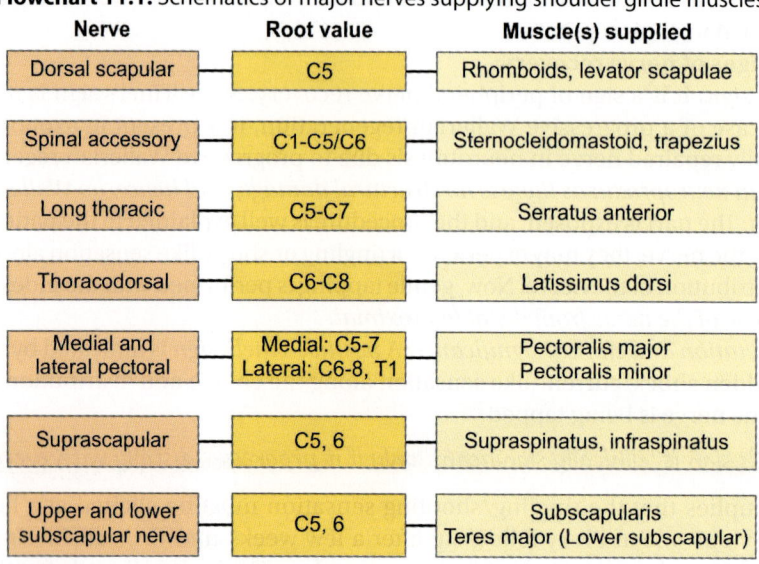

Flowchart 11.1: Schematics of major nerves supplying shoulder girdle muscles.

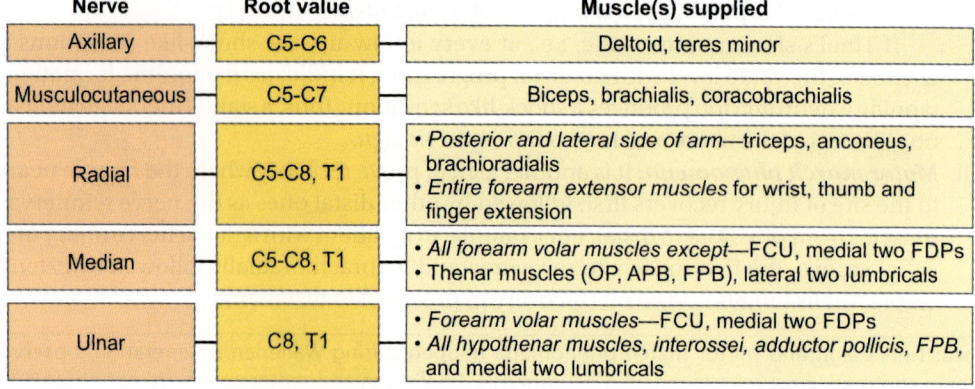

Flowchart 11.2: Schematics of major nerves supplying upper limb muscles.

Note that FPB's superficial head is supplied by recurrent branch of median nerve while deep head is supplied by ulnar nerve.
(FCU: flexor carpi ulnaris; FDP: flexor digitorum profundus; OP: opponens pollicis; APB: abductor pollicis brevis; FPB: flexor pollicis brevis).

The discussion regarding dorsal scapular, spinal accessory, long thoracic and thoracodorsal will remain limited as this chapter is designed to cater undergraduate students.

Individual Peripheral Nerve Examination

Spinal Accessory Nerve (C1–C5, 6)

The spinal portion of the spinal accessory (SA) nerve arises from neurons of the upper spinal cord, specifically C1-C5/C6 spinal nerve roots **(Fig. 11.7A)**. Spinal accessory nerve *supplies sternocleidomastoid and trapezius muscle.* It is often injured in surgeries involving posterior triangle of the neck, such as radical neck dissection or lymph node biopsy.

The motor supply, clinical assessment and features of the spinal accessory nerve paralysis are mentioned in **Table 11.2**.

CHAPTER 11 ♦ Clinical Evaluation of the Peripheral Nerves 249

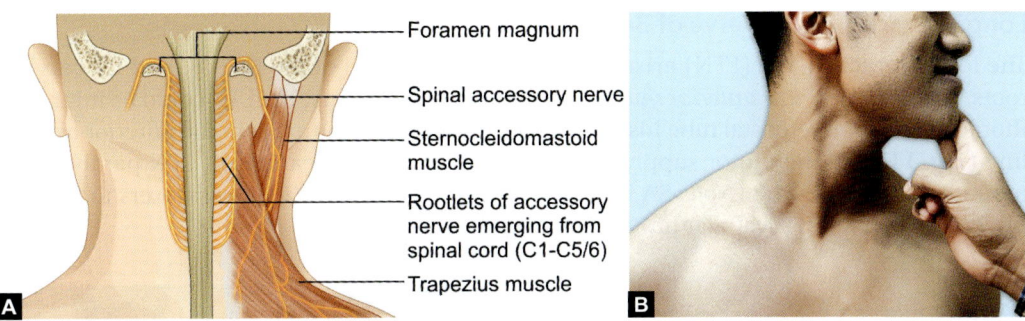

Figs. 11.7A and B

Figs. 11.7A and B: (A) Illustrated figure showing formation and course of the spinal accessory nerve; (B) Test for right side sternocleidomastoid while patient rotates his neck to left side against clinician's resistance.

TABLE 11.2: Muscles supplied by the spinal accessory nerve: its action and evaluation.		
Muscle	Action	How to test function?
Sternocleidomastoid	Rotates the head to the opposite side, tilts the head to same side, and flexes the neck. "Turn-Tilt-Flex"	Ask patient to: • Turn the head to the opposite side (**Fig. 11.7B**) • Tilt the neck to the same side • Flex the neck • Test above movements against and palpate muscle
Trapezius	Elevate and retract scapula	Ask the patient to shrug shoulder against resistance (**Fig. 11.7C**)
Features of spinal accessory nerve paralysis: It results in 'lateral winging' of the scapula (**Fig. 11.7D**) and difficulty to sustain shoulder abduction in the midrange of abduction in the scapular plane		

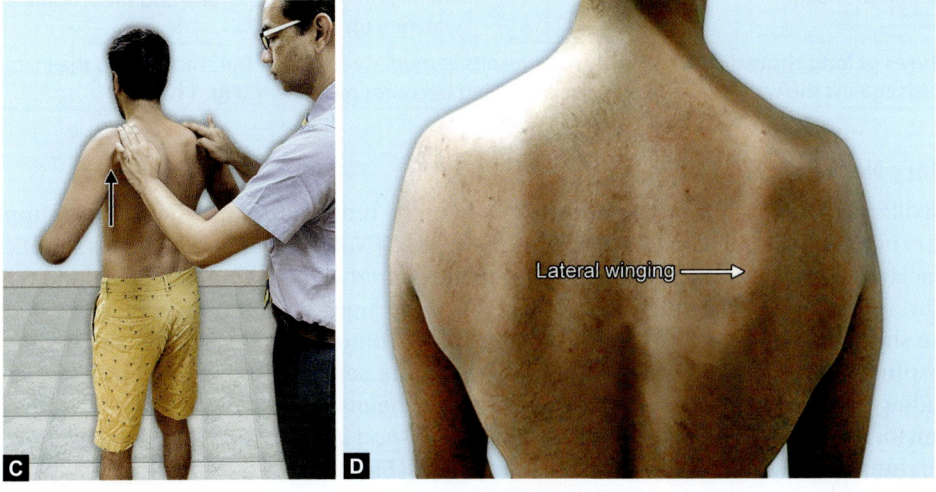

Figs. 11.7C and D

Figs. 11.7C and D: (C) Test for upper trapezius by asking patient to shrug shoulders (black arrow indicates shoulder shrugging by patient); (D) Lateral scapular winging due to weak medial pull (towards spine) of the trapezius.

Long Thoracic Nerve (Nerve of Bell; C5-7)

The long thoracic nerve (LTN) arises from the anterior rami of the C5, C6, and C7 cervical roots. It *supplies serratus anterior muscle*, known as *boxer's muscle*. The LTN could be injured in thoracostomy or intercostal tube insertion as it runs down in the axilla in the anterior axillary line **(Fig. 11.8A)**. The motor supply, clinical assessment, and features of LTN paralysis are mentioned in **Table 11.3** (*Note:* SA is known as boxer's muscle as it allows boxers to throw a forward punch during scapular protraction over the thorax).

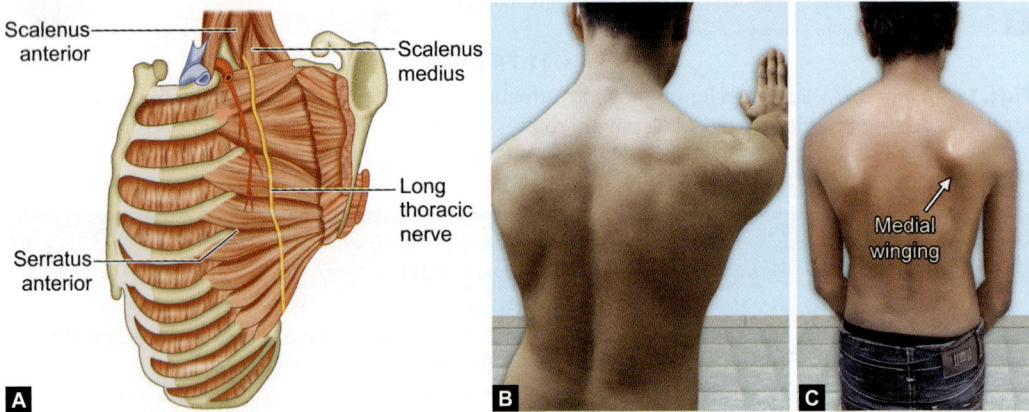

Figs. 11.8A to C: (A) Illustrated figure showing long thoracic nerve; (B) Wall push-up test for serratus anterior; (C) Medial winging in long thoracic nerve palsy.

TABLE 11.3: Muscle supplied by the long thoracic nerve: its action and evaluation.	
The function of serratus anterior (SA)	How to test the function?
SA pulls the scapula forward around thorax, which allows for protraction	The patient is asked to perform repeated push-ups against the wall **(Fig. 11.8B)**, and the scapula is watched for winging
Features of long thoracic nerve paralysis: It results in medial winging of the scapula, and the inability to push against the wall wherein the scapula winging becomes prominent **(Fig. 11.8C)**	

Axillary Nerve (C5, 6)

The axillary nerve arises from the posterior cord of the brachial plexus. The sensory supply of axillary nerve is over the *skin of lower part of the deltoid*. (Note: Upper deltoid skin is supplied by supraclavicular nerves), and motor supply is to the *deltoid and teres minor*. The deltoid muscle has three penna—anterior, middle, and posterior, performing flexion, abduction and extension of the shoulder, respectively. The teres minor inserts onto the greater tuberosity behind the infraspinatus, and is a shoulder external rotator. The sensorimotor functions assessment, including paralysis of the axillary nerve, is discussed below.
 a. **Sensory:** Check sensation over the *lower lateral aspect of the deltoid*. Loss of sensation over this area is known as the "Regimental batch sign" **(Fig. 11.9A)**.
 b. **Motor:** The motor supply, clinical assessment and features of axillary nerve paralysis are mentioned in **Table 11.4**.

TABLE 11.4: Muscles supplied by the axillary nerve: its action and evaluation.

Muscle and its action	Action on shoulder and function assessment
Deltoid: With its tripennate structure, it helps abduct, flex and extend the shoulder joint	• **Anterior penna (Flexion):** With elbow extended and shoulder 90° abducted, the patient is asked to perform horizontal adduction, and the clinician palpates the anterior deltoid fibers • **Middle penna (Abduction):** With the elbow in 90° flexion, the patient is asked to ABduct the shoulder against resistance, while clinician palpates the contraction of the deltoid with the other hand **(Fig. 11.9B)**. • **Posterior penna (Extension):** With elbow extended and shoulder 90° abducted, the patient is asked to perform horizontal extension against resistance, while clinician palpates the posterior deltoid fibers
Teres minor: It is an external rotator of the shoulder	• **Patte's test:** Ask the patient to hold the shoulder in 90° abduction and 90° external rotation while the clinician supports the patient's elbow with one hand. Now, the patient is asked to externally rotate the arm against resistance **(Fig. 11.9C)** • **Hornblower's sign:** Ask the patient to bring his/her hand in front of the mouth, keeping the arm and elbow close to the chest, which requires shoulder external rotation. If the teres minor is paralyzed/completely torn, the patient must lift his elbow by shrugging the shoulder with increased wrist dorsiflexion to bring his/her hand to the mouth **(Fig. 11.9D)**. The attitude of the shrugged shoulder with elevated elbow gives an impression as if the person is attempting to 'blow a horn' giving the name of sign- Hornblower sign!
Features of axillary nerve paralysis: It results in deltoid and teres minor palsy. Deltoid palsy results in loss of contour of the shoulder **(Fig. 11.3C)**, weakness in the shoulder abduction, flexion, and extension. Concomitant paralysis of teres minor results in poor external rotation power (Hornblower's sign). Also, there is loss of sensation over the upper lateral aspect of arm (regimental batch sign)	

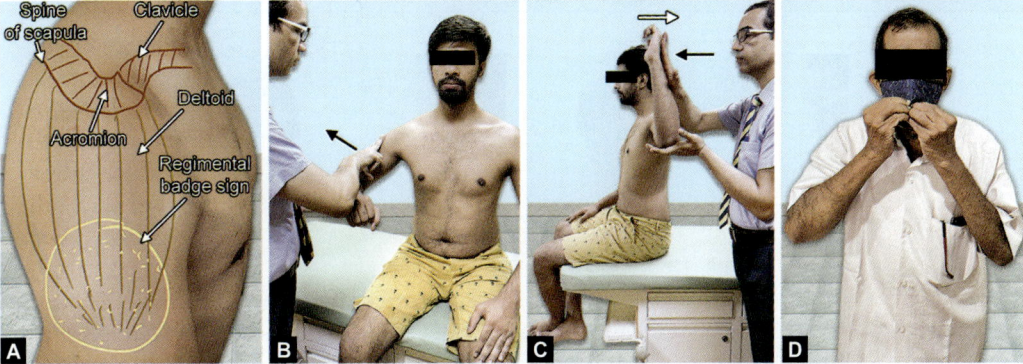

Figs. 11.9A to D: (A) Regimental badge sign; (B) Test for the deltoid middle penna (black arrow depicts abduction by the patient); (C) Patte's test (White arrow shows external rotation attempt by the patient while black arrow depicts clinician's resistance); (D) Hornblower's sign (Right elbow is elevated more than left to reach mouth).

Musculocutaneous Nerve (C5-7)

The musculocutaneous nerve is the terminal branch of the lateral cord of the brachial plexus (C5-7). It innervates the lateral aspect of the forearm via the lateral cutaneous nerve of the forearm for sensation, and motor supply goes to the biceps brachii, brachialis, and coracobrachialis. The nerve can get injured in surgeries around shoulder, such as Laterjet procedure for anterior shoulder instability. The sensorimotor functions assessment of the musculocutaneous nerve is discussed below.

a. **Sensory:** Check for sensations over lateral aspect of the forearm
b. **Motor:** The motor supply, clinical assessment and features of musculocutaneous nerve paralysis are mentioned in **Table 11.5**. Further, one must check biceps reflex in case of musculocutaneous nerve injury.

Radial Nerve (C5-8, T1)

The radial nerve is a terminal branch of the posterior cord of the brachial plexus (C5-8, T1). It provides sensation to the dorsum of the hand (radial 3½ fingers) via the superficial radial nerve.

TABLE 11.5: Major muscles supplied by the musculocutaneous nerve: its action and evaluation.

Muscle	Action	How to test function?
Biceps	• Elbow flexor • Forearm supinator	Keep the patient's elbow in 90° flexion and *forearm supinated*, and ask the patient to flex the elbow against resistance further while the clinician palpates the biceps muscle contraction in the arm (Fig. 11.10A)
Brachialis	Elbow flexion	Keep patient's elbow in 90° flexion and *forearm pronated*, and ask the patient to flex the elbow against resistance further while clinician palpates brachialis medial to the biceps muscle in the arm (Fig. 11.10B)

Features of the musculocutaneous nerve paralysis: It results in loss of elbow flexion, mild loss of supination strength of the forearm, and loss of sensation over the lateral aspect of the forearm.

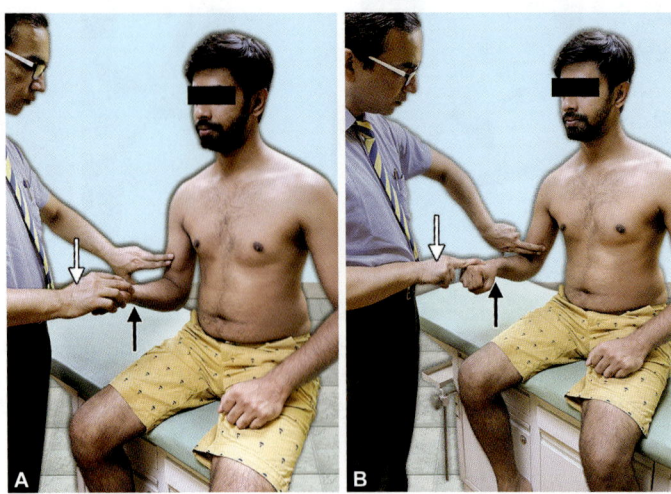

Figs. 11.10A and B: (A) Biceps assessment with forearm supinated; (B) Brachialis assessment with forearm pronated. White and black arrows indicate clinicians resistance and patient's effort, respectively.

Course and motor innervation: The radial nerve innervates the long head of the triceps before entering the spiral groove, while medial and lateral heads of the triceps and anconeus are innervated after entering the spiral groove. After supplying the triceps and anconeus, the radial nerve pierces the lateral intermuscular septum, emerges on the anterolateral aspect of the arm, descends, and supplies brachioradialis and extensor carpi radialis longus (ECRL). Near the elbow joint, the radial nerve divides into two branches—a superficial sensory branch (superficial radial nerve, SRN) and a deep, pure motor branch, posterior interosseous nerve (PIN). After crossing the elbow, PIN enters forearm under the tunnel of supinator. The *PIN* supplies the extensor carpi radialis brevis (ECRB), supinator and muscles of the entire extensor compartment of the forearm. Note that, PIN has no sensory component. The SRN descends in the forearm under the belly of the brachioradialis, innervates the dorsal skin of the thumb and radial 3½ fingers, excluding the dorsum of the thumb and radial 2½ distal phalanx, and radial 1/2 of distal phalanx of the ring finger, which are supplied by the median nerve.

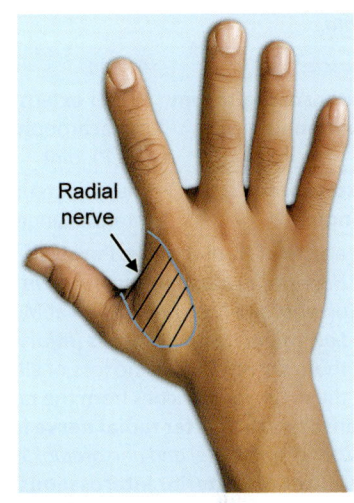

Fig. 11.11A

Fig. 11.11A: Autonomous zone of radial nerve (1st dorsal web space-hashed area)

There are two common areas of injury to the radial nerve; spiral groove (in midshaft fracture humerus) and near the lateral supracondylar ridge (Holstein Lewis fracture or supracondylar fracture). The PIN commonly gets injured in Monteggia fracture dislocation. The sensorimotor function assessment of the radial nerve is discussed below.

a. **Sensory:** Assess the sensation in the autonomous zone of the radial nerve that lies over the *dorsum of the first web space of the hand* (**Fig. 11.11A**).
b. **Motor:** The motor supply, clinical assessment and features of radial nerve paralysis are mentioned in **Table 11.6**. Further, one must check triceps and supinator reflex in case of high and low radial nerve injury, respectively.

TABLE 11.6: Major muscles supplied by the radial nerve: its action and evaluation.

Muscle	Action	How to test function?
Triceps	Elbow extension	Ask the patient to keep the shoulder 90° abduction, internal rotation, and elbow in 90° flexion. Now the patient is asked to extend the elbow against resistance, and the clinician palpates the triceps for contractions (**Fig. 11.11B**)
Brachioradialis	Weak elbow flexor and forearm supinator	With the forearm in mid-prone, ask the patient to flex the elbow against resistance. The brachioradialis stands prominently on the forearm's radial border, palpated by the clinician (**Fig. 11.11C**).
Extensor carpi radialis longus	Wrist extension and radial deviation	Ask the patient to extend his wrist and radially deviate against resistance applied by the clinician on the patient's metacarpals (**Fig. 11.11D**)

Contd...

Contd...

Muscle	Action	How to test function?
Extensor digitorum communis	Finger extension at metacarpophalangeal (MCP) joint	*Keeping PIP and DIP flexed*, ask patient to extend the MCPs against resistance on the proximal phalanx of the fingers and palpate the muscle **(Fig. 11.11E)**
Extensor pollicis longus	Thumb extension at interphalangeal (IP) joint	The patient is asked to extend his thumb against resistance on the terminal phalanx of the thumb **(Fig. 11.11F)**.

Features of Radial Nerve Paralysis
1. **High radial nerve palsy (injury in the axilla):** It results in loss of elbow extension (Triceps palsy), loss of wrist and finger extension at MCP joint leading to "wrist, finger with thumb drop" **(Fig. 11.3A)**.
2. **Low radial nerve paralysis (injury in the radial groove and below):** It results in "Wrist, finger with thumb drop." There is no loss of elbow extension as the long head of the triceps is already supplied by the proximal branches from the radial nerve arising before it enters the spiral groove.

Sensory deficit after radial nerve injury: *Loss of sensation over the dorsum of first web space (autonomous zone) and dorsoradial 3½ fingers.*

Features of Posterior Interosseous Nerve (PIN) Palsy
PIN palsy results only in "finger and thumb drop" while elbow extension and wrist extension-radial deviation are spared due to intact triceps and ECRL, respectively. No sensory loss is observed in isolated PIN palsy as it is a pure motor nerve.

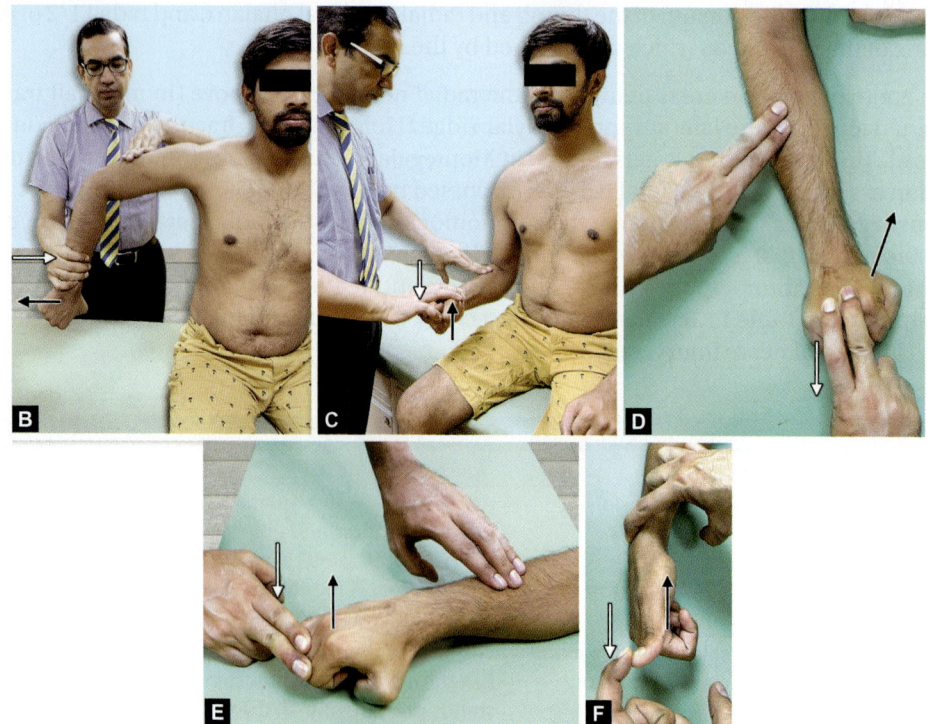

Figs. 11.11 B to F

Figs. 11.11B to F: (B) Test for triceps; (C) Test for brachioradialis (white arrow depicts clinician's resistance while black one depicts patient's push); (D) Test for ECRL; (E) Test for EDC; (F) Test for EPL (ECRL: extensor carpi radialis longus; ECU: extensor carpi ulnaris; EPL: extensor pollicis longus; EDC: extensor digitorum communis). White and black arrows indicate clinicians resistance and patient's effort, respectively.

> **Summary of Radial nerve injury**
> A typical radial nerve palsy results in wrist, thumb, and finger drop **(Fig. 11.3A)** with loss of sensation over the 1st dorsal web space.
> The PIN palsy causes only thumb and finger drop and no sensory loss.

Median Nerve (C5-8, T1)

The median nerve is formed by the unification of the medial and lateral cord of the brachial plexus (C5-8, T1). It carries sensation from the thumb, lateral 3½ volar aspect of fingers and palm area, including the dorsum of the tip of the same fingers and thumb.

The median nerve innervates all forearm flexors except flexor carpi ulnaris (FCU) and medial two tendons of flexor digitorum profundus (FDP), which are innervated by the ulnar nerve. In hand, the median nerve innervates *lateral two lumbricals and thenar muscles* (opponens pollicis, abductor pollicis brevis, and superficial head of flexor pollicis brevis). The deep head of flexor pollicis brevis is supplied by the ulnar nerve. Median nerve injuries are seen in injuries around elbow (supracondylar fracture, elbow dislocation) or around the wrist (lunate dislocation, Smith's fracture). Compressive neuropathy of median nerve is seen in Carpal tunnel syndrome. Median nerve's sensory and motor functions assessment is discussed below.

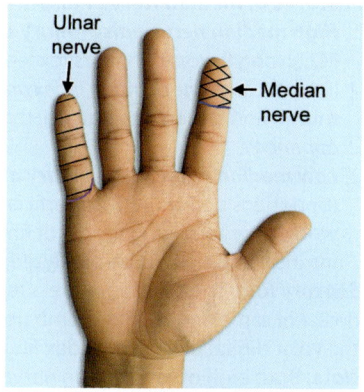

Fig. 11.12A

Fig. 11.12A: Autonomous zones of the median and ulnar nerves

a. **Sensory:** The autonomous zone lies over the volar digital pad of the index finger **(Fig. 11.12A)**.
b. **Motor:** The clinical assessment and paralysis of several muscles supplied by the median nerve are mentioned in **Table 11.7**, while others are mentioned below in detail for better understanding.

TABLE 11.7: Muscles supplied by the median nerve: its action and evaluation.

Muscle	Action	How to test function?
Pronators	Forearm pronation	Keep the elbow in 90° flexion and forearm in mid-prone. Patient is asked to pronate forearm against clinician's resistance who tries to supinate it **(Fig. 11.12C)**
Flexor carpi radialis	Flexion of the wrist, radial deviation	Ask the patient to flex the wrist and radial deviate and apply resistance in the opposite direction (extension and ulnar deviation) **(Fig. 11.12D)**
Flexor pollicis longus	Thumb flexion at IP joint	Ask patient to flex thumb IP joint against resistance and palpate the muscle **(Fig. 11.12E)**
Flexor digitorum superficialis (FDS)	Flexion of the PIP joint	The technique is described below **(Fig. 11.12F)**
Flexor digitorum profundus (FDP)— lateral two tendons	Flexion of the DIP joint	The technique is described below **(Fig. 11.12G)**
Abductor pollicis brevis (APB)	Abduction of the thumb	*Pen test* (described below) **(Fig. 11.12H)**

Contd...

Contd...

Muscle	Action	How to test function?
Opponens pollicis	The opposition of thumb against all fingers	The patient is asked to bring the thumb tip against the little fingertip, and the clinician can try separating it while the patient resists it **(Fig. 11.12I)**

Features of Median Nerve Palsy
1. **High median nerve palsy (injury at the elbow):** It is characterized by *paralysis of wrist flexors* (except FCU), long flexors of fingers (except medial two FDPs), *thenar muscles*, and *lateral two lumbricals*. In such cases, *the pointing index and OK sign* will positively signify paralysis of the long flexor of the thumb and fingers. In addition, thenar muscle palsy would result in a *positive pen test and weak opponens*.
2. **Low median nerve palsy (injury at the wrist):** It is characterized by *paralysis of thenar muscles* (opponens pollicis, APB, superficial head of flexor pollicis brevis) and *lateral two lumbricals*, whereas wrist flexors and long flexors of fingers (FDS, lateral two FDP) are spared. In such a case, only thenar intrinsic muscles will be paralyzed, resulting in a *positive pen test and weak opponens*.

Sensory loss: The sensations are affected over thumb, lateral 3½ fingers and palm on volar aspect and dorsal of same fingers and thumb up to nail beds. The autonomous zone of the median nerve is over the volar digital pad of the index finger.

Note: Both high or low median nerve palsy leads to *"Ape thumb deformity/Simian hand,"* wherein the patient cannot perform opposition due to palsy of opponens pollicis. The thumb lies in the plane of the palm, adducted and rotated, unable to abduct and oppose to the tip of the little finger **(Fig. 11.12B)**. However, it must be noted that classic *"Ape thumb deformity"* is observed in the combined median and ulnar nerve palsy and not in the lone median nerve palsy.

A clinical presentation of the patient with median nerve injury shows wasting of thenar muscles with the *thumb lying in the plane of the palm* with an *inability to oppose and abduct the thumb* **(Fig. 11.12B)**. Other clinical signs associated with median nerve palsy are the *pointing index (Oshner clasping index), pen test, OK sign* and *Benediction sign*.

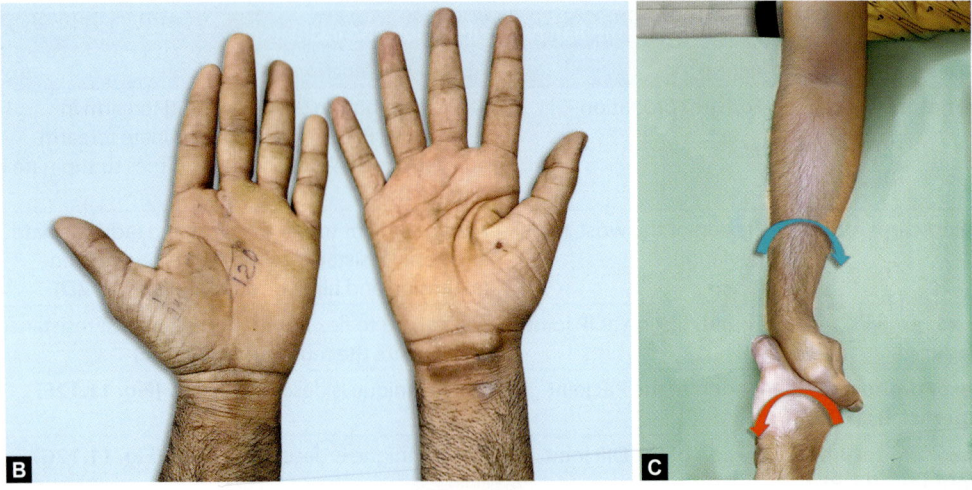

Figs. 11.12 B and C

Figs. 11.12B and C: (B) Wasting of right thenar muscles with thumb adducted to the index finger (Simian hand); (C) Test for pronators. Blue arrow indicates pronation by the patient while red arrow indicates supination resistance by the clinician.

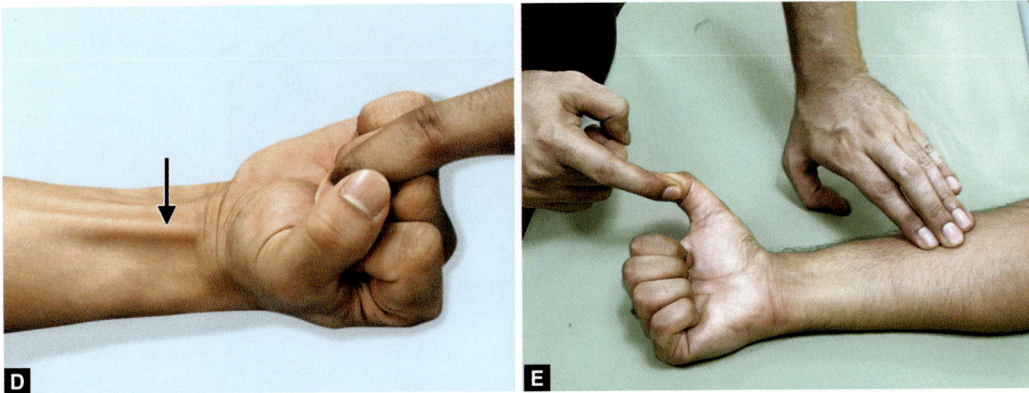

Figs. 11.12D and E

Figs. 11.12D and E: (D) Test for flexor carpi radialis. Black arrow indicates prominent tendon of FCR; (E) Test for flexor pollicis longus.

> **What is anterior interosseous nerve?**
> It is the deep motor branch of median nerve which runs deep in the forearm supplying flexor pollicis longus, pronator quadratus, and lateral FDP. Its paralysis results in inability to flex interphalangeal joint of thumb and DIP joint of index finger causing inablity to make a 'OK' sign. However, thumb muscles remain normal.

The method to test FDS and FDP muscles and other important clinical signs of median nerve palsy (pointing index, pen test, OK sign and Benediction sign) are discussed below.

  i. **Flexor digitorum superficialis (FDS) test:** The FDS is responsible for flexion at the proximal interphalangeal (PIP) joint of four fingers.
    Method: The patient is asked to lay his/her hand flat on the table. The clinician keeps his hand over the other three extended fingers to block FDP action, and "finger to-be-tested" is left free. Then, the clinician asks the patient to flex his "free finger repeatedly." The flexion happens only at the PIP joint of the free finger. The same action is repeated for all four fingers, keeping others blocked **(Fig. 11.12F)**. The rationale of immobilizing three fingers to test the individual FDS power of fourth finger is explained in **Box 11.7**.
  ii. **Flexor digitorum profundus (FDP) test:** The FDP is responsible for flexion at the distal interphalangeal joint (DIP) flexion.
    Method: The patient is asked to lay his hand flat on the table. For a particular finger's FDP to be tested, the clinician holds the middle phalanx from the side and stabilizes it. Then, the patient is asked to flex DIP, and the clinician gives resistance over the fingertip **(Fig. 11.12G)**.

> **Note:** One must avoid holding the middle phalanx in a volar-dorsal fashion as that interferes with the FDP tendon's excursion **(Fig. 11.12G)**.

  iii. **Thumb abduction "Pen test" for abductor pollicis brevis (APB):**
    Method: The patient is asked to lay his hand flat on a table. A pen is held above the thumb, and the patient is asked to touch the pen by abducting his thumb, while APB muscle contraction in the thenar eminence is palpated by the clinician **(Fig. 11.12H)**. If APB is paralyzed, the thumb will not touch the pen.

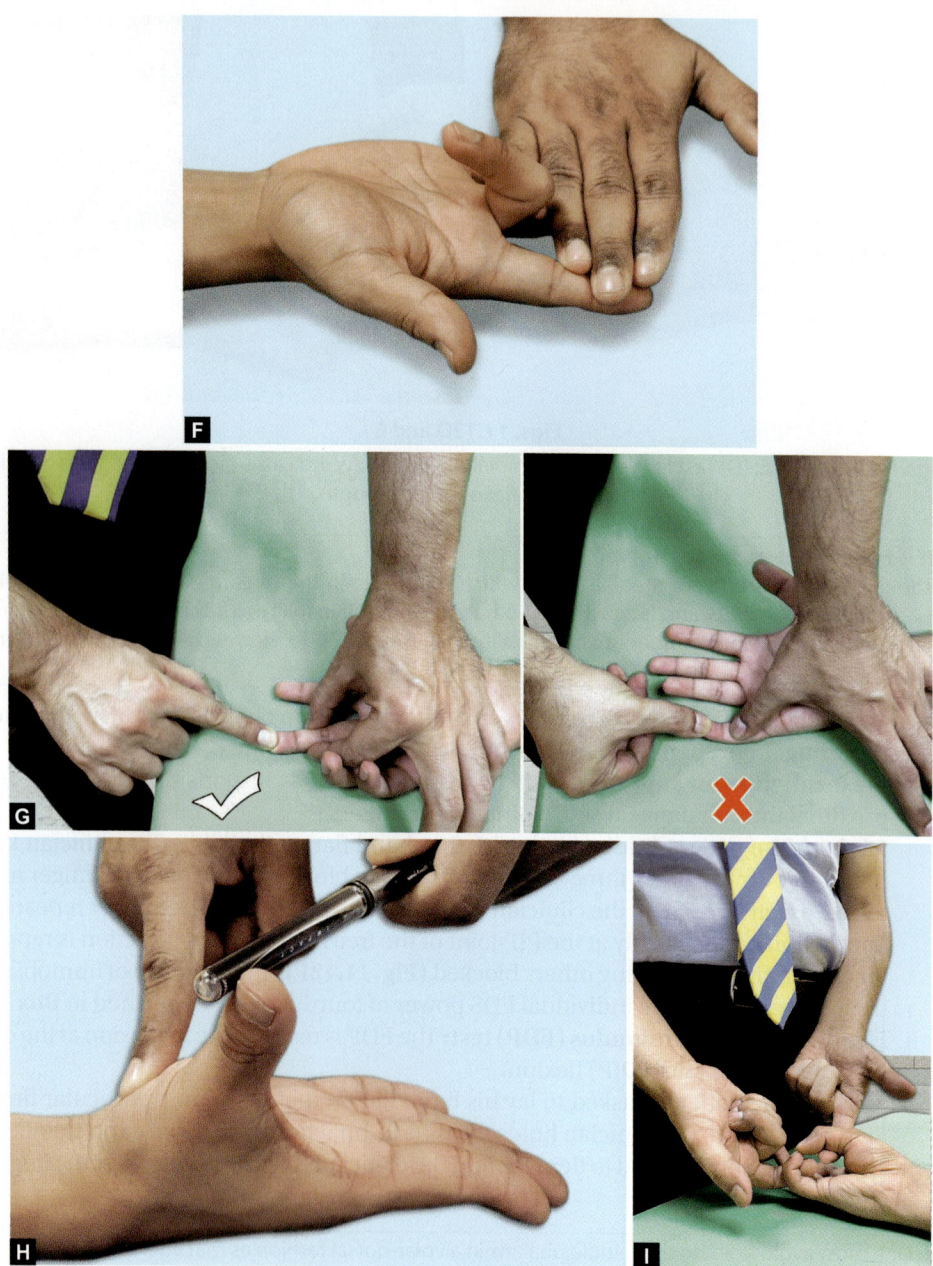

Figs. 11.12 F to I

Figs. 11.12F to I: (F) Test for FDS for PIP joint flexion. Note that FDP action of other three fingers is blocked by keeping them extended; (G) Testing FDP for DIP joint flexion. Left image shows correct method where the clinician holds the middle phalanx from side, whereas right image shows incorrect method of holding middle phalanx wherein the clinician is holding the middle phalanx from above obstructing the FDP excursion; (H) Pen test for APB. The clinician is palpating the contracting APB with his finger; (I) Test for opponens pollicis.

(FDS and FDP: flexor digitorum superficialis and profundus; APB: abductor pollicis brevis; PIP: proximal interphalangeal; DIP: distal interphalangeal).

> **BOX 11.7:** Anatomic basis of FDS test.
>
> FDS tendon inserts over the volar aspect of the middle phalanx base, and is responsible for flexion at the PIP joint. However, FDP while crossing the PIP joint also causes secondary PIP joint flexion. Hence, FDP interferes with the functional assessment of FDS, and therefore, one needs to block the FDP action while assessing the FDS action. Anatomically, FDP tendons share a common muscle belly, especially for medial three fingers. Therefore, by blocking the action of one or more FDP tendons (keeping fingers extended), the other free FDP tendon cannot act in isolation. Hence, *to check the FDS function, the action of FDP has to be blocked by keeping fingers extended!*

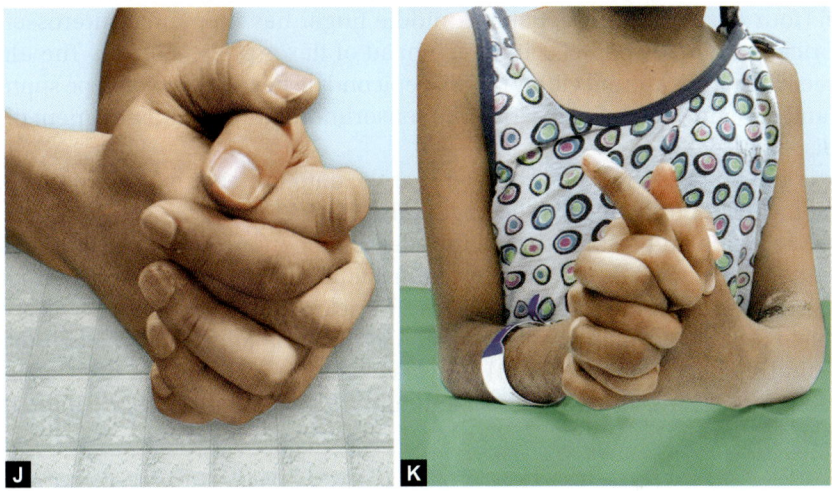

Figs. 11.12 J and K

Figs. 11.12J and K: (J) Normal clasping; (K) Ochsner's clasping or pointing index sign.

iv. **Pointing index sign/Ochsner's clasping sign:** The Ochsner's clasping sign is observed in high median nerve injury due to palsy of long finger flexors (FDS and lateral two FDP).
Method: When a person with intact median nerve is asked to clasp both hands together, all the fingers close easily due to normally innervated long finger flexors **(Fig. 11.12J)**. In a patient with high median nerve injury [affecting the all flexor digitorum superficialis (FDS) and lateral two flexor digitorum profundus (FDP)], the index finger fails to flex at PIP and DIP joint and remains as a "pointing index finger" **(Fig. 11.12K)**.

v. **Benediction sign or Preacher's hand:** Benediction sign is observed in high median nerve palsy. The patient is asked to close the fist of the affected hand. In patients with high median nerve palsy with paralysis of lateral two FDPs, the patient can flex little and middle finger for fist closure as medial two FDPs are supplied by the ulnar nerve. However, the index and middle finger flexion are not possible due to paralysis of lateral two FDPs, and hence fist cannot be closed.

Summary of Median Nerve Injury Signs
1. Wasting of the forearm (volar) and thenar muscles
2. Weak opposition

3. Positive pen test
4. Pointing index sign (positive only in high median nerve palsy)

Ulnar Nerve (C8, T1)

The ulnar nerve arises from the medial cord of the brachial plexus. It carries sensation from volar and dorsal aspects of medial 1½ fingers. Regarding motor supply in the forearm, ulnar nerve innervates flexor carpi ulnaris (FCU) and medial two heads of FDP. Then, the ulnar nerve *crosses the wrist under Guyon's canal* and innervates the muscles of hypothenar eminence (abductor digiti minimi, opponens digiti minimi, and flexor digiti minimi) followed by all interossei (four dorsal and three palmar-middle finger has no palmar interossei), medial two lumbricals, adductor pollicis, and deep head of flexor pollicis brevis. The ulnar nerve injury is seen in injuries around elbow (Medial epicondyle fracture, flexion type supracondylar fracture) and other injuries around wrist. The sensorimotor functions assessment of the ulnar nerve is discussed below.

a. **Sensory:** The sensation must be checked over the autonomous zone of ulnar nerve, which lies over the ulnar border of the little finger **(Fig. 11.13A)**.
b. **Motor:** The action and test for several muscles are mentioned in **Table 11.8**, while others are mentioned below in detail for better understanding. The typical low ulnar nerve palsy results in wasting of hypothenar and interossei muscles and a ***claw hand***. A typical claw hand deformity is characterized by hyperextension at the MCP joint and flexion at the IP joints of little and ring finger **(Fig. 11.13B)**. The claw hand results from an imbalance between paralyzed intrinsic muscles (interossei and lumbricals) and intact extrinsic muscle (long flexors and extensors).

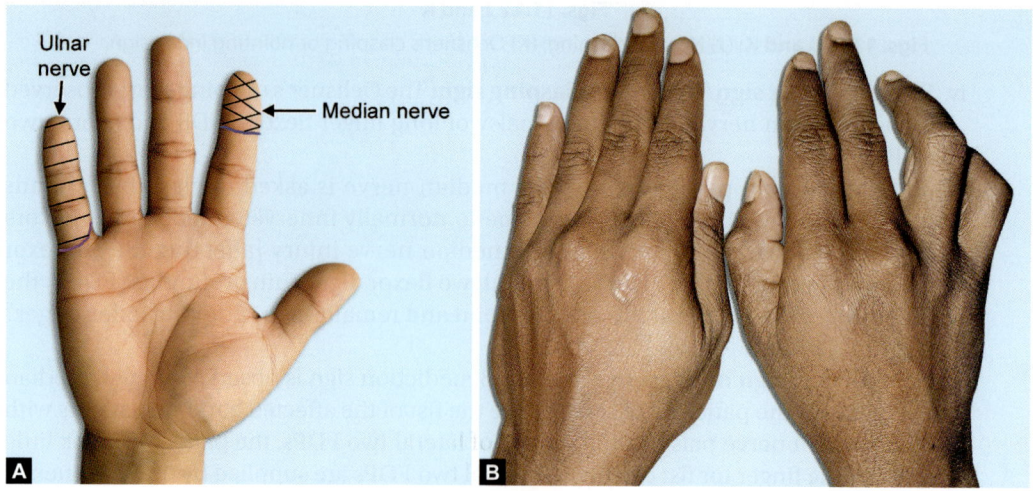

Figs. 11.13 A and B

Figs. 11.13A and B: (A) Autonomous zone of the ulnar nerve; (B) A classic ulnar claw hand showing MCP joint hyperextension and IP joint flexion of little and ring finger along with wasting of interossei muscles in right hand.

(FCU: flexor carpi ulnaris; FPB: flexor pollicis brevis; ADM: abductor digiti minimi; FDM: flexor digiti minimi; ODM: opponens digiti minimi.)

TABLE 11.8: Muscles supplied by the ulnar nerve: its action and evaluation.

Muscle	Action	How to test function?
Flexor carpi ulnaris (FCU)	Flexion and ulnar deviation of the wrist	Ask the patient to flex his wrist and ulnar deviate against resistance. The taut FCU tendon can be palpated on the ulnar side of the wrist **(Fig. 11.13C)**
FDP of medial two fingers	Flexion at the DIP joint	The method to assess the FDP tendon is already described in the median nerve section (vide supra)
Abductor digiti minimi	Abduction of the little finger	The patient is asked to abduct his little finger against resistance while the clinician palpates the taut ADM over the hypothenar eminence **(Fig. 11.13D)**
Dorsal interossei	• Abduction of fingers • MCP joint flexion and IP joint extension	Ask the patient to abduct his index finger against resistance and palpate the first dorsal interosseous muscle between the thumb and index finger **(Fig. 11.13E)**
Palmar interossei	• Adduction of fingers • MCP joint flexion and IP joint extension	***Card test:*** The patient is asked to hold a card in between his fingers as tightly as possible, and the clinician tries to pull it off with the same fingers of his same side hand. For example, if the patient holds the card between the index and middle finger of the left hand, the clinician should also hold the card between the index and middle finger of his left hand. In case of weak interossei, it is easy to pull out the card **(Fig. 11.13F)**.
Adductor pollicis	Adduction of thumb	***Book test/Froment's sign:*** The patient is asked to hold a book between his thumb and index finger, and the clinician also holds it in the same way. Then, the clinician tries to pull the book away from the patient while the patient is asked to resist slipping the book away from his/her hand. In a normal adductor pollicis, the book is held between the adducted thumb and index finger with thumb IP join extended (green arrow, **Fig. 11.13G**). In the case of adductor pollicis palsy, the patient uses his flexor pollicis longus (supplied by median nerve) to hold the book resulting in a thumb flexed at the IP joint (red arrow) **(Fig. 11.13G)**. *Note: It is vital to hold the book between thumb and index finger, which are kept parallel, rather than holding the book in a pinch fashion.*

Features of Ulnar Nerve Palsy
1. ***High ulnar nerve palsy (injury at the elbow):*** In high ulnar nerve affection, there is palsy of wrist flexors (FCU) and long-finger flexors (medial two FDP), hypothenar muscles, medial two lumbrical, interossei, and adductor pollicis. Further, high ulnar nerve injury results in classic *ulnar paradox is observed.*
2. ***Low ulnar nerve palsy (injury at the wrist):*** In low ulnar nerve injury, *FCU and medial two FDP are spared, whereas* hypothenar muscles, medial two lumbrical, interossei, and adductor pollicis are paralyzed.
   Low ulnar palsy results in classic *"claw hand" deformity (intrinsic minus hand)* characterized by *hyperextension at MCP and flexion at IP joints of little and ring finger* **(Fig. 11.3B)**.
3. ***Sensory loss:*** There is loss of sensation over the medial 1½ fingers and corresponding palm area on both dorsal and volar aspects **(Fig. 11.13H)**.

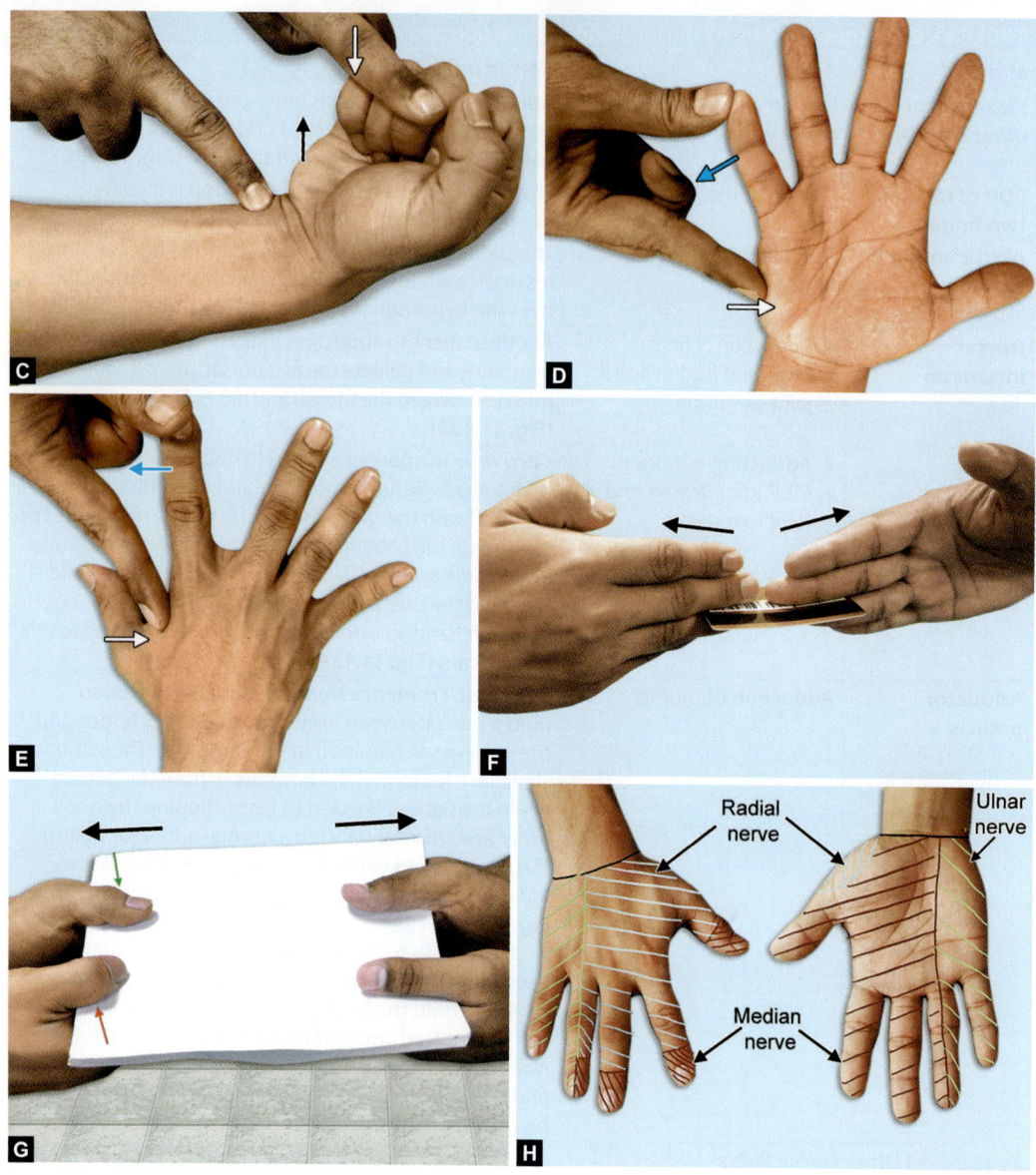

Figs. 11.13 C to H

Figs. 11.13C to F: (C) Test for flexor carpi ulnaris; (D) Test for abductor digiti minimi (ADM). Blue arrow indicates little finger abduction against resistance and white arrow indicates palpation of ADM by the clinician; (E) Test for first dorsal interosseous muscle. Blue arrow indicates abduction by index finger interosseous, and white arrow indicates palpation of 1st dorsal interosseous by the clinician; (F) Card test for interosseous; (G) Book test or Froment's sign for adductor pollicis. Black arrows in opposite direction show patient's and clinician's attempt to pull the book to their side. Green arrow indicates intact left adductor pollicis while red arrow shows paralysed adductor compensated by thumb flexion at the IP joint; (H) Sensory innervation of the hand by all three nerves on dorsal (left image) and volar aspect (right image).

Several other vital signs and phenomena associated with ulnar nerve palsy are discussed below.
i. **Ulnar paradox:** An important phenomenon associated with ulnar nerve palsy is the ulnar paradox characterized by mild deformity in hand with higher ulnar nerve injury and severe deformity of the hand with low ulnar nerve injury **(Box 11.8)**.

BOX 11.8: Ulnar paradox.

Typically *higher the neurological lesion*, severe is the paralysis, and consequently, a *more apparent deformity is observed in the affected extremity*. However, there is a paradox in patients with ulnar nerve lesions where the *deformity in hand is milder in higher lesions* near the elbow and *severe in lower lesions* near the wrist! The explanation is discussed below.
- **In lower-level lesion of the ulnar nerve near the wrist:** It leads to classic claw hand with MCP hyperextension and IP flexion. In such patients, only intrinsic muscles of the hand supplied by the ulnar nerve (interossei and lumbricals) are paralyzed, whereas long-finger flexors are intact. Typically, lumbricals and interossei cause MCP joint flexion and IP joint extension. Since interossei and lumbricals are paralyzed, the unopposed action of long finger MCP extensors (from the radial nerve) and long finger flexor (by median and ulnar nerve) hyperextend MCP joint and flex the IP joints, respectively giving the hand a typical claw appearance.
- **In higher-level lesion of the ulnar nerve near the elbow:** In higher lesions of ulnar nerve, along with palsy of the interossei and lumbrical palsy, FDP to the fourth and fifth finger is also paralyzed, leading to decreased flexion at IP joints. Meanwhile, finger extensors extend the finger. Therefore, clawing is "not so prominent or obvious".

This is the paradox in ulnar nerve injuries that higher ulnar nerve lesions at the elbow level result in lesser clawing than lower lesions at the wrist level causing prominent clawing.

---

ii. **Tardy ulnar nerve palsy:** Sometimes, certain conditions around the elbow, such as the non-union of lateral condyle fracture, can result in *late-onset ulnar nerve palsy*, known as "Tardy ulnar nerve palsy" **(Box 11.9)**.

BOX 11.9: Tardy ulnar nerve palsy.

It is a condition wherein there is delayed (Tardy) or gradual onset neuropathy of the ulnar nerve after several months or years of the initial pathology. It commonly occurs after non-union of the lateral condyle humerus fracture, leading to gradual cubitus valgus deformity. A progressive cubitus valgus results in stretching and friction neuritis of the ulnar nerve followed by peri- and intra-neural fibrosis, affecting its sensorimotor function.

Summary of Ulnar Nerve Signs
1. Wasting of hypothenar and interossei muscles. 1st web space interosseous wasting is the earliest sign of ulnar nerve injury.
2. Ulnar clawing
3. Card test
4. Froment's sign

Examination of the Lower Limb Nerves

Three important nerves innervate the lower limb—femoral, obturator, and sciatic. The latter divides into common peroneal and the tibial nerve.

Femoral Nerve (Dorsal Division of Anterior Primary Rami of L2, L3, L4)

The femoral nerve originates from the dorsal division of the anterior primary rami of L2-4 nerve roots. It descends through the substance of psoas major, innervates iliacus muscle, and

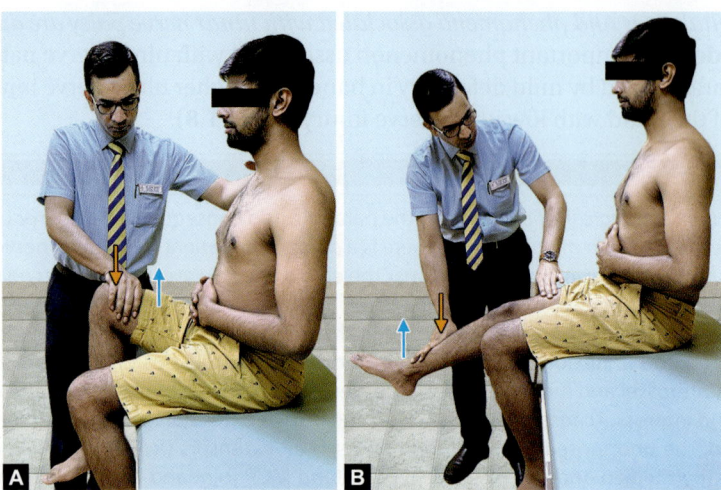

Figs. 11.14A and B: (A) Test for hip flexor- patient attempting hip flexion against resistance; (B) Test for knee extensors (quadriceps). Patient is attempting knee extension against resistance while clinician is palpating quadriceps. Blue arrow denotes patients attempt while orange arrow denotes clinician's resistance.

divides into anterior and posterior divisions. The anterior division has anterior cutaneous branches and supplies pectineus and sartorius, while posterior division innervates quadriceps and gives rise to the saphenous nerve. The femoral nerve injury can occur in anterior hip dislocation, anterior surgical approach to the hip, hysterectomy, urogynecological surgeries, or penetrating injuries to groin or thigh. The sensorimotor function assessment of the femoral nerve is discussed below.

a. **Sensory:** Assess sensations over *anteromedial aspect of the thigh* and *anteromedial aspect of the leg and foot* (saphenous nerve).
b. **Motor:** It involves assessment of hip flexor and knee extensors.
   i. *Hip flexor strength assessment:* With the patient sitting on the couch, ask him/her to flex the hip against the resistance **(Fig. 11.14A)**.
   ii. *Knee extensor (Quadriceps) strength assessment:* With the patient sitting on the couch, ask him/her to extend the knee against resistance while the clinician palpates quadriceps for contraction **(Fig. 11.14B)**.

Paralysis of the femoral nerve: It would result in weakness of the quadriceps muscle. Consequently, patient would be unable to extend his/her knee.

Obturator Nerve (Ventral Division of Anterior Primary Rami of L2, L3, L4)

The obturator nerve originates from the ventral division of anterior primary rami of L2-4 nerve roots. It supplies all hip adductors (adductor longus, adductor brevis, adductor part of adductor magnus), gracilis, and obturator externus. The sensory and motor function assessment of obturator nerve is discussed below.

a. **Sensory:** Middle part of medial aspect of the thigh
b. **Motor:** Ask the patient to adduct his thigh against resistance, while clinician palpates adductor group of muscles on the medial aspect of the thigh for contraction **(Fig. 11.15)**.

Sciatic Nerve (L4, L5, S1-3)

The sciatic nerve is derived from the lumbosacral plexus and runs from the gluteal region to the back of the thigh innervating, and supplying all hamstring muscles (semitendinosus, biceps femoris, semimembranosus, and hamstring part of adductor magnus), which are knee extensors.

Further, the sciatic nerve descends at the back of the mid-thigh and divides into the common peroneal and tibial nerve at the superior angle of the popliteal fossa. The common peroneal nerve descends inferolaterally, stays just behind the biceps femoris tendon, winds around the neck of the fibula and divides into the superficial and deep peroneal nerve, while the tibial nerve descends into the calf. Sciatic nerve injury could occur in posterior hip dislocation or posterior surgical approach to the hip. The sensory and motor function of the sciatic nerve and its division are discussed below.

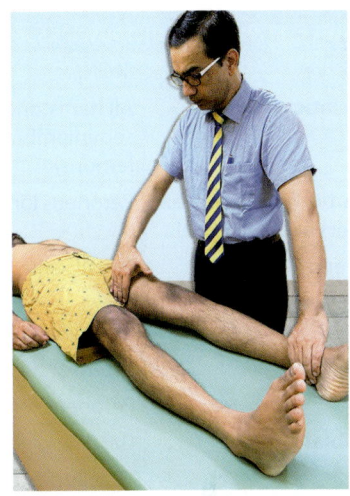

Fig. 11.15: Test for obturator nerve. Patient is attempting hip adduction against resistance while clinician is palpating adductors.

a. **Sensory:** Except for the saphenous nerve area on the medial aspect of the foot, the rest of the sensation over the foot is supplied by various divisions of the sciatic nerve, i.e., superficial and deep peroneal nerve, tibial nerve, and sural nerve **(Fig. 11.16)**.
   The specific areas over the foot supplied by various nerves are mentioned below.
   - *Tibial nerve:* It carries sensation from the entire plantar aspect of the foot. Under the flexor retinaculum, the tibial nerve divides into the medial and lateral plantar nerve, which supplies the medial 3½ and lateral 1½ plantar aspect of the foot and toes, respectively.
   - *Superficial peroneal nerve:* It supplies the entire dorsum of the foot except for the first web space.
   - *Deep peroneal nerve:* It supplies the first dorsal web space.
   - *Saphenous nerve:* It supplies the medial border of the foot up to the ball of the great toe. Note that the saphenous nerve is the largest branch of the femoral nerve and innervates the medial portion of the lower leg and the foot.
   - *Sural nerve:* It supplies the lateral border of the foot.

b. **Motor:** After innervating hamstrings, the sciatic nerve

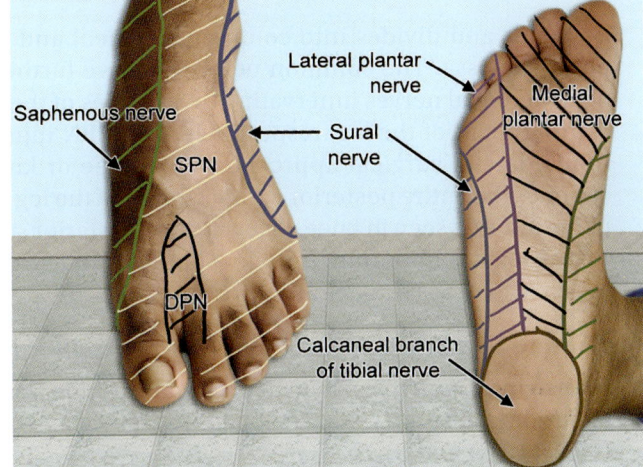

Fig. 11.16: Sensory innervation of the foot.
(SPN: superficial peroneal nerve; DPN: deep peroneal nerve).

TABLE 11.9: Important muscles supplied by the sciatic nerve and divisions: its action and evaluation.

Nerve	Muscles	Action
Sciatic nerve	All hamstrings (semitendinosus, semimembranosus, biceps femoris)	Hamstrings are responsible for knee flexion
Superficial peroneal nerve (L4, 5, S1, 2)	Peroneus longus and brevis	Eversion at subtalar joint and plantar flexion at the ankle joint
Deep peroneal nerve (L4, 5, S1, 2)	Tibialis anterior	Ankle dorsiflexion, inversion at subtalar joint
	Extensor hallucis longus	Great toe extension (both MTP and IP joint)
	Extensor digitorum longus	Lesser toes extension (MTP and IP joints)
	Peroneus tertius	Dorsiflexion at the ankle joint and eversion
Tibial nerve (L4, 5, S1-3)	Gastrocsoleus	Ankle plantar flexion, minor knee flexor
	Tibialis posterior	Ankle plantar flexion, subtalar inversion
	Flexor hallucis longus	Great toe plantar flexion (MTP, IP joints)
	Flexor digitorum longus	Lesser toes plantar flexion (MTP, IP joints)

Features of Sciatic Nerve Palsy
a. *Sciatic nerve palsy at the hip:* It results in a loss of knee flexion and ankle-foot is rendered flail.
b. *Sciatic nerve injury just above popliteal fossa:* It results in flail ankle and foot. However, knee flexion is spared.
c. *Common peroneal nerve palsy:* It results a 'typical foot drop' characterized by loss of dorsiflexion at the ankle, eversion of the subtalar joint, and toe dorsiflexion.
d. *Tibial nerve palsy:* It results in gross weakness in ankle plantar flexion, weak inversion, and loss of toe plantar flexion.
c. *Sensory loss:* Almost all sensations are lost in the lower limb except the areas supplied by the femoral, obturator and saphenous nerve.

descends and divides into common peroneal and tibial divisions at the apex of the popliteal fossa. The common peroneal nerve further divides into the superficial and deep peroneal nerves innervating the muscles of the lateral compartment and anterior compartment of the leg, respectively. The CPN injury can occur due to fracture neck fibula, lateral surgical approach to the knee or knee dislocations. The tibial nerve supplies the entire posterior compartment of the leg and all the sole muscles. The tibial nerve injury is seen in knee dislocation or posterior surgical approach to the knee. **Table 11.9** discusses important muscles supplied by the sciatic nerve, its divisions, and their palsy. Also, assess ankle reflex (S1,2).

Method to Test Key Muscles Innervated by Sciatic Nerve and its Divisions

1. **Hamstrings:** With the patient in the prone position, ask the patient to flex the knee (50–70° of flexion) while the clinician applies resistance and palpates the contracting hamstrings **(Figs. 11.17A and B)**.

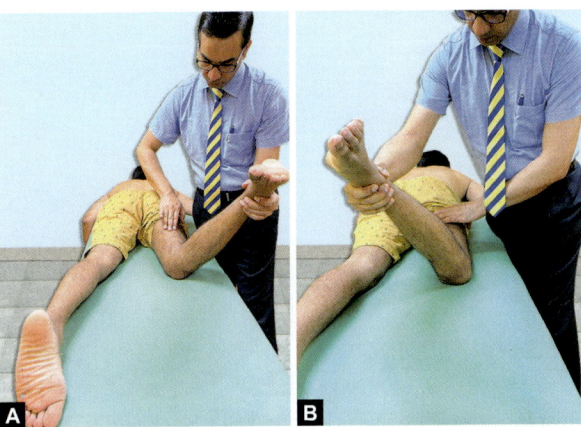

Figs. 11.17A and B: Test for hamstrings. (A) Test for medial hamstrings (hip and leg in internal rotation); (B) Test for lateral hamstrings (hip and leg in external rotation). Patient is attempting knee flexion against resistance while clinician is palpating medial and lateral hamstrings.

Test of Muscles of Anterior Compartment of the Leg (Innervated by Deep Peroneal Nerve)

1. **Tibialis anterior (TA):** While the patient is sitting/supine, he/she is asked to dorsiflex his ankle, invert at the subtalar joint, and the clinician gives resistance to the medial border of the foot against inversion and feels for the taut TA tendon in the front of the ankle **(Fig. 11.18)**.
2. **Extensor hallucis longus:** With the patient sitting/supine, the clinician holds the proximal phalanx of the great toe from the side with his thumb and index fingers, and the patient is asked to dorsiflex his great toe. The clinician gives resistance to dorsiflexion with his index finger on the tip of the great toe and feels for the taut EHL tendon **(Fig. 11.19A)**.
3. **Extensor digitorum longus:** While the patient is sitting/supine, the ankle is held in slight plantar flexion, and the patient is asked to dorsiflex his second to the fifth toe. The clinician gives resistance to dorsiflexion with his fingers on the tip of the toes and feels for the taut EHL tendon **(Fig. 11.19B)**.

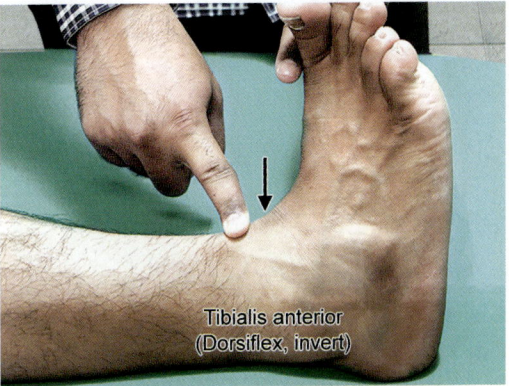

Fig. 11.18: Test for tibialis anterior. Black arrow shows taut TA tendon palpated by the clinician.

Test of Muscles of Lateral Compartment of the Leg (Innervated by Superficial Peroneal Nerve)

1. **Peroneus longus and brevis:** With the patient is in a sitting/supine position and ankle free in plantar flexion, the patient is asked to evert the foot, and the clinician gives resistance to the lateral border of the foot. The taut peroneus longus is palpated behind the lateral malleolus **(Fig. 11.20)**.

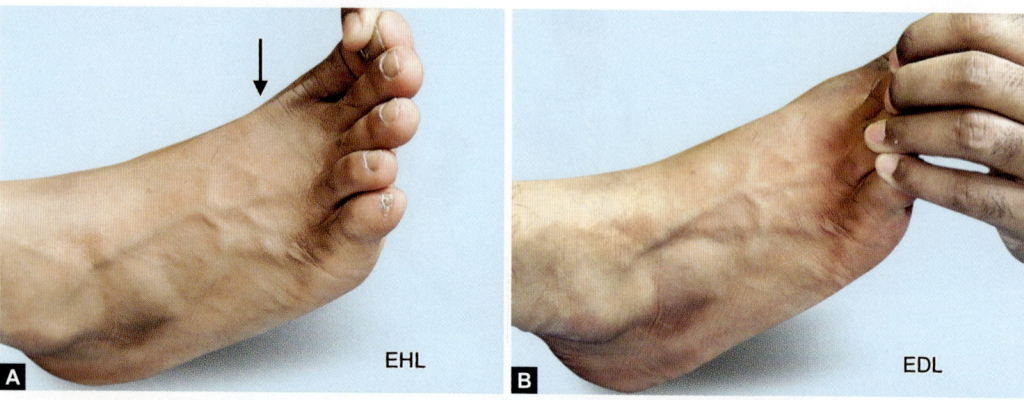

Figs. 11.19A and B: (A) Test for extensor hallucis longus (EHL). Black arrow shows taut EHL tendon; (B) Test for extensor digitorum longus (EDL).

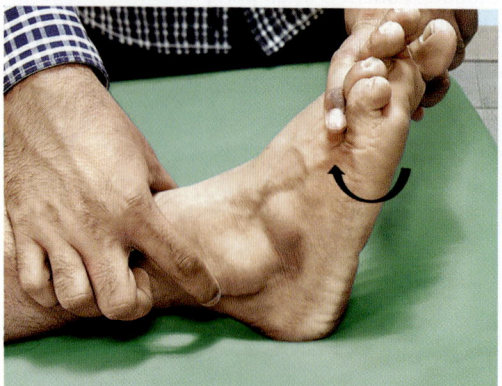

Fig. 11.20: Test for peroneus longus and brevis where patient is attempting eversion while clinician is palpating evertors behind the lateral malleolus (curved black arrow indicates eversion at the subtalar joint).

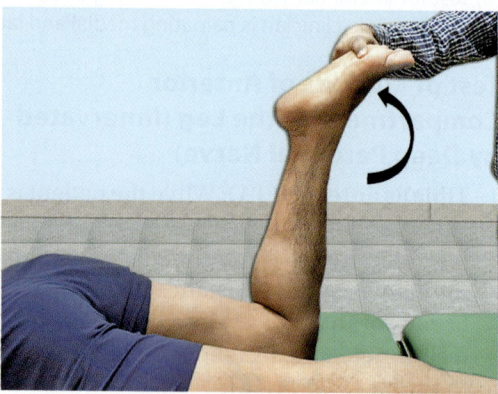

Fig. 11.21: Test for soleus muscle (with knee flexed). Curved arrow indicates ankle plantar flexion against clinician's resistance.

Test of Muscles of Posterior Compartment of the Leg (Innervated by Tibial Nerve)

1. **Soleus:** The patient is asked to lie prone with the knee flexed to 90° (knee flexion relaxes gastrocnemius and its action). The patient is asked to plantarflex his ankle, and the clinician provides resistance against plantar flexion **(Fig. 11.21)**.
2. **Gastrocnemius:** With the patient in the prone position, keep the patient's knee extended and ask him/her to plantarflex the ankle against resistance applied by the clinician over the plantar aspect of the foot while the clinician palpates the gastrocnemius **(Fig. 11.22)**. Another

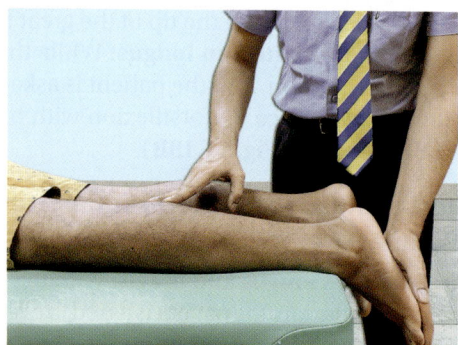

Fig. 11.22: Test for gastrocnemius with knee extended. Ankle plantar flexion is assessed against clinician's resistance.

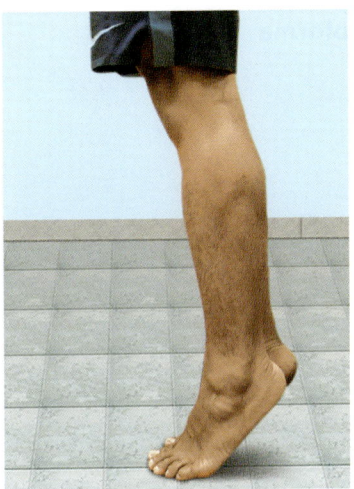 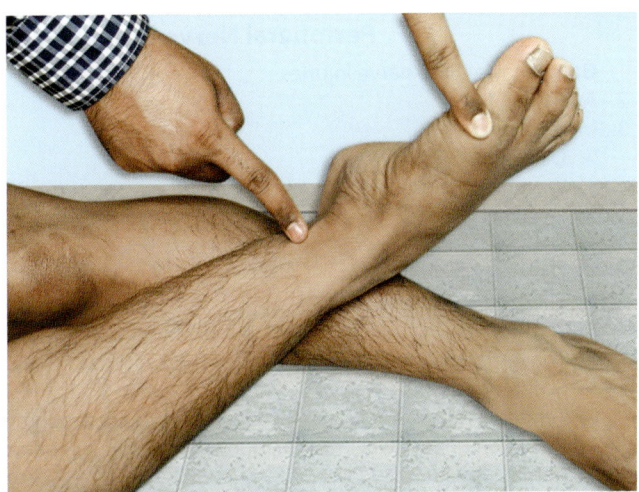

Fig. 11.23: Test for gastrocnemius muscle against gravity wherein patient stands on tip toe.

Fig. 11.24: Test for tibialis posterior (TP) with ankle in plantar flexion and inversion against clinician's resistance and clinician palpating contracting TP just above the medial malleolus.

method is to ask the patient to stand on his forefoot by plantar flexing his ankle where gastrocnemius is tested against gravity **(Fig. 11.23)**.

3. **Tibialis posterior (TP):** While the patient is sitting/supine, he/she is asked to plantarflex at the ankle, invert at the subtalar joint, and the clinician gives resistance to the medial border of the foot against inversion and feels for taut TP tendon behind the medial malleolus **(Fig. 11.24)**.

Note: Both the tibialis anterior (TA) and posterior (TP) are invertors at the subtalar joint; the former is a dorsiflexor, whereas the latter is a plantar flexor of the ankle joint. To test TA, the ankle is dorsiflexed, which stretches the TP and nullifies TP's action. To test TP, the ankle is plantarflexed, which stretches the TA and nullifies TA's action.

4. **Flexor hallucis longus:** Ask the patient to plantarflex the great toe against resistance.
5. **Flexor digitorum longus:** Ask the patient to plantarflex the toes against resistance.

Notes

Peripheral Nerve Examination Proforma

1. **Gait:** In lower limb nerve injuries
2. **Attitude**
3. **Inspection:**
    - Deformity
    - Wasting of muscles
    - Swelling
    - Scars
    - Dysmorphic changes
    - Skin and nail changes
4. **Palpation:**
    - The temperature difference between the two sides
    - Scar tenderness
    - Tenderness throughout nerve: generalized/point tenderness
    - Palpation of any swelling, scar, bony irregularity, or characteristics for the etiology responsible for nerve palsy
5. **Movements:**
    - Assessment of any fixed deformity
    - Active and passive movement of paralyzed joints
    - Active movement of normal joints
6. **Measurements:** Limb length, muscle wasting
7. **Neurological examination:**
    a. Sensory examination
    b. *Motor examination:* Bulk, tone, power, reflexes (superficial and deep), coordination, abnormal movements
    c. Individual nerve examination
    d. *Nerve recovery sign:* Tinel's sign, motor march
    e. *Autonomic system examination:* Anhidrosis, nail changes, axon reflex
8. **Lymph node examination:** In case of infective/tumorous cause of nerve palsy

Common Deformities following Specific Nerve Injuries and Other Conditions

1. **Foot drop:** Foot drop occurs either due to sciatic nerve injury (posterior hip dislocation, posterior surgical approach, gluteal injections) or common peroneal nerve injury (fracture neck fibula, posterolateral knee dislocation). Various other causes such as infection/tumor/lumbar disc prolapse affecting these nerves or root forming these nerves can also cause foot drop.
    - ***Sciatic nerve injury:*** If the sciatic nerve is injured near the hip or at the upper end of the posterior aspect of the thigh, the patient loses knee flexion (hamstring) as well as foot and ankle movements (dorsiflexion, plantar flexion, inversion, and eversion), leading to *flail foot and ankle*. However, Sciatic nerve injury just above the popliteal fossa spares the hamstrings but results in flail foot. The sciatic nerve injury results in loss of sensation over the foot except the medial border, which is supplied by the saphenous nerve.
    - ***Common peroneal nerve injury:*** It results in classic foot drop with loss of dorsiflexion and eversion. However, plantar flexion and inversion are possible due to spared tibial nerve. Further, there is sensory loss only over the dorsum of the foot.
    Note that tibial nerve injury does not result in foot drop. It causes loss of plantar flexion at the ankle and toes, weak inversion, and sensory loss over the plantar aspect of the foot. However, the patient will perform dorsiflexion and eversion due to intact dorsiflexors and evertors.

2. **Wartenberg syndrome or Cheralgia paraesthetica:**
   - ➢ *Definition:* Compressive neuropathy of the superficial sensory radial nerve (SRN) at the wrist.
3. **Cubital tunnel syndrome:**
   - ➢ *Definition:* Ulnar nerve compression near the elbow behind the medial epicondyle.
4. **Guyon's canal compression:**
   - ➢ Ulnar nerve compression in the Guyon's canal. Often seen in long-distance cyclists with drop-down handlebar where the hand is rested for long.
5. **Meralgia paraesthetica:**
   - ➢ *Definition:* Compressive neuropathy of the lateral cutaneous nerve of the thigh (LCNT)
   - ➢ *Etiology:* Entrapment under the inguinal ligament due to pregnancy, tight clothing, obesity, tool belts worn by carpenters. Rarely, traumatic.
   - ➢ *Presents with:* Pain and paraesthesia over the lateral aspect of the thigh. Standing and walking may aggravate while sitting may relieve pain.
6. **Tarsal tunnel syndrome:**
   - ➢ *Definition:* Compressive neuropathy of the posterior tibial nerve (PTN). The tunnel lies posterior to the medial malleolus beneath the flexor retinaculum.
7. **Hansen's disease:**
   - ➢ *Definition:* Chronic infectious disease caused by the acid-fast bacteria *Mycobacterium leprae* and *M. lepromatosis*, characterized by skin lesion (s) and involvement of peripheral nerves.
   - ➢ *Risk factors to contract leprosy:* Contact with a known patient, poor socioeconomic status
   - ➢ *Pathology:* The mode of transmission is uncertain. However, entry through the respiratory route appears most likely.
   - ➢ *Classification:* (A) *Ridley and Jopling:* This classification considers the clinical spectrum that correlates with the level of the immune response to *Mycobacterium leprae*. At one end of the spectrum, patients with tuberculoid leprosy (TL) are resistant to the pathogen with the localized, while patients at the other end of spectrum are more susceptible to the pathogen and suffer with lepromatous leprosy (LL), which can disseminate systemically. The borderline type of leprosy lies in between TL and LL type.
     (B) *WHO classification:* Based upon the number of skin lesions and skin smear findings.
      (a) *Multibacillary (MB):* Six of more skin lesions and positive skin smear
      (b) *Paucibacillary (PB):* Up to five skin lesions and negative skin smear
   - ➢ *Clinical presentation:*
     - ♦ *Skin lesions* (macule, papules, or nodules); ill-defined, hypopigmented, or erythematous patch with anesthesia.
     - ♦ *Involvement of the nerves* such as greater auricular, ulnar, median, superficial radial, tibial, and common peroneal resulting in motor weakness and sensory loss.
     - ♦ *Eye symptoms* (iridocyclitis, corneal ulcers, lagophthalmos)
     - ♦ *Immunological reactions* (type 1 or 2 lepra reactions)
   - ➢ *Investigations:* Skin smear, skin and nerve biopsy
   - ➢ *Treatment:* Multidrug therapy (Dapsone, Clofazimine, Rifampicin) for six months (PB) and 12 months in MB type. Prednisolone is administered in lepra reactions. Treatment of paralytic disabilities by splinting, tendon transfer, joint fusion. Non-healing ulcers require debridement and skin grafting or flap coverage.

CHAPTER 12

Clinical Evaluation of the Bone Tumors

Bone tumors are commonly encountered in orthopedic outpatient practice. The knowledge of eliciting a good history and performing a comprehensive examination is key to establishing a bone tumor diagnosis. However, before we proceed to the basics of history taking and examination of bone tumors, understanding a pertinent clinical classification of the bone tumor and difference between benign and malignant bone tumors is important.

CLASSIFICATION OF BONE TUMORS

Bone tumors can be classified into benign, malignant and tumor-like lesions. The malignant bone tumors can be further classified as primary (sarcomas) and secondary bone tumors (metastatic tumors). Clinical classification of bone tumors is shown in **Flowchart 12.1**. **Table 12.1** illustrates the difference between a benign and malignant bone tumor.

HISTORY TAKING IN BONE TUMORS

The patients with bone tumors commonly present with the following complaints:
1. Swelling
2. Pain
3. Deformity, shortening
4. Pressure symptoms

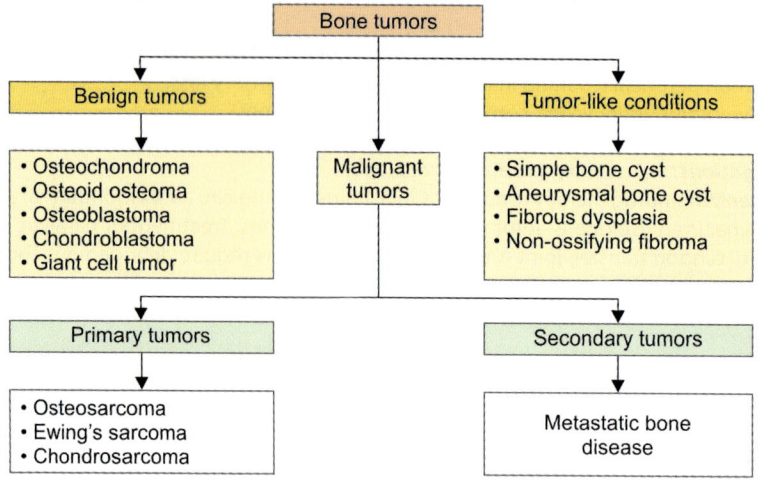

Flowchart 12.1: Clinical classification of bone tumors.

TABLE 12.1: Difference between benign and malignant bone tumors.

Characteristics	Benign	Malignant
Growth	Slow, may stop at maturity	Rapid
Duration	Long	Short
Pain character	Localized, subsides with rest	Constant, present even on rest and night
Constitutional features (weight and appetite loss, fever)	Rare	Common
Spread	Remains mostly local	Infiltrates the adjacent tissues and can involve distant organs
Swelling surface	Smooth	Irregular
Local temperature	Normal	Raised
Consistency	Firm/hard	Variable
Metastasis	Rare	Yes
Radiograph	Limited geographic growth	'Moth-eaten' or 'permeative' appearance
	• Well-defined margins • Narrow zone of transition	• Ill-defined margins • Wide zone of transition
Histopathology	No features of malignancy	• Numerous mitotic bodies • Anisocytosis • Anisonucleosis • Hyperchromatism

5. Constitutional symptoms
6. Symptoms due to metastasis from bone
7. Symptoms due to a 'primary' in case of a metastatic bone lesion
8. Effect on activities of daily living

Certain must-know facts about the bone tumor are listed in **Box 12.1**.

BOX 12.1: Must-know facts about the bone tumor during history assessment.

- Age of the patient
- Duration of symptoms
- *Site in the body:* Flat bone/long bone/short bones
- *Location in the bone:* Epiphysis/metaphysis/diaphysis
- Single/multiple

Demographic Data

1. **Age:** Age plays a significant role in assessing a bone tumor as most benign and malignant tumors are common in specific age groups. The important bone tumors (or tumor-like lesions), which are usually encountered in daily practice with its most common age group, are mentioned in the **Table 12.2**

TABLE 12.2: Relevance of age and common tumors and tumor like lesions in the bone	
Age (years)	Tumors
10–20	Simple bone cyst, aneurysmal bone cyst, chondroblastoma, Ewing's sarcoma, and osteosarcoma
21–40	Giant cell tumor (osteoclastoma), malignant fibrous histiocytoma
>50	Metastatic bone disease, multiple myeloma, secondary osteosarcoma, and chondrosarcoma

2. **Gender:** Certain bone tumors have a predilection for males, while some have a predilection for females.
   - *Osteosarcoma* is common in males in a ratio of 2:1.
   - *Ewing's tumor* has a slight male predilection with a ratio of 3:2.
   - *Giant cell tumor* of bone is common in females in a ratio of 2:3.

History of Present Illness

1. **Swelling:** Swelling is one of the most common presenting symptom in patients with bone tumor. It may or may not be associated with pain **(Fig. 12.1)**. The characteristics (location, onset, duration, progression, associated symptoms) of the swelling must be further evaluated.
   - *Location of the swelling:* The location of the bony swelling could give a clue to the possible diagnosis. For example, bony swelling at the end of a long bone in a skeletally mature patient in the third-fourth decade of life is likely to be osteoclastoma, while a bone tumor in a flat bone-like pelvis or scapula in an elderly be chondrosarcoma.

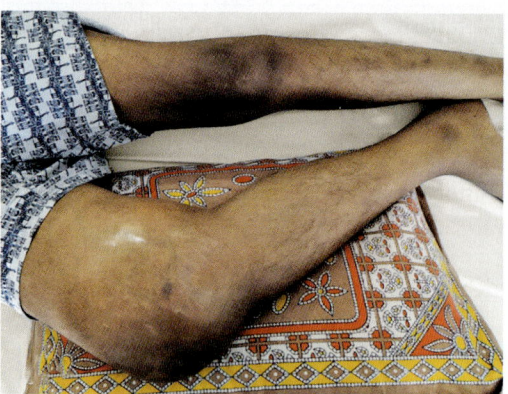

Fig. 12.1: A painful, progressive swelling at the lower end of the right thigh.

   - *Onset:* Acute or insidious. An insidious onset swelling suggests a slow-growing tumor or probably a benign bone tumor.
   - *Duration:* It could be in days, months, or years. Chronicity of the swelling favors a benign swelling (e.g., osteochondroma), whereas a shorter duration with quick enlargement in size may suggest malignant pathology.
   - *Progression:* Static or progressive. A static swelling or a slowly progressive tumor suggests a benign course of the tumor, whereas a tumor with rapid progression may indicate malignant disease.
   - *Associated symptoms of swelling* such as pressure symptoms over the artery, vein and nerves such as distal limb swelling, tingling, numbness, and weakness of muscles.
   - *History of similar swellings* elsewhere in the body is observed in multiple exostosis, metachronous osteosarcoma, polyostotic fibrous dysplasia, and multiple enchondromatosis.
2. **Pain:** Pain is a common symptom in patients with bone tumors. One must assess several pain characteristics of a tumor, which are mentioned in **Table 12.3**.
3. **Deformity, shortening:** A tumor gives rise to a deformity or shortening in the limb due to affection of the growth plate or occasionally due to a pathological fracture.

TABLE 12.3: Characteristics of pain in benign vs. malignant tumor.

Pain Characteristics	Benign	Malignant
Onset	Insidious	Could be sudden (Always consider the possibility of associated pathological fractures)
Duration	Chronic/long standing	Acute
Character	Dull aching	Throbbing
Diurnal variation	Rarely seen	Very common
Rest pain	Rarely seen	Very common
Relieved by NSAIDs	Diagnostic of osteoid osteoma	—

4. **Symptoms of joint involvement:** Presence of swelling over the joint and restricted movement indicate the joint involvement. However, sometimes, the restricted movement may be due to muscle spasm and pain.
5. **Pressure symptoms of tumor:** A tumor in a limb may compress upon surrounding nerve or vascular structure (vein/artery), giving rise to several compression features such as distal swelling, claudication, sensory disturbance, or limb weakness. A spinal tumor (metastasis/multiple myeloma) could result in a sensorimotor loss in the limbs and bladder bowel involvement.
6. **Constitutional symptoms:** Symptoms of fever, weight loss, and loss of appetite are relevant in malignant bone tumors and would be absent in benign bone tumors.
7. **Symptoms suggestive of metastasis from bone tumor:** Bone-to-bone metastasis occurs in osteosarcoma, Ewing's sarcoma, multiple myeloma, and neuroblastoma, which could result in bone pain, swelling, or pathological fracture. Certain malignant bone tumors, such as osteosarcoma can metastasize to the lung, and such patients can present with cough or hemoptysis.
8. **Symptoms of a primary (not bony) causing metastatic bone lesion:** While eliciting a history that is suggestive of a malignant bone tumor, it is essential to understand that occasionally the 'malignant bone tumor' is a result of metastasis from some other soft tissue tumor and one must elicit appropriate history to confirm the source of the primary. The most common cancers (80%) which metastasize to bone are lungs, prostate, breast, and kidney. Other tumors which rarely metastasize are thyroid, melanoma, sarcomas, genitourinary and gastrointestinal. Almost always, the metastasis occurs in the areas of bone rich in red marrow, such as the spine, pelvis, proximal femur, proximal humerus and skull.
9. **Effect on activities of daily living:** Disabilities and limitations of activities of daily living should be elicited in individuals with bone tumors irrespective of their benign or malignant nature.

Past History

It includes history of DM, hypertension, and other relevant medical and surgical history.

Personal History

- History of loss of appetite/weight and bone pain in elderly women (those with severe osteopenia) could be symptoms of multiple myeloma.
- *History of smoking:* Chronic smokers could present with lung cancer with bony metastasis.

- History of prostatism (decreased urinary force due to obstruction of flow through the prostate gland) must be probed further in older males to ascertain that there is no prostatic carcinoma causing urinary obstruction.
- History of bladder and bowel habit, disturbed sleep due to pain, especially in malignant tumors.

Treatment History

Detailed treatment history may suggest the nature of the tumor in question, benign or malignant, as the latter requires chemo- or radiotherapy. History of radiation therapy for other tumor is important. For example, radiotherapy given for soft organs of the pelvis may later result in secondary osteosarcoma of the pelvic bones. A patient who present with bone pain, swelling, etc., with a history of tumor elsewhere in the body (cured/under treatment) could be due to metastasis from tumor (treated/under treatment).

Occupational History

Certain tumors could be an occupational hazard, such as plutonium exposure could result in osteosarcoma and chondrosarcoma. The radium exposure could result in osteosarcoma (radial dial painters of the past).

Family History

It may be positive in tumors such as multiple exostoses.

EXAMINATION

General Examination

Detailed general and systemic examinations are required in cases of bone tumors, especially if it is a case of malignant bone tumor. One must check pulse, temperature, respiratory rate, and blood pressure as a part of the examination in patients with a bone tumor. Several examples of the importance of general examination are mentioned here.
- *Pallor:* Anemia is quite common in multiple myeloma and malignant bone tumors.
- *Lymph node enlargement:* Bone sarcomas spread through the hematogenous route. Few sarcomas spread to lymph nodes such as synovial sarcoma, epithelioid sarcoma, and rhabdomyosarcoma.
- *Edema:* Compression of the veins can cause bilateral or unilateral limb edema.
- *Stature:* Patient with short stature and multiple swellings over the body (axial and appendicular skeleton) with deformities could be suffering from diaphyseal aclasis (Multiple exostoses).

Systemic Examination

- A systemic examination should be undertaken to look for signs of metastasis in other major systems, especially lungs and other bones in the body. The patients with metastasis to the lung can present with features of a collapse or pleural effusion of the lung. Other organs spread from the bone tumor is uncommon. However, one must examine all areas to look for any evidence of metastasis.
- Likewise, a thorough systemic examination of the neck, chest, and abdomen-pelvis should be undertaken to locate the primary in case of metastatic bone disease. The primaries which commonly cause bone metastasis are breast, lung, kidney, and prostate.

- Per-rectal or per-vaginal examination may be required in case of suspicion of local malignancy of pelvis.
- Examination of other parts of the skeletal system may be required in conditions where multiple bones may be involved, like exostoses, bony metastasis, etc.
- Sternal tenderness could be present in multiple myeloma.

Local Examination

Gait

It should be described in standard fashion in patients with lower limb and spine tumors. However, avoid gait assessment, if there is suspicion of impending pathological fracture or neurological deficit.

Attitude

It should be described in standard fashion.

Inspection

The swelling arising from the bone should be looked for, the following specifics:
- **Site (location):** The location of the bone tumor is the most critical inspection finding, and can give a fair clue about the clinical diagnosis. There are bone tumors that occur specifically in the epiphysis, metaphysis, and diaphysis of long bones **(Fig. 12.2)**. Flat bones such as the pelvis and scapula are more prone to chondrosarcoma, while red marrow areas are prone to metastasis from other organs. Multiple myeloma is common in flat bones and the red marrow area of long bones.
- Other swelling features, such as size, shape, surface, extent, number, etc., must be described on the lines of a standard swelling examination protocol.
- **Overlying skin:** Must be observed for:
  - *Stretched and glistening skin* suggests a rapidly growing tumor.
  - *Dilated veins* over the skin of the swelling suggest an aggressive growth.
  - *Puckered skin* is observed in case of skin infiltration by the tumor, usually malignant.
  - *Ulcerations or fungation* in the overlying skin suggest malignant growth.
- **Any scars, sinuses** overlying the swelling have to be highlighted upon. Examination of surgical scars (of biopsy or other surgery) is essential part of the tumor examination.

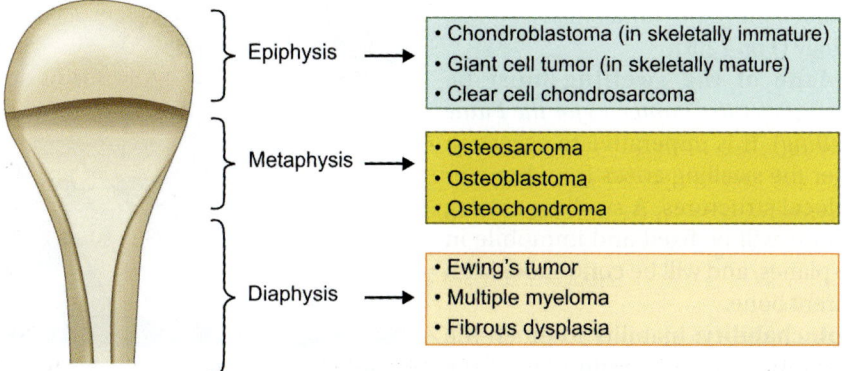

Fig. 12.2: Location of common tumors in a long bone.

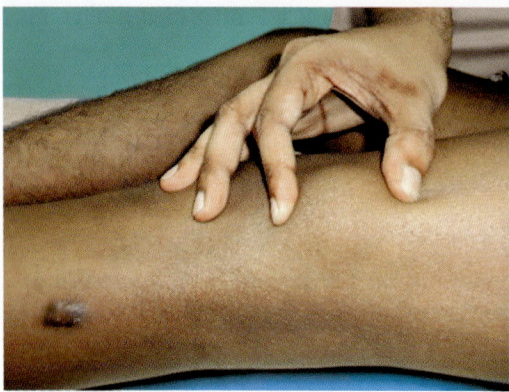 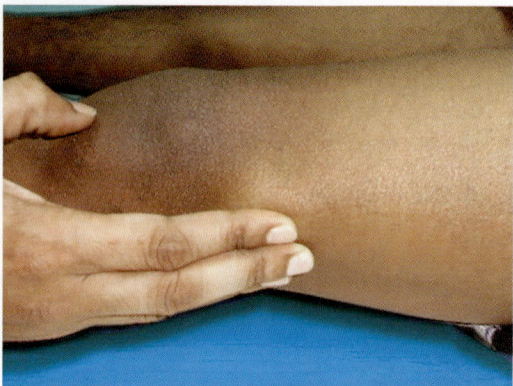

Fig. 12.3: The site, size, shape, and extent of the swelling along with the mobility of the swelling should be assessed in palpation.

Fig. 12.4: Tenderness, surface, and consistency of the swelling should be elicited as depicted in the figure.

- **Look for any bony deformity and shortening**, indicating an underlying pathological fracture.
- Observe **any distal swelling** that may indicate the tumor's pressure features over the vessels.

Palpation

- **Local rise of temperature** over the swelling: Malignant tumors can have a rise in local temperature.
- Confirm **site, size, shape, surface, and edge** of the swelling **(Fig. 12.3)**.
- **Tenderness** over the swelling **(Fig. 12.4)**
- **Consistency:** Variable consistencies from soft to firm in a centrifugal pattern may suggest a malignant tumor as central necrosis may turn a tumor soft.

- Hard consistency suggests the predominance of bony elements.
- Firm consistency suggests the predominance of cartilaginous elements.
- Soft consistency suggests the pre-dominance of fibrous or vascular elements.

- **Surface:** *Smooth or bosselated*—smooth surface may indicate benign tumor, whereas bosselated surface may be appreciated in malignant bone tumors **(Fig. 12.5)**.
- **Edge:** An ill-defined edge may suggest a malignant bone tumor rather than a benign pathology **(Fig. 12.5)**.
- **The plane of the swelling** must be assessed (*Refer to Chapter 15 for the Plane of Swelling*). It is imperative to ascertain whether the swelling arises from bone or other local structures. A swelling arising from bone will be fixed and immobile in all the planes, and will be continuous with the parent bone.
- **Skin pinchability:** Inability to pinch the overlying skin suggests infiltration of the skin, which might be observed in malignant lesions.

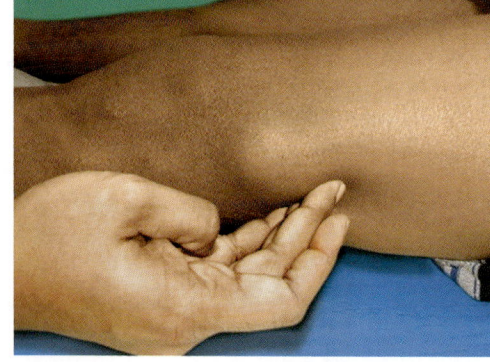

Fig. 12.5: The margin or edge is well-defined when the tumor and the surrounding bone can be palpated as discrete entities as depicted in this figure.

Movements

Assess any preexisting deformity at the joint followed by active and passive ROM. In case of compressive or infiltrative nerve palsy, the active ROM at the distal joint will be decreased or absent. The ROM may also be restricted if:
- The *lesion is in the proximity of the adjacent joint and may act as a bony block* in the movement. For example, osteochondroma arising from the posterior aspect of the tibia or femur would restrict flexion of the knee.
- The *intra-articular spread of the tumor* would restrict joint movement or local muscle spasm.

Measurements
- Pediatric bone tumors affecting the physis or in the vicinity of the physis are known to cause limb length discrepancies (shortening or lengthening). Any surgery in the past for a bone tumor could affect the length either by affecting the growth plate or by resecting a part of the long bone. A pathological fracture could also result in shortening of the limb.
- Adjacent muscle wasting might occur in long-standing bone tumors, which has to be quantified.

Neurovascular Examination

It is important to assess the neurovascular status of the limb as tumors can compress the local nerve, artery, and vein.

Lymph Node Assessment

Although uncommon in bone tumors, lymph node enlargement is observed in rhabdomyosarcoma, epithelioid cell sarcoma, and synovial cell sarcoma.

Bone Tumor Examination Proforma

1. **General and systemic examination**
2. **Gait (if the tumor is in the lower limb or spine)**
3. **Attitude of the limb**
4. **Inspection of the tumor:**
   a. Site, size, shape, number, extent, surface and other points for a swelling examination
   b. Overlying skin
   c. Scar, sinuses, ulcers, fungation
   d. Any deformity, shortening, proximal and distal muscle wasting
   e. Distal swelling
5. **Palpation:**
   a. Local rise of temperature
   b. Confirm the inspection findings such as size, shape, margin, surface, and edge. Palpate for overlying skin pinchability and other applicable palpatory finding for a swelling
   c. Tenderness, consistency
   d. Plane of the swelling
6. **Movement of joint adjacent to the tumor**
7. **Measurement of the limb (length), girth of the limb**
8. **Neurovascular status:**
   a. *Distal vascular status:* Pulses, skin temperature, any venous engorgement
   b. *Neurological status:* Sensory and motor status
9. **Examination of lymph nodes**

Important Bone Tumors (in Brief)

1. **Osteochondroma:**
   - **Affects:** Most common benign bone tumor affecting the pediatric population.
   - **Site:** It usually affects the metaphyseal region of the long bones and grows away from the joint.
   - **Clinically:**
     - Slow growing and painless exophytic swelling arising at the ends of long bones.
     - Usually asymptomatic and hence neglected by patients for a long time.
     - Solitary or multiple
     - Multiple osteochondromas are associated with the autosomal dominant syndrome called hereditary multiple exostoses (Diaphyseal aclasis).
     - The growth of the tumor stops once skeletal maturity is attained. If it continues to grow or if there is sudden growth, it may suggests a malignant transformation.
   - **Pathologically:** Cartilage tumor. Cartilage-capped tumor with underlying trabacular bone.
   - **Diagnosis:** X-ray shows an excrescent growth with or without a pedicle (*sessile or pedunculated*) usually disproportionately smaller to the clinical picture, which is due to the cartilage cap not evident in the radiographs **(Fig. 12.6)**.
   - **Treatment:** Extraperiosteal resection of symptomatic osteochondromas is recommended.
   - **Complications:** Bursa formation leading to bursitis (a most common cause of the pain), mechanical block to the joint movement, pathological fracture of the stalk, neurovascular compression, and malignant transformation into chondrosarcoma (1% and 5% chance of malignant transformation in solitary vs. multiple exostoses, respectively).

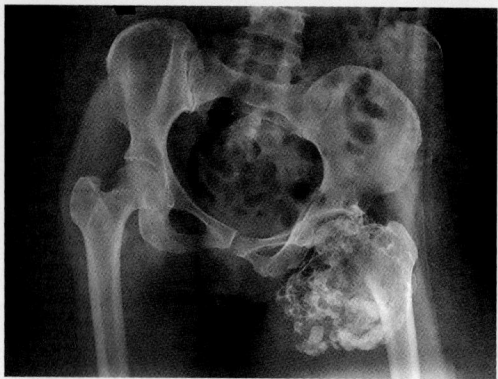

Fig. 12.6: X-ray of osteochondroma femur.

2. **Giant cell tumor (Osteoclastoma):**
   - **Affects:** Skeletally mature adults: 20–40 years, females are more likely to be affected.
   - **Site:** Epiphysis of a long bone.
   - **Clinically:** Gradually progressive swelling and dull aching pain.
   - **Pathologically:** A benign tumor but locally aggressive.
   - **Diagnosis:** X-ray reveals a well-defined *eccentric, expansile geographic* lytic lesion at the epiphysio-metaphyseal region of the bone **(Fig. 12.7A)**. The "soap-bubble appearance" on the radiograph is characteristic of GCT **(Fig. 12.7B)**.
   - **Treatment:** Extended curettage and reconstruction with bone graft/bone cement/combination

3. **Osteosarcoma:** Most common primary bone malignancy
   - **Affects:** Common between 10–20 years of age.
   - **Site:** Metaphyseal tumor. Commonly affects the growing end of bone-especially around the knee in 70% of cases.

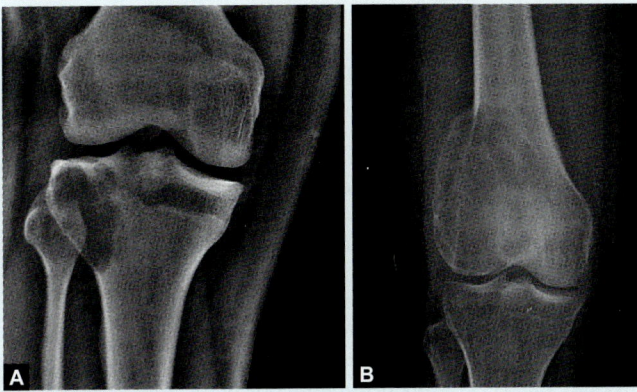

Figs. 12.7A and B: (A) Plain X-ray of the knee with GCT showing an eccentric, epiphyseal lesion of the lateral tibial condyle; (B) Expansile, eccentric and epiphyseal lesion with soap-bubble appearance of distal femur lateral condyle.

- ➢ **Clinically:**
  - ♦ Vague, dull aching pain which may occur at rest.
  - ♦ Pain may precede a swelling associated with restricted mobility.
  - ♦ Diffuse swelling along with tenderness and local rise of temperature, overlying dilated veins
  - ♦ Restriction of movements of the adjoining joint may be noted.
- ➢ **Diagnosis:** Radiograph may show an osteosclerotic and osteolytic lesion in the metaphyseal region of the bone. Characteristic radiographic findings of the lesion are periosteal reaction in the form of "Codman's triangle" and "sunburst appearance" **(Figs. 12.8A and B)**.
  - ♦ *Magnetic resonance imaging (MRI)* may help to stage the tumor, intramedullary spread (skip lesions) and to reveal the involvement of the neurovascular structures.
  - ♦ *Bone scan:* Three-phase ^{99m}Tc bone scan. PET scan is preferred as it can reveal both bony and soft tissue metastasis.
- ➢ **Treatment:** Neoadjuvant chemotherapy followed by limb-salvage surgery followed by adjuvant chemotherapy. The commonly used chemotherapy drugs are ifosfamide, methotrexate, cisplatin, and adriamycin.

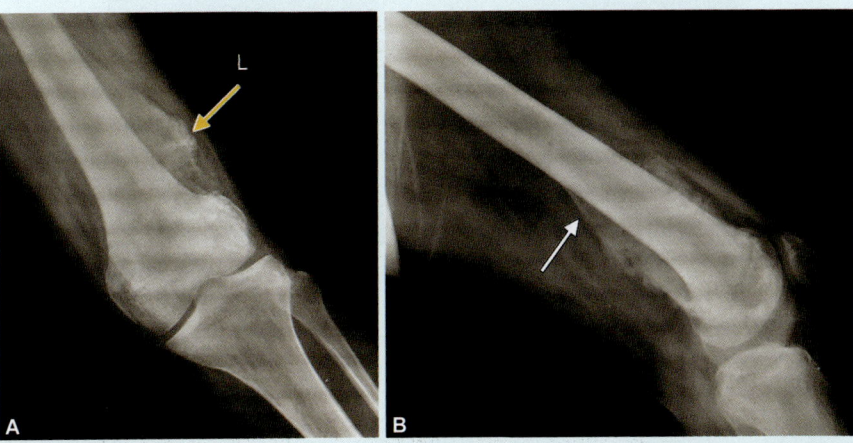

Figs. 12.8A and B: Plain X-rays of left femur showing osteosarcoma of distal femur. (A) AP view of distal femur with yellow arrow shows sunburst appearance; (B) Lateral view of distal femur with white arrow shows Codman's triangle.

4. **Ewing's sarcoma (Primitive neuroectodermal tumor group of malignancies):**
    - **Affects:** Second most common primary malignant bone tumor. Age group 5–15 years
    - **Site:** Diaphysis; the most common site is the lower extremity (most common—femur) with an incidence of 45%, followed by the pelvis and the upper extremity.
    - **Clinically:**
        - Moderate-to-severe pain of short duration with rapidly increasing swelling **(Fig. 12.9)**.
        - Child may present with acute onset fever, associated pain, and swelling. It is very important to note that Ewing's may be mistaken for acute or chronic osteomyelitis and vice versa. Only histopathological examination can confirm the diagnosis.
        - Metastasis is common in 10% of individuals at the time of presentation, and it commonly occurs in the lungs.
    - **Diagnosis:** X-ray of the area concerned shows moth-eaten, permeative lucent lesion affecting the bone. Aggressive periosteal reaction characterized by "onion-peel appearance" is characteristically seen in a radiograph of Ewing's sarcoma **(Fig. 12.10)**. Further, MRI of local growth and PET-CT scan is required for both skeletal and extraskeletal metastasis.
    - **Treatment:** Neoadjuvant chemotherapy (Vincristine, doxorubicin, and ifosfamide) followed by surgery followed by adjuvant chemotherapy.

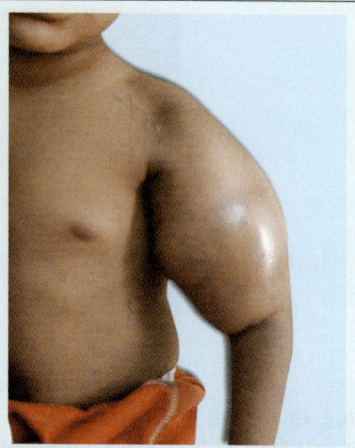

Fig. 12.9: Large diaphyseal swelling of left humerus.

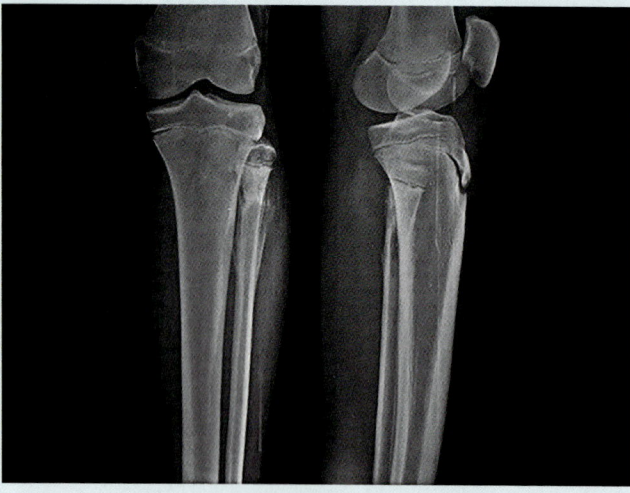

Fig. 12.10: Plain X-ray of the fibular Ewing's sarcoma shows a typical 'onion-peel' appearance.

CHAPTER 13

Clinical Evaluation of the Amputation Stump

INDICATIONS FOR AMPUTATION

Alan Apley highlighted the indications as "three Ds."

1. **Dead (or Dying):** It includes dry gangrene due to peripheral vascular disease, which is the most common indication. Other examples of a dead limb are severely traumatized limb, burns, and frostbite.
2. **Deadly:** It includes conditions, which if not eradicated by amputation immediately, might prove fatal. Examples include gas gangrene, severe sepsis, malignant tumors, and crush injuries of the limb leading to crush syndrome.
3. **Damned nuisance:** Retaining the limb may be worse than having no limb at all because of:
   - Unrelenting pain in the limb
   - Gross malformation wherein any attempt of reconstruction is futile, while an amputated stump can give a better function with prosthesis, instead.
   - Recurrent local septic focus such as chronic osteomyelitis with failed multiple repeated attempts of medical and surgical treatment.
   - Severe loss of function such as Charcot's foot and ankle along with non-healing ulcer and osteomyelitis where multiple attempts of treating bone and soft tissue infection have failed. An amputation would offer a better quality of life or cosmesis.

THE SCHEME OF HISTORY TAKING IN A PATIENT WITH AMPUTATION STUMP

Demographic Details

It includes name, age, sex, occupation, and place of residence. If the upper limb is involved, one must ascertain the dominant limb.

Chief Complaints

The common complaints include:
- Pain in the stump or the nearby joint
- Swelling over the stump
- Wound over the stump, with or without discharge
- Deformities of the neighboring joints
- Tingling/numbness/burning sensation while touching the stump or while donning the prosthesis

History of Presenting Complaint(s)

This part elaborates on the presenting complaints and their associated problems.
i. **It begins with the circumstances leading to the amputations.** The causes of the amputations can be broadly divided into traumatic and atraumatic.

a. ***Traumatic amputations*** are usually seen in young individuals following motor vehicle accidents and work-related injuries (the distal extremities of the upper limb, in particular).
b. ***Atraumatic amputations*** include those due to peripheral vascular disease (seen in older individuals) and those due to tumors.

ii. **The present state of the limb:** Next, the focus should be on the present state of the limb, and questions should be directed to know whether the patient is having any problems with the stump.

a. ***Pain at the stump*** may be due to a nonhealing wound, ill-fitting prosthesis, continuous claudication, recurrence of a tumor, and infection.
b. ***Phantom limb sensation*** may also lead to pain at the stump, and the description is typical.
c. ***Tingling/numbness/burning sensation*** while touching the stump or donning the prosthesis.
d. ***Presence of any wound (sinus or ulcer):*** It may be due to persistent infection or an ill-fitting prosthesis

iii. **Fitting of the prosthesis:** Questions related to the fitting of the prosthesis should be asked. An ill-fitted prosthesis may be the reason for constant discomfort, pain, and nonhealing wound.

iv. **The overall general complaint of the patient:** One must ask the patient regarding any overall fatigue, weakness, endurance, lack of coordination, and balance which would hinder the mobility of the patient.

v. **Present disability of the patient:** Further, the present disability of the patient should be discussed. The disability may stem from pain, weakness, deformity of the neighboring joint, and ill-fitting prosthesis.

Past History

This part elaborates on the past medical and surgical histories. The medical history includes questions regarding diabetes mellitus, hypertension, and ischemic heart disease, and is especially important in amputations secondary to peripheral vascular disease.

The past surgical history should include details on attempts at limb salvaging procedures such as vascular bypass surgeries, surgeries done for treatment of multiple nonhealing wounds over an insensate limb with underlying osteomyelitis (in Charcot's arthropathy), etc.

Personal History

This includes the personal habits and daily routine of the patient. It is imperative to take a detailed history of tobacco consumption in any form (smoking, chewing) as there is a direct cause-effect relationship between smoking and peripheral vascular disease (Buerger's disease). Alcohol history is equally important as chronic alcoholism leads to atherosclerosis.

Family History

Family history of peripheral vascular disease, musculoskeletal tumors, diabetes, etc., is important.

Psychological Evaluation due to Amputation

A general psychological assessment of the patient, such as depression, anxiety, coping mechanism suicidal thoughts, etc., is important to understand how amputation has affected him/her. Assessment by a psychologist/psychiatrist is vital in the patient's overall well-being.

After these points mentioned earlier are asked, it is imperative to determine the patient's expectations, as the treatment should be planned to tailor to his/her needs.

Keeping these points in mind, let us now go through a general scheme of examination of a patient presenting with an amputation stump.

EXAMINATION

General and Systemic Examination

It is essential in amputations secondary to peripheral arterial occlusive disorder.
- The *general examination* includes a head-to-toe evaluation to look for signs of an underlying systemic condition(s).
- The *systemic examination* includes a brief examination of the cardiovascular system, respiratory system, central nervous system, and abdomen-pelvis. The cardiovascular examination is critical in peripheral vascular disease.

Local Examination

The examination of the affected limb (in case of lower limbs) begins with an assessment of the following:

Functional Mobility and Gait

- **Functional mobility** must be assessed and commented upon, especially in the case of lower limb amputee, such as—
  - Balance in sitting
  - Mobility in bed
  - Ability to transfer and mobilize
  - Standing balance, and tolerance with prosthesis
- **Gait:** The patient is made to walk (as he normally does), and gait is observed from front, sides, and behind. Mostly, gait is assisted with orthosis or prosthesis **(Fig. 13.1)**. However, the foot amputee may walk without a prosthesis (Syme's or forefoot amputee).

Following the gait assessment, the patient is then made to lie supine (position of rest) to comment upon other factors.

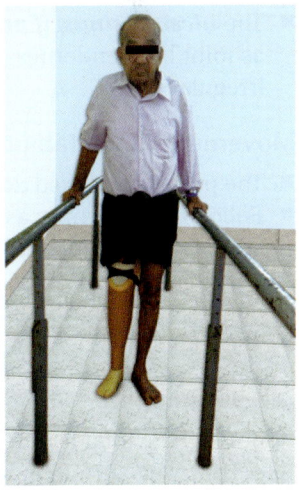

Fig. 13.1: Patient walking with a below-knee prosthesis.

Attitude

The attitude of the limbs: It is described as the position assumed by each joint at rest.

Inspection of Stump

Inspection should include the following points **(Fig. 13.2)**:
- The **shape** of the stump: Cylindrical, conical, bulbous, or irregular.
- **Scar of the stump should be assessed with the following points:**
  - State of the surgical incision— healed or the presence of gaping.

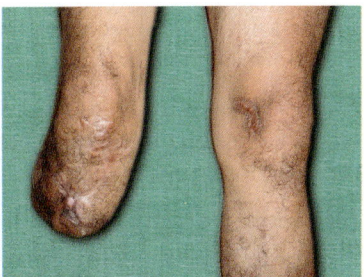

Fig. 13.2: Below-knee amputation stump shows badly scarred stump.

- ❏ Whether scar has healed with the primary intention or secondary intention
- ❏ Any hypertrophic scar/keloid formation
- **Swelling** of the stump
- **Wasting** of the muscles of the proximal part of the limb
- Presence or absence of **sinus, discharge** from the wound, *excoriation, erythema, ulcer, or callosities*
- **Protruding or impinging bony ends**.

Palpation of Stump

Palpation should be gentle and should confirm the findings obtained from inspection.
- **Local temperature:** A rise in local temperature is suggestive of infection/inflammation.
- The presence/absence of **tenderness over the stump** and site of tenderness should be noted.
- The bony stump is palpated to assess the **edge, the protruding prominence, and the soft tissue covering**.
- Whether **scar** is mobile or adherent to underlying tissues or bone.
- A detailed examination of **ulcer or sinus, if present** should be done accordingly.
- The **ulcer or sinus, if present** should be palpated to assess the degenerative changes, such as joint line tenderness, synovial hypertrophy, joint effusion, bony deformities, and bony irregularities.

Movements and Stability of Neighboring Joints

- The presence of fixed deformities or contractures should be noted at the proximal joints.
- Following deformity assessment, the ROM at the joint proximal to the stump should be assessed and compared to that of the normal limb.
- Further, it is important to note the presence of pain during movement and joint crepitus, both of which may indicate degenerative changes.
- The stability of the joint should be assessed on the standard pattern for that joint.

Measurements

Routinely, the total length of the stump is measured from a fixed proximal landmark or joint line. However, current guidelines advise clinical measurement of the stump from soft tissue landmarks mentioned here:

Above-knee stump: The stump of an amputated thigh will be measured from the perineum, at the origin of the adductor tendons, to the bony end of the stump, with the amputee recumbent and the stump lying parallel with the other lower limb.

Below-knee stump: From the insertion of the internal hamstring muscles to the bony end of the stump with the patient recumbent and the knee flexed at 90°.

Above-elbow stump: From the anterior axillary fold to the bony end of the stump, with the stump hanging parallel to the chest wall. Indicate whether the amputation site is above or below the insertion of the deltoid muscle.

Below-elbow stump: From the insertion of the biceps tendon to the bony end, with the elbow flexed at 90°. Indicate if the amputation site is above or below the attachment of the pronator teres.
- Amputation of fingers should be described as the level of amputation, such as through the distal, middle, or proximal phalanx or metacarpophalangeal joint.

- Also, report the fraction of hand remaining in a hand amputee.
- Similarly, foot bone loss must be recorded as to what level of amputation has been performed. Always report loss of metatarsal head, if any.
- Next, the girth of the limb proximal to the stump should be measured and compared to the normal limb to assess muscle wasting.

Neurovascular Status of Stump and Adjoining Areas

- **Vascularity of the stump** is assessed by skin temperature and the level of dependent rubor.
- The stump is then examined for the **presence of neuroma** (pain and localized paresthesia on percussion) by tapping the stump, **sensory deficits, and paresthesia**. Presence of protective sensation can be confirmed using 10 g Semmes–Weinstein monofilament (it represents the pressure threshold to protect the skin from ulcerations), 128 Hz tuning fork test, and Pinprick sensation test. Also, assess the proprioceptive sensation on the joints of residual limb and contralateral limb.
- The **motor power and reflexes** of the amputated limb should be examined and recorded.
- Always assess the patient's **overall coordination and balance**, which would ensure adequate mobility when the prosthesis is donned.

Prosthesis Examination

Once the amputated limb is examined, it is imperative to examine the prosthesis (if the patient is using one) to look for wear, loosening, breakage, etc.

Upper Limb, Spine, and Pelvis Examination in Case of Lower Limb Amputee

A quick overall examination of the upper limb, spine, pelvis, and core stability for movement, power, and balance is essential to ensure the patient's overall ability to mobilise with the prosthesis.

Principles of Amputation

The following principles should be borne in mind while performing an amputation to create an ideal stump:
- The scar should be well healed and mobile, away from the subcutaneous bony edges.
- The skin should remain sensate.
- The stump should have a cylindrical or conical shape at closure.
- Traumatized tissue must be adequately debrided.
- Myoplastic techniques may be attempted in nonischemic limbs (Myoplasty: Suturing muscle-tendon to opposite group muscle; Myodesis: Suturing muscle-tendon to the bone via a predrilled hole).
- Nerves should be gently sectioned and allowed to retract into proximal soft tissues to prevent neuroma formation in inappropriate places.
- The bone should be beveled to avoid sharp edges, which may cause dependent skin necrosis.

  The characteristics of an ideal stump are mentioned in **Box 13.1**.

> **BOX 13.1:** Ideal stump characteristics.
>
> - Adequate length
> - *Ideal shape:* Preferably conical or cylindrical
> - Appropriately placed surgical scars healed with primary intention, which are non-adherent
> - No keloid or painful hypertrophic scars
> - The bony ends well covered with muscles with no prominent/sharp bone ends
> - Free from any soft tissue or bony infection, no sinuses/ulcers
> - No neuroma
> - Full range of movement at the proximal joint, no fixed deformity
> - Normal sensation at the stump
> - Muscle power more than grade 3

Complications of Amputation

The following are the common complications seen after amputation:
- Infection
- Wound necrosis
- Pain
- Joint contractures
- Phantom limb sensation: Mirror therapy should be done
- Neuroma formation
- Painful scars
- Bone overgrowth (in growing children)

Special Amputation Stumps

1. **Lisfranc's amputation:** Foot amputation *through the tarsometatarsal joint* while retaining the mid and hindfoot (calcaneus, talus, and heel pad) **(Fig. 13.3)**.
2. **Chopart's amputation:** Foot amputation *through the midtarsal joint* while retaining the hindfoot (calcaneus, talus, and heel pad).
3. **Syme's amputation:** Ankle disarticulation, removal of malleoli, *but* heel pad is retained. It works if there is a patent posterior tibial artery. The retained heel pad gives an excellent weight-bearing surface, and the patient can walk without a prosthesis **(Fig. 13.4)**.

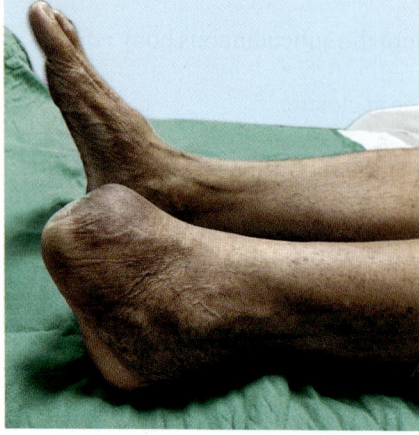

Fig. 13.3: Lisfranc's amputation stump.

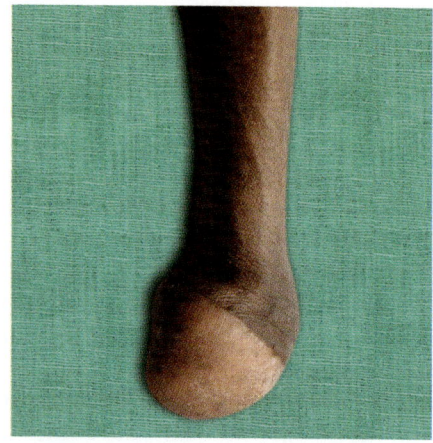

Fig. 13.4: Syme's amputation stump.

4. **Pirogoff amputation:** It is a Syme's variant where in ankle disarticulation, and malleoli are removed; but along with the heel pad, the posterior part of the calcaneum is retained.
5. **Hindquarter amputation or external hemipelvectomy:** Entire lower limb with the same side innominate bone is removed.
6. **Forequarter amputation:** Entire upper limb with scapula and clavicle is removed.

Box 13.2 discusses several features of disarticulation.

BOX 13.2: A note on disarticulation.

Disarticulation: When amputation is done through the joint
Advantages:
- Long lever prevents contractures and allows consequently the better muscle and movement control due to longer lever arm
- Maintains muscle length and strength
- Preferred in children as it preserves the growth plates
- Candidates for end-bearing prosthesis
- Better proprioception and distribution of pressure

Disadvantages:
- Bulky prosthesis
- Poor cosmesis
- More demanding surgical procedure with the risk of increased wound complications

---

Amputation Stump Examination Proforma

1. **General and systemic examination**
2. **Gait**
3. **Attitude**
4. **Inspection of the stump:**
   a. Shape
   b. Scar
   c. Swelling
   d. Sinuses, ulcers, callosities, discharge
   e. Bony protrusions
   f. Proximal muscle wasting
5. **Palpation:**
   a. Local rise of temperature
   b. Tenderness of the stump, bony end, swelling, scar
   c. Swelling if present—bony (e.g., recurrence of tumor) and soft tissue (e.g., neuroma)
   d. Scar—mobile or fixed to the underlying bone
   e. Detailed examination of sinuses and ulcers, if present
   f. Palpate the proximal muscles to confirm wasting
   g. Palpation of joint proximal to stump
6. **Movement of joint proximal to stump**
   a. **Measurement of the stump**
   b. **Neurovascular status:**
      i. Vascular—skin temperature, capillary refill, skin rubor
      ii. Neurological—examine for the presence of neuroma (localized paresthesia of percussing around the scar); sensory deficits; motor deficits of the muscles controlling the proximal joint
   c. **Examination of lymph nodes draining the stump**
   d. **Examination of the prosthesis**

CHAPTER 14

Clinical Evaluation of Gait and Various Patterns of Gait

INTRODUCTION

In layman's term, gait is the manner or style of walking. Its analysis is an important part of examining the lower limb and spine as it reflects the biomechanical compromise of the spine, hip and lower limbs, thereby understanding the pathological process that has affected the primary function and how the patient has compensated for it. Gait disturbances are described as deviations from normal walking.

DEFINITION OF GAIT

A normal gait is an energy-efficient, series of rhythmical, alternating movements of the trunk and limbs, which results in the forward progression of the center of gravity, allowing bipedal mobility from one place to another. A normal gait depends on a complex interplay between nervous, musculoskeletal, and cardiopulmonary systems.

PHASES OF GAIT

The gait cycle is divided into two phases—*stance and swing*, which are described below.
1. **Stance phase:** It is the time during which the limb is *in contact with the ground* while supporting the weight of the body. *The stance phase occupies 60% of the gait cycle.*
2. **Swing phase:** It is the time when the limb is advancing, and *not in contact with the ground* while body weight is supported by the contralateral limb. *The swing phase occupies 40% of the gait cycle.*

Various sequences in the stance and swing phase are illustrated in **Figure 14.1**.

ETIOLOGY OF GAIT DISTURBANCE

Gait disturbances are described as any deviations from normal walking. Numerous etiologies may result in gait disturbances. Detailed history taking and examination helps in identifying

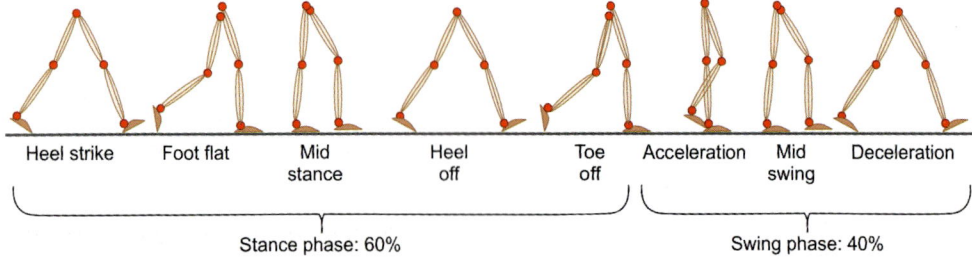

Fig. 14.1: Illustration of stance and swing phase in the gait cycle.

the accurate etiology. The gait disturbance cannot be corrected unless the correct etiology is identified and treated. Various etiologies are mentioned below.
1. **Neurological diseases:** Diseases affecting the central and peripheral nervous system can cause gait disturbance. Various common causes are cerebrovascular accident (Hemiplegia), Parkinson's, cerebellar disorders (Motor ataxia), subacute combined degeneration (sensory ataxia), cerebral palsy, poliomyelitis, peripheral nerve affections, muscular dystrophies, and Charcot–Marie–Tooth disease.
2. **Conditions affecting musculoskeletal integrity of the lower limbs:** Any cause which affects the pelvis-hip-rest of the lower limb biomechanics would cause gait disturbance, such as conditions causing painful hip, hip with altered lever mechanism (developmental dysplasia of the hip, non- or mal-union of hip fractures, coxa vara, coxa valga, etc.), and a short limb.
3. **Electrolyte imbalance:** Various electrolyte imbalances such as hyponatremia, hypokalemia, and hypomagnesemia can cause gait disorders.
4. **Vitamin deficiency:** Vitamin B_{12} deficiency could result in subacute combined degeneration, contributing to gait disturbances.
5. **Others:** Psychological causes (anxiety, depression) and malingering should be ruled out. Note that patients with psychological disturbance or malingering would not have a consistent gait pattern.

History

1. Gait analysis is mainly observational. However, the patient may present with specific complaints concerning his gait. The most common of these are:
   - Pain while walking
   - Stiffness
   - *Limp:* It may be painful or painless *(Note: Limp is a symptom, while lurch is a sign).*
2. The onset, duration, and progression of the complaint (mainly, limp) have to be noted, and the disability resulting from an altered gait has to be analyzed. For example, a person with a stiff hip gait may complain of difficulty getting into or out of a vehicle.
3. The history should also detail the use of a walking aid and the change of footwear.
4. Various neurological and structural conditions influence the gait. The pertinent history detailing these disorders affecting the gait must be evaluated.
   - *Neuromuscular:* Cerebrovascular accident (CVA), cerebral palsy, poliomyelitis, Parkinson's disease, peripheral nerve injury or affection, and myopathy
   - *Structural:* Limb length discrepancy, developmental dysplasia of the hip, congenital talipes equinovarus, malunited intertrochanteric femur, stiff hip or knee, etc.
5. Assessment of gait disturbance on activities of daily living and patient's quality of life, including psychological disturbance, must be noted.

Examination

As mentioned before, gait analysis is observational in routine clinical practice. Specific prerequisites are to be followed while commenting on gait.
1. Gait should be observed from the front, behind, and sides.
2. The patient should be made to walk barefoot.
3. The shoulder, entire spine, pelvis, and lower limbs should be exposed, with only the private parts covered.
4. A walkway of sufficient length (20 feet) and width should be available.

5. The following structural and functional features should be observed while evaluating the gait:
   a. Head position
   b. Position of the shoulders
   c. Trunk position
   d. Arm swing
   e. Pelvic tilt
   f. The swing of the lower limbs
   g. Time spent in the stance and the swing phase
   h. Base (distance between the two feet) and other temporal parameters of the gait.

   For example, in a child with right side DDH (malfunctioning abductor mechanism), the gait is described as "head is central in position, the arm swing is alternate and rhythmic, bipedal, unaided painless gait with the patient lurching to the right side and the pelvis dropping on the left side. This is a description of a Trendelenburg gait on the right side."

COMMONLY ENCOUNTERED GAIT PATTERNS

Antalgic (Coxalgic) Gait
- It is observed in conditions causing *pain in any of the lower limb bones and joints*.
- The patient walks with a shortened stance phase on the affected side, with a decreased swing of the normal side. However, the pelvis remains at the same level (c.f. Trendelenburg gait where the pelvis drops).

   Further, the patient *lurches on the affected side* as it helps move the body's center of gravity toward the painful hip, which decreases the moment arm of body weight to hip joint, reducing total force on the hip **(Fig. 14.2A)**. Therefore, the total amount of reactionary force over the hip decreases, which helps in reducing the pain.

Trendelenburg Gait
- It is observed in conditions causing *dysfunction of the abductor mechanism of the hip, such as* DDH, coxa vara, and Perthes' disease, etc.
- Typically, in a single-leg stance, due to gravity, the unsupported side of the pelvis (swing side) tends to drop down, which is prevented by contraction of the hip abductors of the contralateral limb that is in the stance phase. However, when the abductor mechanism on the stance side is dysfunctional, the contralateral pelvis (swing side) drops down, and, in an attempt to lift the pelvis, the *patient lurches on the side of the stance (or affected side)* **(Fig. 14.2B)**. This action of lurching on the affected side moves the center of gravity nearer to the fulcrum on the weak side, shortening the moment arm from the center of gravity to the hip joint and reducing the effort required by the hip abductors.
  Therefore, during the Trendelenburg gait, the pelvis rocks up and down with the patient lurching to the affected side.
  When observed from the side—stride length is short and step length is reduced.
- A bilateral Trendelenburg's gait is called a *Waddling gait*. It is observed in bilateral DDH.

High-stepping Gait
- It is observed in *foot drop*.
- In footdrop, the *'ankle dorsiflexor's weakness'* results in two characteristic pathological events during the gait cycle.

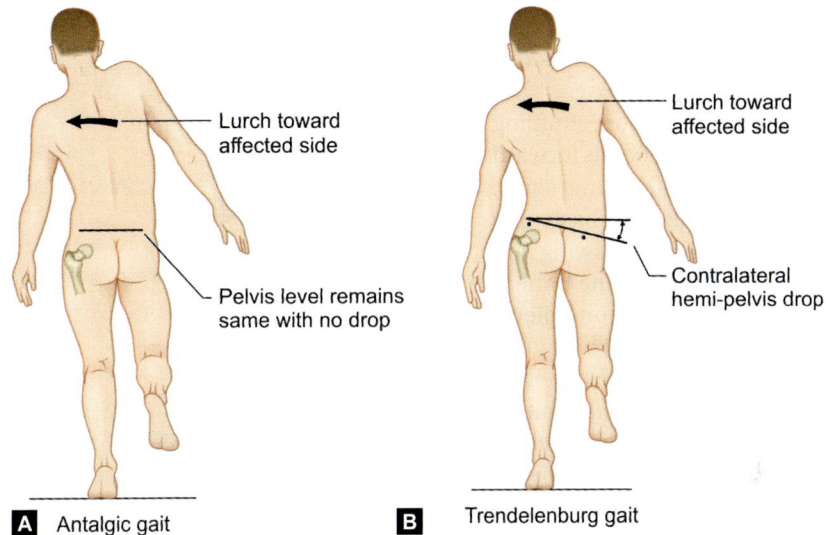

Figs. 14.2A and B: (A) Antalgic/coxalgic gait; (B) Trendelenburg gait.

Note: The Trendelenburg gait is very similar in appearance to a antalgic gait except drop in the level of the pelvis.

a. To clear the foot off the ground, the patient will have to hyperflex his/her hip and knees resulting in high stepping.
b. At the beginning of the stance phase, instead of heel striking the floor first, the forefoot strikes the floor (as ankle dorsiflexors are paralyzed), giving a "high-stepping phenomena."

Extension Lurch or Gluteus Maximus Gait or Rocking Horse Gait

- It is seen in *paralysis of the gluteus maximus*, an extensor of the hip.
- Typically, the gluteus maximus begins to contract at the moment of heel-strike, slowing forward motion of trunk by arresting flexion of the hip and initiating extension. However, when the gluteus maximus is weak, the trunk lurches backward (gluteus maximus lurch) at heel-strike on the weakened side to interrupt the forward motion of the trunk. The patient's trunk moves forward and backward too much, giving a rocking horse gait appearance **(Fig. 14.3)**.

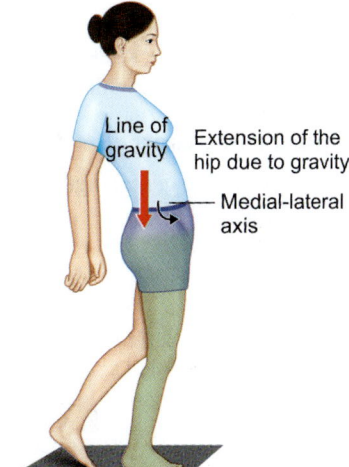

Fig. 14.3: Extension lurch/gluteus maximus gait.

Scissoring Gait

- Typically, it is observed in *spastic cerebral palsy* due to *adductor contracture/spasm*.
- Here, the leg in the swing phase crosses anteriorly over the leg in the stance phase like a scissor **(Fig. 14.4)**. It appears as if the patient is walking through waist-deep water.

Festinant Gait

- It is observed in basal ganglia lesions leading to *Parkinson's disease*.
- It is characterized by a "short, shuffling gait" where the patient bends forward (stooped posture) while taking short, quick steps with involuntary hastening (festination), reduced arm swing and trembling of extremities. The patient turns around stiffly 'all in one piece', and also has poor posture control (retropulsion) **(Fig. 14.5A)** (*The gait is something like how a fast bowler bends forward in his initial run-up with small steps!*).

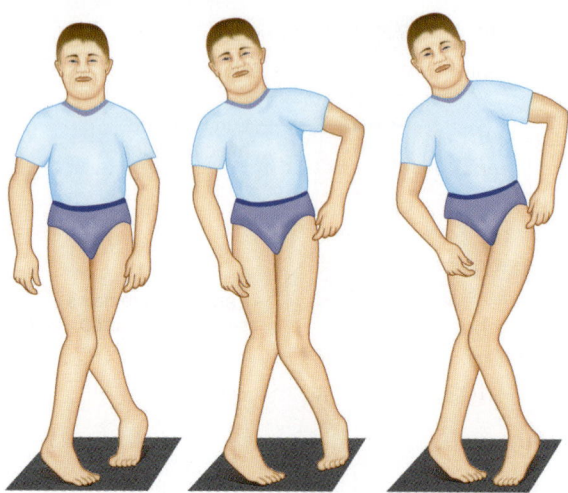

Fig. 14.4: Scissoring gait.

Quadriceps Weakness

It is classically described in *patients with poliomyelitis affecting quadriceps muscle resulting in hand-to-knee gait*. In this type of gait, the patient bends forward to let the center of gravity fall in front of the knee and let the knee lock in extension due to posteriorly directed joint reaction force. In extreme quadriceps weakness, the patient may adopt a *hand-to-knee gait* wherein the patient pushes the knee posteriorly with his hand to extend and lock the knee so that he/she can propel forward with a locked-extended knee **(Fig. 14.5B)**.

Knock Knee Gait

It is observed in *genu valgus deformity* wherein both knees knock with each other while walking **(Fig. 14.5C)**.

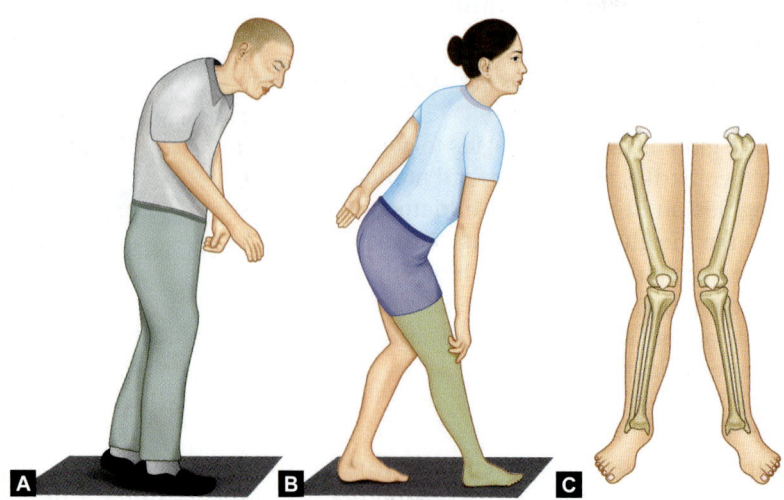

Figs. 14.5A to C: (A) Festinant gait (in Parkinson's); (B) Quadriceps weakness—hand-to-knee gait; (C) Knock knee gait (in severe genu valgum).

Hemiplegic Gait/Circumduction Gait

It is classically observed in a *hemiplegic patient recovering after an episode of a cerebrovascular accident (CVA)*. During the swing phase, the patient tries to *circumduct the hip, makes a half-circle stiffly outwards and forwards to* clear the ground.
- **Upper limb:** Arm in adduction, flexion, internal rotation; elbow flexed, forearm pronated, and wrist-fingers are flexed held closely to the chest.
- **Lower limb:** Hip in extension, adduction, medial rotation; knee extension, ankle plantar flexion, and inversion.

These spastic muscles are synergistically activated into hip and knee extension during the stance phase of walking, and the abnormal spastic activation does not allow the hip and knee to flex for foot clearance. The patient also leans the trunk to the contralateral side to clear the affected limb off the ground during walking.

Ataxic Gait

Ataxic gait is often characterized by difficulty to walk in a straight line, poor balance, lateral veering, a broad base of support, inconsistent arm motion, variable cadence, and lack of repeatability. These symptoms often resemble gait seen under the influence of alcohol. Typically, it is observed in two situations: *'cerebellar disorder'* and *'sensory ataxia'* due to lesions of the posterior column of the spinal cord.

a. **Cerebellar ataxia gait:** Gait is staggering, unsteady impaired balance wherein the patient adopts a *wide base of support (BOS)*. This wide BOS creates large side-to-side swaying due to deviation of the center of gravity. The patient cannot stand with both feet together with eyes closed or open. Other cerebellar signs may be present such as dysmetria/dysdiadochokinesia, nystagmus, slurred speech, hypotonia, and intentional tremor.

b. **Sensory ataxia gait or stomping gait:** It is observed in disorders of the posterior column of the spinal cord. It is characterized by an unsteady and wide-based gait, wherein patients throw their feet outwards and forward and bring them down first in the heel and then on the toes, with a double-tapping/stomping sound (c.f. foot drop wherein forefoot strikes first followed by the heel). With eyes open, patients try to balance their gait by watching the ground, whereas with eyes closed, they cannot stand with feet together (Rhomberg sign positive), and staggering worsens.

Notes

CHAPTER 15

Clinical Evaluation of the Swelling, Scar, Sinus, and Ulcer

HISTORY AND EXAMINATION OF A SWELLING

Relevant History
Swelling is one of the common complaint in patients. One must probe the swelling on the following aspects: Onset, duration, progression, painless or painful, associated sinus, similar swelling elsewhere, exacerbating and relieving factors and other associated symptoms.

Onset
- **Acute onset:**
  - *Following trauma:* Fracture displacement of the bone, dislocation of joint, and hematoma
  - *Spontaneous:* Acute osteomyelitis, tumor (mostly malignant), acute inflammation of a joint, acute infections, bursitis.
- **Insidious onset:** Tumor (primarily benign), inflammatory or chronic infective origin, ganglion, and Baker's cyst.

It is possible that the patient may have noticed the swelling recently. However, the size might indicate that it could have been present for a much longer period and yet remained unnoticed by the patient. Such swellings are also described as insidious in onset.

Duration
- **Since birth:** Congenital (e.g., meningocele)
- **Short duration (days to weeks):** Acute osteomyelitis, tumor (mostly malignant), and inflammatory
- **Long duration (months to years):** Tumor (primarily benign), ganglion.

Progression
- **Growing slowly:** Benign swellings (tumor, ganglion, lipoma)
- **Growing rapidly:** Malignant swellings (osteosarcoma and Ewing's sarcoma)
- **Suddenly increasing in size after remaining stationary for some time:** Malignant transformation of benign swellings
- **Fluctuation in size:** Inflammatory swelling (gout), ganglion
- **Reduction in size or disappearance:** It is observed if swelling ruptures, or regresses if primary cause subsides. This is a typical phenomena associated with Baker's cyst whose size can reduce after it ruptures, or it decreases in size if the primary pathology in the knee subsides. Sometimes, swellings can be accentuates with a particular joint posture, while attenuates with another.

> Note that Baker's cyst is almost always secondary to a primary pathology in the knee such as osteoarthritis, rheumatoid arthritis. Further, rupture of Baker's cyst is associated with acute pain and swelling in the calf, which mimics deep vein thrombosis.

Pain

- **Painless:** Most benign tumors are painless. However, they may turn painful if there is any malignant change.
- **Intermittently painful:** Ganglion, Baker's cyst.
- **Painful:**
  - *Dull aching pain:* Degenerative origin swelling such as Bouchard, Heberden nodes, slowly growing benign tumor
  - *Throbbing pain:* Inflammatory swellings, abscess, malignant tumors
  - *Pain followed by swelling:* Inflammatory conditions and malignant tumors
  - *Initially painless swelling, which becomes painful later:* Malignant transformation of a benign tumor, sudden hemorrhage in tumor, pathological fracture, and nerve entrapment/compression by a swelling.

  In swellings associated with pain, history should be obtained regarding characteristics of pain as well. Malignant transformation is associated with continuous and progressively severe pain, while nerve compression is associated with shooting pain, tingling and paresthesia along the distribution of the nerve.

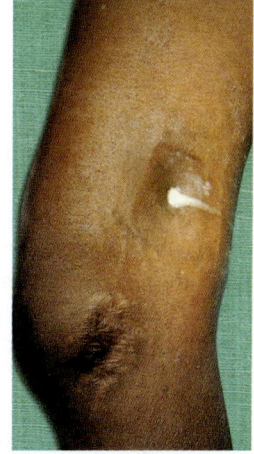

Fig. 15.1: Sinus with purulent discharge and swelling of the distal thigh.

Associated Sinus

Primarily, a sinus around the bone indicates chronic osteomyelitis. *Nevertheless, not all sinuses need to arise from the bone.* It is important to note that the presence of a sinus indicates that underlying the sinus, there is a dead and infected tissue or material. Ask for the type of discharge from the sinus; hemorrhagic, serous, seropurulent, or purulent **(Fig. 15.1)**.

Similar Swellings Elsewhere

- **Multiple swellings:** Diaphyseal aclasis (multiple exostosis), neurofibromatosis **(Fig. 15.2)**
- **Multiple asymptomatic subcutaneous swellings:** Multiple lipomas and neurofibromatosis (associated café-au-lait spots)
- **Multiple bony swellings at epiphyses:** Multiple exostoses
- **Lymph nodes in neck, axilla or groin** may suggest an underlying infection or malignancy.

Exacerbating or Relieving Factors

Vascular swellings, especially of venous origin may increase in size with dependency.

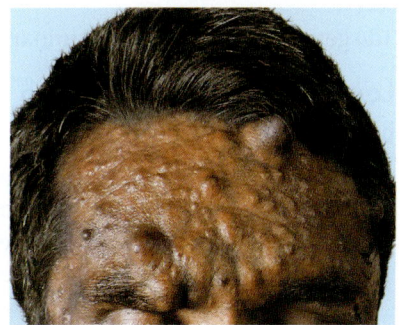

Fig. 15.2: Multiple swelling over forehead in neurofibromatosis.

Other Associated Symptoms

- ***Constitutional symptoms:*** Constitutional symptoms such as significant loss of weight, loss of appetite, fever, malaise, and cachexia are observed in malignant tumors, chronic infection (tuberculosis), and occasionally in inflammatory disorders (rheumatoid arthritis).

It is essential to understand that constitutional symptoms indicate sinister pathologies, and the clinician must probe further to diagnose the condition.
- **Compressive symptoms:** Symptoms of compression of neurovasculolymphatic structures is a feature of tumors. These symptoms are observed distal to the compression.
  - *Nerve compression*: Manifested by shooting pain, paresthesia, numbness, and motor weakness (distal to compression) depending upon amount of compression.
  - *Vascular compression*: Venous congestion or thrombus produces distal edema, whereas arterial compression (e.g., cervical rib) produces ischemic features.
- **Growth disturbance/angular deformities:** Lesion damaging growth plate (juxtaphyseal tumors such as diaphyseal aclasis/osteomyelitis).
- *Functional disability:* Difficulty in using the limb-affecting activities of daily living.
- **Symptoms of a primary in case of a secondary metastatic tumor (swelling) is suspected:** If there is a suspicion of bony metastasis and concomitant swelling in the limb (with/without pathological fracture), one must probe and look for a primary. For example, urinary complaints (prostate tumor), breathing difficulty, cough, hemoptysis (lung tumor), neck swelling (thyroid carcinoma), and breast lumps (malignant breast tumor).

Past History
- History of infection elsewhere (must be asked in the case of children and immunocompromised patients) in patients with *acute or chronic osteomyelitis.*
- **History of excision in the past:** Incomplete excision of cysts in the past, if the cyst wall was not completely removed, can result in recurrence (e.g., ganglion).

Family History
To rule out hereditary disorders such as osteogenesis imperfecta, achondroplasia, and multiple exostoses.

EXAMINATION

The general and systemic examination should be done in the standard fashion.

Local Examination of Swelling

Inspection

The inspection of swelling is done under following headings: site, size, shape, number, extent, surface, edge, overlying skin, pressure effects, neighboring joints, surrounding muscle wasting and limb length discrepancy. The description is mentioned below.
1. **Site:** Often, a site may suggest the etiology of the swelling **(Table 15.1)**. Several examples of swelling as per characteristic location are mentioned below.
   - *Epiphysis*: Osteoclastoma and chondroblastoma
   - *Metaphysis*: Bone cyst, osteoid osteoma, osteosarcoma, and acute pyogenic osteomyelitis
   - *Diaphysis*: Ewing's sarcoma, multiple myeloma, and syphilitic osteomyelitis
   - *Small bones of the hand*: Enchondroma, spina ventosa (tubercular dactylitis).

> **Note:**
> - Ganglions are very common over the dorsum of the wrist/around the wrist **(Fig. 15.3A)**.
> - Rheumatoid nodules are seen over the extensor surface of the long bones, especially in the forearm **(Fig. 15.3B)**.

TABLE 15.1: Differential diagnosis of swellings based on anatomical site.

Epiphyseal	Metaphyseal	Diaphyseal	Flat bones	Vertebral body	Posterior spinal elements
• Giant cell tumor • Chondroblastoma • Chondrosarcoma • Osteomyelitis	• Osteochondroma • Osteosarcoma • Chondromyxoid fibroma • ABC • Enchondral bone cyst • Nonossifying fibroma • Osteomyelitis	• Fibrous dysplasia • Ewing's sarcoma osteoid osteoma • Chronic osteomyelitis • Osteoblastoma • Lymphoma • Adamantinoma • Eosinophilic granuloma	• Ewing's sarcoma • Chondrosarcoma • Multiple myeloma • Metastasis from other primaries	• Metastasis from other primaries • Multiple myeloma • GCT • Ewing's sarcoma	• Metastasis from other primaries • ABC • Osteoid osteoma

(ABC: aneurysmal bone cyst; GCT: giant cell tumor)

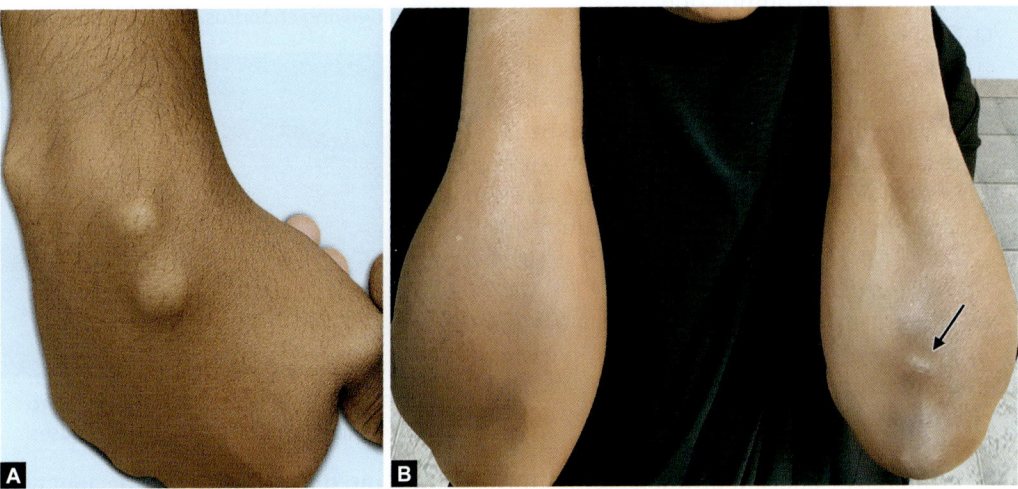

Figs. 15.3A and B: (A) Ganglion over the dorsum of the wrist; (B) Rheumatoid nodule over the extensor aspect of the left forearm.

2. **Size:** Approximate length and width of the swelling.
3. **Shape:** Spherical/oval/irregular/other. The swelling usually tends to attain a spherical shape, but this growth is hindered by unyielding fascia or bone.
4. **Number:**
   ❑ *Solitary:* Osteomyelitis, ganglion, and most tumors.
   ❑ *Multiple:* Diaphyseal aclasis, neurofibromatosis.
5. **Extent:** The vertical and horizontal extent of the swelling must be described using bony landmarks.
6. **Surface:**
   ❑ *Smooth:* Usually, benign tumors or other benign swellings line ganglion, lipoma
   ❑ *Irregular:* Malignant tumors and chronic infection.

7. **Edge:**
   - *Well defined:* Usually pedunculated swelling
   - *Indistinct:* Sessile swelling.
8. **The skin overlying the swelling:**
   - *Edematous and congested:* Acute osteomyelitis
   - *Stretched, shiny with dilated veins:* Malignant tumors and hypervascular soft tissue sarcomas **(Fig. 15.4).**
   - *Sinus:* Chronic pyogenic and tubercular osteomyelitis
   - *Scarred:* Chronic osteomyelitis or previous surgery **(Fig. 15.5).**
9. **Pressure effects (limb distal to the swelling):**
   - *Edema:* Due to venous compression, lymphatic obstruction
   - *Paresis:* Nerve compression
   - *Pulsations:* If the swelling is right over the artery compressing it, the feel of pulse might alter while palpating it proximal or distal to the swelling. While pulsation could be feeble distal to the swelling, it could prominent (or bounding) proximal to the swelling as swelling compresses the artery resulting in rebound flow *(Note: Theoretically, this finding to be confirmed during palpation)*
   - Veins proximal to the compression might appear engorged due to distal compression.
10. **Neighboring joints:**
    - Diffuse swelling seen in acute osteomyelitis over the adjacent joint is usually due to sympathetic effusion or when the pus breaks down into the joint cavity associated with metaphysis, leading to septic arthritis
    - *Angular deformities:* Sequelae of osteomyelitis and diaphyseal aclasis.
11. **Muscle wasting**
12. **Shortening/lengthening of bone:** Often observed in chronic osteomyelitis, trauma (malunion, non-union), and diaphyseal aclasis.

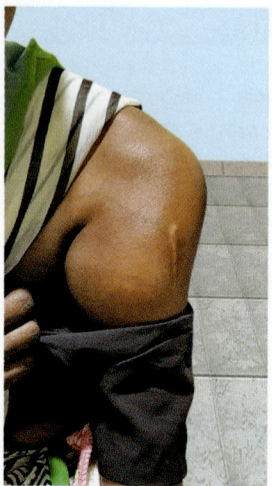

Fig. 15.4: Stretched shiny skin due to underlying chondrosarcoma of humerus.

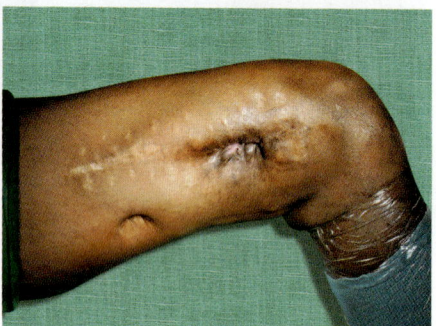

Fig. 15.5: Chronic scarred limb due to previous surgeries and healed sinuses.

Palpation

The inspectory findings must be confirmed by palpatory methods systematically under the following headings: Local temperature, tenderness, and swelling specific characteristics—site, size, extent, surface, edge, overlying skin pinchability, consistency, pulsatility, the plane of the swelling, fluctuation, fluid thrill, reducibility, compressibility, translucency and impulse on coughing. Also, assess underlying bony irregularity, associated ulcer and sinus, and any pathological fracture of the underlying bone.

1. **Local temperature:** It is assessed by the dorsum of the fingers.
   - Raised in inflammatory, infective, and malignant swelling
2. **Tenderness:**
   - *Tender:* Inflammatory swellings, malignant tumors, infection, and acute trauma
   - *Nontender:* Chronic degenerative condition
3. **Swelling-specific characteristics:**
   - *Site:* Confirm the exact the site of the swelling by palpating all around with respect to the bone.
   - *Size, shape and extent:* Confirm the size and shape by palpating the swelling. The vertical and horizontal extent of swelling is better appreciated during palpation.
   - *Surface*
     - *Smooth and lobulated:* Benign tumors, Baker's cyst, ganglion
     - *Nodular or matted:* Mass of lymph nodes in TB
     - *Irregular:* Malignant tumors and chronic infection.
   - *Edge:*
     - *Well-defined:* Benign tumors, ganglion
     - *Ill-defined:* Indistinct or ill-defined implies that the margins imperceptibly merge into the surrounding tissues. It is observed in inflammatory/infective/malignant swellings.
     - *Initially well-defined and later rapidly progressing to ill-defined:* Benign turning malignant.
   - *Overlying skin pinchability:* One must try to gently lift the skin above the swelling. A swelling arising from the skin would be adherent to the skin. A swelling which is not arising from the skin would be adherent in case of chronic infection, inflammation or malignant tumors infiltrating the skin. It is adherent with underlying swelling in chronic infections, inflammation, scars and malignant tumors (due to infiltration).
   - *Consistency:*
     - *Soft:* "Like the feel of the earlobe." For example, lipoma, acute osteomyelitis with subcutaneous abscess (soft tissue over the swelling), are soft in feel
     - *Cystic:* Cysts and chronic abscessess.
     - *Firm:* "Like the feeling of the tip of the nose." For example, fibroma
     - *Bony hard:* "Like the feel of the forehead." For example, osteoma, exostosis, giant cell tumor (eggshell crackling—must not be elicited), and irregular new bone over chronic osteomyelitis area
     - *Variable consistency (soft-firm-hard):* Certain tumors can have variable consistency due to variable amounts of cartilage, fibrous and osteogenic components in the tumor mass along with tumor necrosis. For example, osteosarcoma, chondrosarcoma.
   - *Pulsatility:* Apart from arterial swellings (aneurysm), highly vascular tumors, such as vascular secondaries (from thyroid and renal adenocarcinoma), telangiectatic osteosarcoma, and highly vascular osteoclastoma can be pulsatile.
     Further, it is essential to understand the difference between pulsatile swelling and transmitted pulsation. A *'swelling arising from an artery (aneurysm)'* is pulsatile, while *'swelling lying over an artery'* only transmits the pulsation of underlying artery. The method to differentiate between the two is discussed below **(Figs. 15.6A to C)**.
     - *Pulsatile swelling*: When a pair of fingers kept over the swelling as far apart move away from each other, it indicates a pulsatile swelling **(Fig. 15.6B)**.

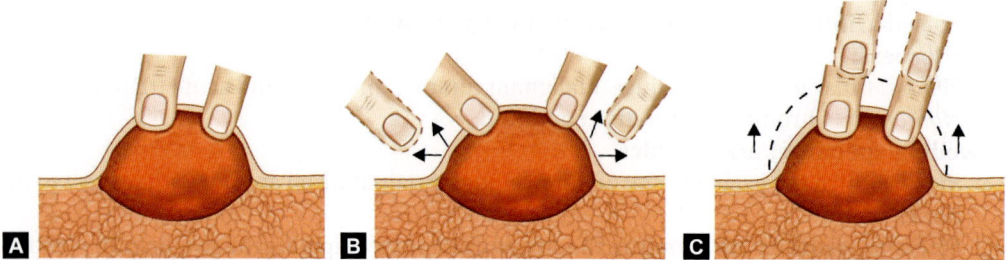

Figs. 15.6A to C: Clinical method to differentiate between pulsatile swelling transmitted pulsation. (A) Two fingers kept over the swelling as far apart; (B) Diverging fingers indicating pulsatile swelling; (C) Vertically upward and parallel movement of the fingers indicate transmitted pulse.

- *Transmitted pulsation*: When fingers move only vertically parallel to each other and not away from each other, it indicates transmitted pulsation **(Fig. 15.6C)**.
- **Plane of the swelling:** It is imperative to identify the plane of the swelling. Also, the swelling may possess some characteristic features when it arises from a particular structure. In relation to a muscle, swelling may be submuscular, intramuscular, or supramuscular. The swelling may also arise from nerve, muscle, tendon, bone, vascular structure, or fat cells. Characteristics features of the plane of swelling are mentioned in **Box 15.1**.

BOX 15.1: Characteristic features of the plane of the swelling and other swellings.

- A **submuscular swelling** becomes less prominent when the muscle is contracted
- An **intramuscular swelling** remains the same when the muscle is contracted
- A **supramuscular swelling** becomes prominent when the muscle is contracted
- A **swelling arising from the tendon** does not move much along the axis of the tendon but can be moved in the plane perpendicular to it, especially when the tendon is made to contract
- A **swelling arising from the nerve** may cause sensorimotor symptoms. Also, when the swelling is percussed, it may cause shooting pains/tingling along the course of the nerve
- **Difference between arterial and venous origin swelling:** An arterial swelling is pulsatile, whereas venous swelling is nonpulsatile. With limb elevation, venous swelling decreases in size and fills slowly when emptied by milking it. Arterial swelling does not decrease in size with limb elevation and fills quickly after it is emptied by milking
- **Lipoma** edges slip under the finger
- **Bony swellings** are hard in consistency and fixed to the bone if they arise from the same.

- **Fluctuation:** It should be evaluated in two planes, perpendicular to each other.
  - Fix the swelling by placing the thumb and index finger of one hand at the opposite poles (or as far from each other as size allows) of the swelling (watching fingers). Now press the swelling at the summit with the other hand's index finger (displacing finger) and feel for the fluctuation with the index finger and thumb of the other hand **(Fig. 15.7)**. Now, repeat the test by placing the watching fingers on the plane perpendicular to the first ones. A positive fluctuation implies fluid or gas in the cavity.
- **Fluid thrill:** It is performed in case of swelling containing fluid. Tap the swelling with two fingers on side side and feel the percussion wave on other side of the swelling with finger of other hand.

- **Reducibility:** Reducibility implies that *gentle pressure over the swelling makes it reduce in size and disappear into a cavity*. This is a feature of swellings which are connected to a cavities of abdomen, pleural space, spinal canal, or cranium. Typically, it is a feature of hernia. However, it is also observed in meningocele.
- **Compressibility:** In contrast to reducibility, compressibility implies that *swelling can be reduced in size but will not disappear completely*. A compressible swelling will immediately reappear as soon as pressure is taken off, while reducible swellings do not reappear till the 'cavity pressure' increases by coughing, etc. Compressible swellings are filled with a fluid and are usually vascular swellings of either arterial/venous/capillary/lymphatic origin.

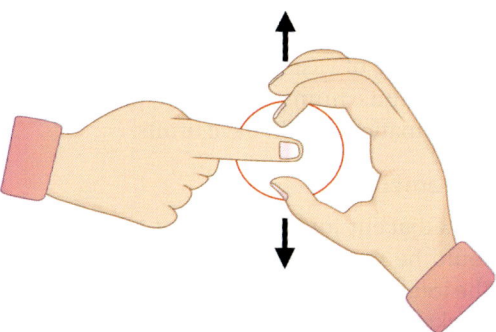

Fig. 15.7: Fluctuation elicitation in a swelling.

Difference between swelling of arterial origin vs. venous.
An arterial swelling is usually pulsatile, whereas venous swelling is non-pulsatile. With limb elevation, arterial swelling does not decrease in size, whereas venous may gradually decrease. After emptying an arterial swelling by milking with a hand, it fills up quickly once the hand is removed. In contrast, the venous swelling fills slowly. Arterial swelling may have a thrill and bruit, whereas venous may not possess such characteristics.

Note: Compressible and reducible are different terms!
- **Compressible** means that the swelling reduces in size when external pressure is applied over the swelling and gradually reappears once pressure is taken off.
- **Reducible** means that once the swelling is reduced with external pressure, it reappears only once intracavity (intra-abdominal) pressure is elevated, e.g., hernia.

- **Translucency:** In swellings with clear fluid, a torchlight would pass through it and create a flare of light in the swelling. To conduct this test, room may need to be darkened, or a tube of folded X-ray or a thick dark paper may be used. Shine a cold light on one edge of the swelling and watch for transillumination through the other end of the tube. Light seen emerging from the other side is termed as "transillumination." Transillumination confirms air or clear fluid (serum, lymph, plasma) within the swelling.
- **Impulse on coughing:** In orthopedic conditions, it may be observed in meningocele. Swelling is held by the hand or hand is kept over the swelling and patient is asked to cough. An impulse if felt by the hand.
4. **Bony irregularity:** It is felt in areas where the bone is superficial and not covered by muscles. It is due to subperiosteal new bone formation classically seen in chronic osteomyelitis, Brodie's abscess, and united fracture.
5. **Ulcer and sinus** (Read section on sinus examination)
6. **Presence of fracture:** Abnormal mobility at the bone is suggestive of pathological fracture or non-union.

Auscultation

In swelling of vascular origin, listen for arterial bruits and venous hums. An aneurysm or arteriovenous malformations could have bruits.

Movement

The adjacent joint movement should be assessed. It could be normal or decreased (painless or painful). The joint movement might be limited if the pathology is blocking the joint movement (exostosis) or has spread to the joint, muscles crossing the joint, or to the other adjoining local soft tissues.

Measurement and Examination of the Contralateral Limb

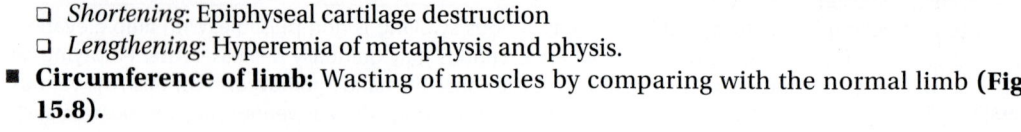

Fig. 15.8: Wasting of right side thigh muscle.

- **Length of bone:** Limb length discrepancy (seen in osteomyelitis) and tumors (diaphyseal aclasis)
  - *Shortening*: Epiphyseal cartilage destruction
  - *Lengthening*: Hyperemia of metaphysis and physis.
- **Circumference of limb:** Wasting of muscles by comparing with the normal limb **(Fig. 15.8).**

Neighboring Joint Swelling

The neighboring joint could be swollen because of sympathetic effusion. Rarely, the infective swelling from the vicinity of a joint could result in septic arthritis. In case of sympathetic effusion, the joint movements are nearly complete and painless, whereas movements are grossly restricted and painful in septic arthritis.

Examination of Regional Lymph Nodes and Other Organs

- It is mandatory in case of infective and tumorous lesions. "If you are considering a possibility of a malignant swelling, always visualize a possibility of a distant metastasis; thus do not fail to examine possible organs where it might have metastasized". One must palpate neck for associated thyroid swelling and adjacent lymph nodes. Palpate abdomen for any mass (hepatosplenomegaly and renal lump) and ascites.
- Chest examination may be required to assess the presence of lung pathology (collapse, pleural effusion) if there is suspicion of lung primary or metastasis or any infective pathology (TB).
- Per rectal or per vaginum examination in a relevant case
- Skull, spine, and long bone examination to look for secondaries and pathological fractures, if any.
- Distal neurovascular assessment.

The characteristics of benign and malignant swellings are mentioned in **Table 15.2**.

TABLE 15.2: Characteristic differences between benign and malignant swellings.

	Benign	Malignant
Skin	• Not stretched • Not shiny • No discoloration	Usually stretched, shiny, loss of hair
Temp	Normal	May present with warmth
Tender	Nontender	Rest pain, night cries, pain usually precedes the swelling
Edge	Well-defined	Ill-defined
Surface	Soft	Variable
Infiltration to adjacent tissue	No	Yes
Neurovascular compression	No	Yes
Lymph nodes	Not enlarged	Enlarged
Metastasis	No	Yes
Constitutional symptoms	Absent	Present (fever, weight loss, loss of appetite cachexia, anemia)
Histology		
Encapsulated	Almost always	Not encapsulated
Anaplasia	Not present	Present
Cell differentiation	Present	Undifferentiated

HISTORY AND EXAMINATION OF A SCAR

Relevant History

- **Etiology:** Trauma, history of infection or previous surgery, history of radiation or steroid exposure
- **The growth of scar:** The keloids can grow fast and irregularly and then attain a plateau of growth.
- **Associated symptoms:** Pain, itching, and recent ulceration

Examination

Inspection of the Scar

Inspect a scar for the following characteristics:
1. **Anatomical parameters:** Describe the site, extent, orientation, contour and color of the scar. Contour implies that whether scar is elevated from the nearby skin or not. For example, a 6 cm long pinkish horizontal scar is present over the tibial shin, which is 3 cm below the tibial tuberosity extending from the pes anserinus area to the anterolateral aspect of the knee. The scar appears slightly elevated from the rest of the normal skin.
2. **Healing status:** Healing/healed.
3. **Method of healing:** Primary or secondary intention
   - ❏ Healing by primary intention refers to the healing of a wound in which the edges are closely re-approximated surgically. In this type of wound healing, epithelialization occurs

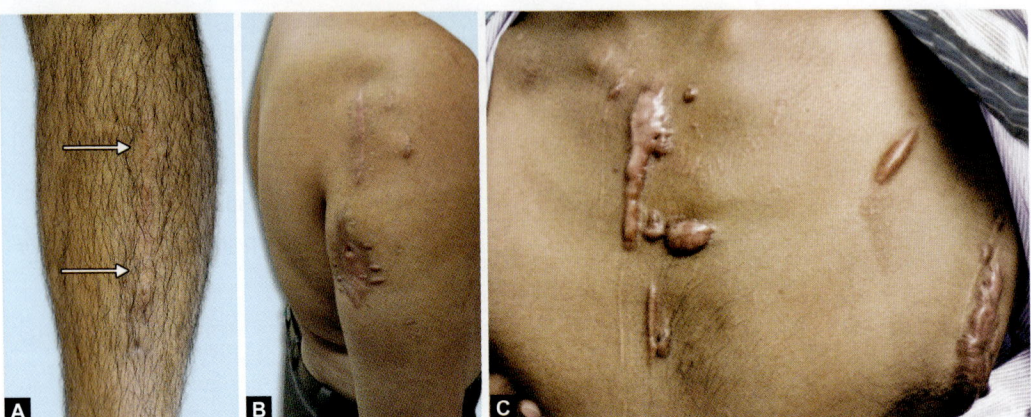

Figs. 15.9A to C: (A) Scar healed with primary intention; (B) Scar healed with secondary intention; (C) Multiple keloid over the sternum and chest.

with no/minimal granulation tissue and scar formation. It works best with wounds or incisions where there has been little loss of tissue and have been neatly approximated. Further, the level of the scar healed by primary intention is almost at the same level as of the surrounding **(Fig. 15.9A)**.

- Healing by secondary intention refers in which a gap is left between the edges of the wound for natural healing to occur. A scar healed by secondary intention is usually irregular and is always at a lower level than the surrounding skin due to extensive scarring and contraction of wound **(Fig. 15.9B)**. *Note that contraction in scars healed by secondary intention occurs due to presence of myofibroblast in the wound, which result in contraction of the wound.*

4. **Any evidence of pathological scarring:** Hypertrophic scar or a keloid. Hypertrophic scar is defined as an abnormally raised, pink, persistent scar tissue *within the boundaries of the original wound,* whereas keloid scars are significantly abnormally raised, persistent scars that *extends beyond the wound's boundaries* **(Fig. 15.9C)**. The key characteristics of keloid are itchy, tendency to spread, tender and vascular. **Table 15.3** depicts the differences between the two types of pathological scars.
5. **Any presence of skin breakdown** *over the scar, a sinus, or an ulcer over the scar.*
6. **Skin surrounding the scar:** One must note about the condition of surrounding skin whether there has been extensive scarring around the main scar, which may indicate a major injury. Also color of the surrounding skin must be noted—hypo- or hyperpigmented.
7. **Any sign of surgical correction** *(Z- or V-Y plasty).*

Palpation of the Scar

1. **Feel for tenderness over the scar:** Pathological scars are often tender to palpate.
2. **Mobility of the scar:** Is it fixed to the underlying tissues? This may be really important for those scars, which are overlying the joints as an adherent scar may limit the joint movement.

Associated Functional Impairment

Assess the function of local joint and muscles whether their function and movement is hampered by the presence of the scar.

TABLE 15.3: Differences between hypertrophic scar and keloid.

	Hypertrophic scar	Keloid
Genetic predisposition	No	Yes
Racial predisposition	No	Yes. Common in darker complexion than fair ones. Common in people of African origin
Predilection to surfaces	Extensor surface	Ear lobe, chest, sternum, shoulder, back, cheek, and knees
Non-traumatic occurrence	No	Yes
Time to develop	Within 1–2 months of injury	Months to years after the injury
Tendency to spread beyond the original wound	No	Yes
Appearance	Red/pinkish, rarely thicker than 4 mm	Hyperpigmented, skin stretched and shiny
Tender	+	++
Pruritic	+	++
Ulcerations	Rare	Possible
Vascular	No	Yes
Chance of regression	May regress over time, especially after six months	Never regresses
Chance of recurrence after excision	Less	High
Histologically	Parallel pattern of collagen	Random, whorl pattern of collagen
	Myofibroblasts +	No myofibroblast

HISTORY AND EXAMINATION OF A SINUS

Definition

The sinus is defined as a blind track lined by granulation tissue that connects the surface to a cavity in the tissue.

> **Note:** A fistula is a communicating tract between two epithelial surfaces, commonly between a hollow viscera and the skin or between two hollow viscera.
> - The most common cause of a persistent sinus in orthopedic patient is 'chronic osteomyelitis.' Therefore, most of the history and examination is directed towards the evaluation of bony pathology.
> - **Why does a sinus persists?:** Most important reason for a persistent sinus is presence of a foreign body or a necrotic dead tissue (sequestrum, suture material) in the deeper plane from where the sinus is connected. Other causes are chronic infections such as tuberculosis, inadequate drainage of abscess, and a epithelialized tract.

Relevant History

- **Onset and progression:** A patient with chronic osteomyelitis gives a typical history of the cyclical development of fever, swelling, and pain followed by the bursting of the abscess, resulting in the formation of a discharging sinus. There might be a history of extrusion of

bone chips or pieces. Ask for any history of trauma, open fractures, surgery, etc. Often, there is a periodical history of quiescence and exacerbation of sinus activity.
- **Pain:** It is suggestive of an inflammatory etiology or may be due to the blockage of the sinus, leading to increased intrasinus or cavity (from where the sinus is originating) pressure.

> **Note:** One must remember that *presence of the sinus in an orthopedic case does not always naturally imply osteomyelitis!* The presence of a sinus implies that there is a *dead tissue (sequestrum, other tissue)/ dead material (foreign body, non-absorbable suture material) inside*, which is harboring the infection. The infected material (pus) keeps coming out via the sinus and discharges over the surface. As long as the dead tissue or material persists, the sinus will continue! Further, a weeping sinus may indicate an underlying malignancy.

- One must always probe into other systemic conditions such as diabetes or other immunocompromised states, which is a known cause for higher chance of deeper infection.
- Also, ask any history of tuberculosis anywhere else in the body.

Examination

Inspection

- **Site:** It could be anywhere along the length of the bone. However, the level of external opening of sinus might not correspond with the level of the cavity in the bone.
- **Number:** Look for number of sinuses around the affected site. Some may be active, while others may be quiescent.
- **Margins:**
    - Pouting granulation tissue at the margin of the sinus is suggestive of a dead material (sequestrum, foreign body) in the depth of the sinus **(Fig. 15.10)**. Exuberant granulation tissue can also suggest the presence of a foreign body within.
    - Undermined sinus with a thin bluish margin is seen in the tubercular sinus.
- **Discharge:** The sinus would discharge either fluid or occasionally bone pieces (sequestrum). The various type of fluid discharges from sinus are:

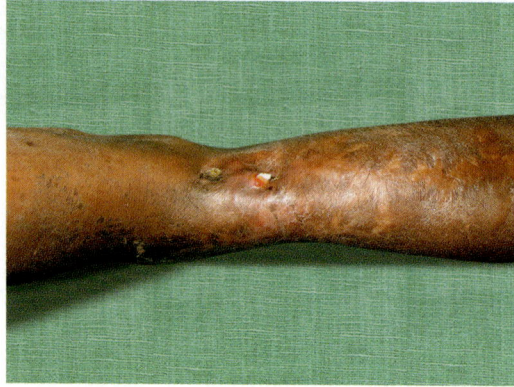

Fig. 15.10: Pouting granulation over the sinus. White sequestrum is also present at the sinus opening.

  - *Serous:* Serous drainage is composed mainly of plasma. It is often thin and watery and will usually have a clear to yellowish or brownish appearance. Continuous serous drainage is a sign that there are high levels of bacterial load in the wound.
  - *Seropurulent:* As the name suggests, seropurulent drainage is a combination of serous drainage and purulent drainage. Seropurulent wound drainage appears as a light, green, or yellow fluid and is often indicative of a developing or clearing infection.
  - *Purulent discharge:* Purulent drainage often appears as slightly thicker, milk-like malodorous liquid. The color of purulent drainage may vary from a grayish-yellow to

green or brown. Purulent drainage is caused by the number of living and dead infectious cells in the area (bacteria, immune cells). It is an indicator of active infection in the cavity.
- ❏ *Sanguineous:* Sanguineous wound exudate is composed of blood and viscous serum and does not signal the presence of localized or systemic infection.
- ❏ *Serosanguinous:* Often observed in tuberculous osteomyelitis.
- ❏ Sulphur granules in actinomycotic sinus.

Note that discharge of a sequestrum is a hallmark of osteomyelitis.
- **Surrounding skin:** Scarring of the surrounding skin is frequent in chronic osteomyelitis. It happens due to recurrent infection, multiple surgeries, or a history of trauma.

Palpation
- **Tenderness:** A sinus could be tender in case of active infection of bone with associated purulent discharge. However, it is usually the underlying infected bone that is tender.
- **Fixity to the bone:** Hold the base of the sinus and move it side to side. A sinus arising from bone (in chronic osteomyelitis) is fixed to the underlying bone, while a sinus arising from soft tissues retains its side–side mobility. *Assessment of sinus fixity to the underlying bone is an essential characteristic of an osteomyelitis sinus.*

Standard Assessment of Movement at Neighboring Joint and Examination of Regional Draining Lymph Nodes

The neighboring joints may be stiff due to chronic scarring, muscle wasting and multiple surgeries coupled with immobilization. One must also palpate the regional lymph nodes, which might be swollen and tender due to chronic infection. A hard, immobile lymph node may indicate malignancy.

HISTORY AND EXAMINATION OF AN ULCER

Definition
An ulcer is defined as a break in the continuity of the skin or mucous membrane with loss of surface tissue, disintegration, and necrosis of the epithelial tissue with superadded infection.

Relevant History

1. **Onset:** One must probe into the onset of ulcer—traumatic or insidious, if present, should be considered. Following trauma, an open wound can get infected and result in an ulcer. Similarly, trauma sustained several weeks or months priorly can result in an ulcer that fails to heal. An ulcer due to arterial/venous insufficiency or sensory deficit might be atraumatic or associated with minor trauma. A Marjolin's ulcer may develop in a chronic scar of a burn.
2. **Location:** Location of an ulcer may often indicate the possible etiology.
   - ❏ *Ulcer over the malleolus with surrounding congested, dark skin*: Most likely, a venous ulcer **(Fig. 15.11)**

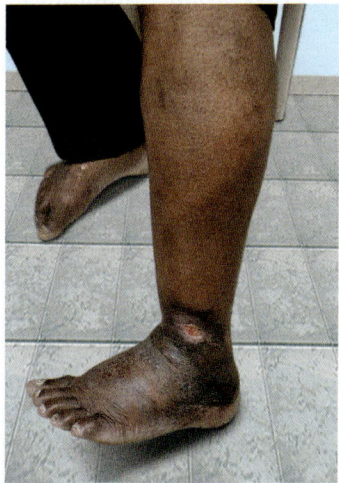

Fig. 15.11: Venous ulcer over the lateral malleolus with surrounding hyperpigmented, congested skin.

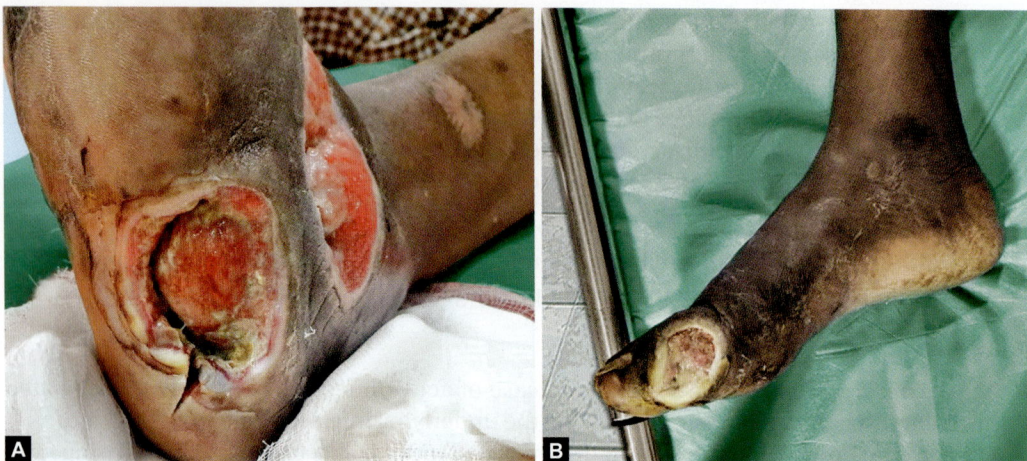

Figs. 15.12A and B: (A) A healing ulcer with sloping edge over the plantar aspect of the foot and medial malleolus, surrounded with darkened skin; (B) A non-healing ulcer over the great toe in a diabetic surrounded with darkened skin.

- *Ulcer over the plantar aspect of foot*: The ulcers on plantar aspect are often due to diabetes or peripheral nerve lesions (trophic ulcer). *Note that diabetic ulcers are usually due to combined micro- and macroarterial insufficiency and peripheral neuropathy.* Diabetic ulcers are often surrounded by darkened skin, indicating a chronic arterial insufficiency **(Figs. 15.12A and B)**.
3. **Duration:** An arbitrary definition is to consider ulcers with a duration of less than 6 weeks as acute and more than 6 weeks as chronic. A long-standing nonhealing ulcer with peripheral fibrosis and a hard indurated base is called a ***callous ulcer***.
4. **Progression:** Chronic ulcers do contract due to fibrosis but tend to stay stagnant after that. Malignant ulcers progress relentlessly. Other than the size of the ulcer, association with symptoms such as pain and discharge should also be considered in progression. A healing ulcer is characterized by shrinking of the size and depth.
5. **Pain:** Acute ulcers are usually excruciating, and the severity of pain relates directly to the site of the ulcer (ulcers on the ventral aspect of the leg or forearm tend to be more painful than the dorsal ones), depth, and presence of associated inflammation. Chronic ulcers with underlying fibrosis can gradually become painless. It is also important to note that painless/minimally painful ulcers (to start with) are often associated with diseases such as diabetic neuropathy, peripheral nerve diseases, and tabes dorsalis. Malignant ulcers are classically painless unless there is infiltration of the nerves.
6. **Discharge:** Color and quantity of discharge must be considered. Purulent discharge indicates active infection. Serous/serosanguinous discharge usually means a healing ulcer (if previous was purulent). A bloody discharge portends a malignancy. Bony chips extruding along with the discharge should also be asked for, as it may suggest osteomyelitis of the underlying bone.
7. **Associated diseases:** History of associated causes leading to nonhealing ulcers and painlessness should also be asked for, including diabetes mellitus, peripheral neuropathy, Hansen's disease, peripheral arterial disease, syringomyelia, spina bifida, and transverse myelitis. Immunocompromised (HIV/AIDS) or immunosuppressed status (chronic steroid

therapy, immunosuppressant drugs) would also result in chronicity of an ulcer due to poor immunity and healing tendency.

> **Note:** A *Marjolin's ulcer* arises in a chronic scar **(Fig. 15.13)**. It represents a malignant degeneration and is mostly a well-differentiated squamous cell carcinoma. Albeit rare, it is essential not to miss this entity, especially in chronic lower extremity wounds (although originally described in burn scars). The latent period is around 20–25 years. Clinically, they are painless ulcers, which become painful as they extend beyond the confines of the scar. Due to chronicity induced extensive fibrosis around the ulcer and previous obliteration of local lymphatic vessels, there is a very little chance of metastasis into other organs or regional lymph node involvement.

Examination

Inspection

The inspection of an ulcer involves assessment of number, site, size, shape, floor, edge, discharge and condition of surrounding skin.
- **Number:** Single/multiple
- **Site:** Describe the site of the ulcer with respect to a bony landmark.
- **Size:** One must assess the size of the ulcer.
- **Shape:** Mostly irregular.
- **Floor:** The exposed surface of the ulcer is called the floor *(Note: The floor is seen while the base is felt!)*
  One must describe the contents of the floor such as granulation tissue, bone, muscle, fascia, subcutaneous tissue, or dead tissue **(Fig. 15.14)**.
- **Edge (Fig. 15.15):** The type of edge could give a clinical clue to the type of the ulcer.
  - *Sloping edge:* Healing ulcer [with three zones from center to periphery; red in the center of the ulcer followed by a narrow blue zone due to a thin epithelium, followed by an outer white zone due to a fibrotic scar **(vide supra—Fig. 15.12A)**
  - *Punched out edge:* Trophic ulcer (neuropathic ulcer and syphilis)
  - *Undermined edge:* Tuberculosis (undermined edges because subcutaneous tissue is destroyed faster than skin)
  - *Everted edge:* Squamous cell carcinoma.
  - *Rolled-out edge:* Basal cell carcinoma.
- **Discharge:** Serous or seropurulent or purulent
- **Surrounding skin and part of the limb:**
  - Glossy red or edematous in acutely inflamed ulcers

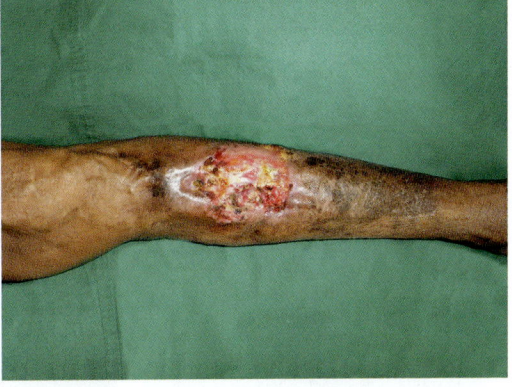

Fig. 15.13: Marjolin's ulcer over the leg due to a chronic non-healing ulcer in a scar.

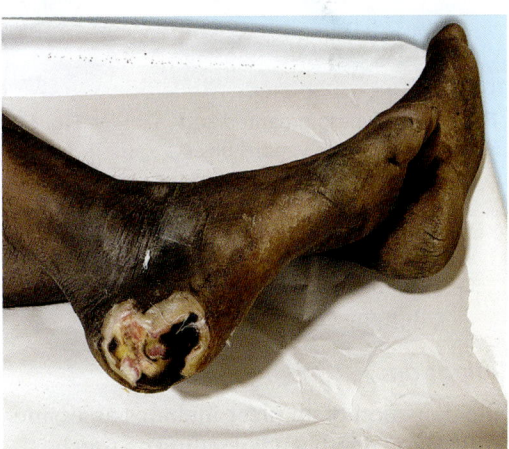

Fig. 15.14: A non-healing ulcer over the heel with unhealthy granulation and dead tissues.

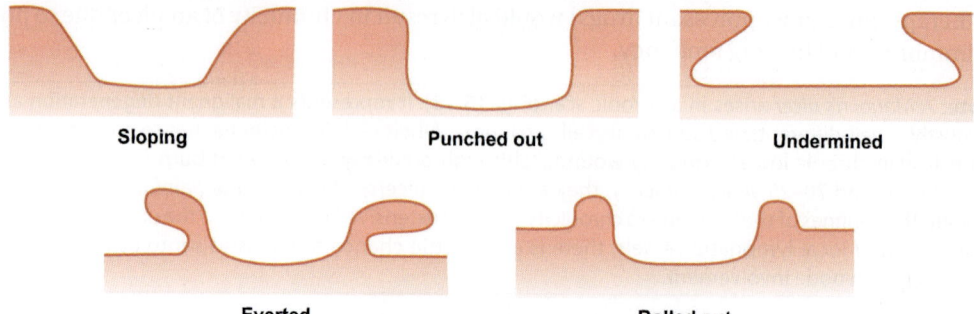

Fig. 15.15: Various types of ulcer edge.

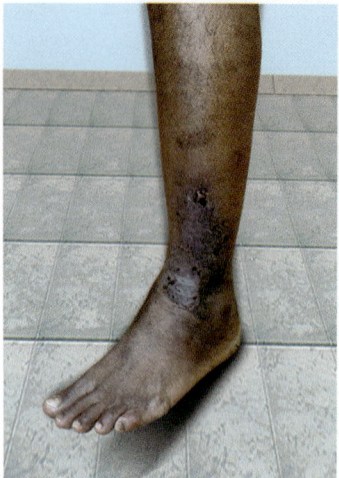

Fig. 15.16: Hyperpigmented and eczematous skin in venous ulcer.

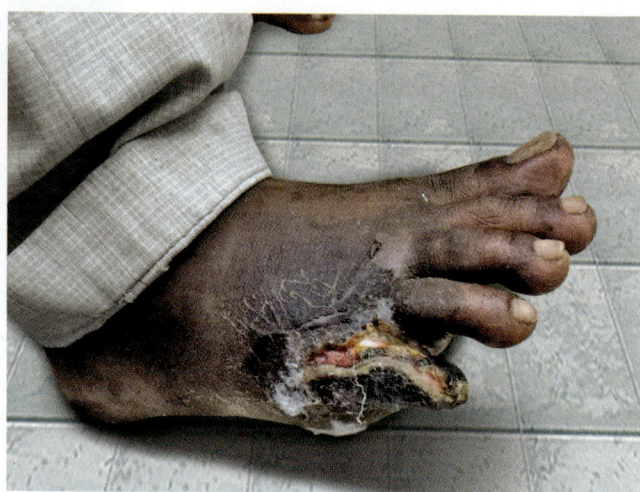

Fig. 15.17: Ulcer over the toe with gangrene of the toe in a diabetic.

- Eczematous and pigmented in varicose ulcers (**Fig. 15.16**)
- Dark, hyperpigmented skin in arterial ulcers
- Toes or fingers may show evidence of advanced arterial insufficiency in the form of gangrene (**Fig. 15.17**).

Palpation

The palpation of an ulcer includes assessment of local temperature, tenderness, base, fixity, induration, depth, and bleeding on touch.
- **Local temperature:** A rise in local temperature indicates acute inflammation, whereas cold surrounding skin is suggestive of arterial insufficiency or a chronic ulcer.
- **Base, fixity and induration of ulcer:** It refers to the state of the tissue underneath the floor of the ulcer. Induration and fixity to the underlying tissue are felt in inflammatory and malignant ulcers.
- **Tenderness:** Acute ulcers may be tender, while chronic ulcers are lesser painful.

A *painless ulcer* may indicate *underlying neuropathy*, such as Charcot's arthropathy or neuropathic ulcers in spina bifida. In such a situation, a complete neurological examination is vital.
- **Depth**
- **Bleeding on touch:** It is often a feature of a malignant ulcer.

Draining Regional Lymph Node

Tender lymph nodes are a feature of acute ulcers. Several mobile, slightly enlarged (tender/non-tender) may indicate chronicity of an ulcer, which intermittently gets infected. Hard and fixed lymph nodes are seen in malignant ulcers.

Feel for the Pulse and Assess the Neurological Status of the Limb

The pulse could be feeble or absent in ulcers due to arterial insufficiency (diabetics, thromboangiitis obliterans or other cause of arterial insufficiency). The sensations are reduced in diabetics or other causes of trophic ulcers such as peripheral neuropathy, spina bifida.

Notes

Index

Page numbers followed by *b* refer to box, *f* refer to figure, *fc* refer to flowchart, and *t* refer to table.

A

Abbreviated injury scale 18
Abdomen 276
    examination of 228
Abduction 62*f*, 63*f*, 130, 132, 133*f*, 251
    deformity 130
Abductor digiti minimi 260, 261
    rests for 262*f*
Abductor mechanism 140, 140*f*
    abnormal responses of 141*f*
    normal responses of 141*f*
Abductor pollicis
    brevis 99, 248, 255, 257, 258
    longus 96, 97
Abductor
    neuromuscular affections of 141
    post-surgery weakness of 141
Above-elbow stump 286
Above-knee stump 286
Abrasion 23
Abscess, paraspinal 214*f*
Accident, site of 22
Acetabular labrum 120, 121*f*
Achondroplasia 36, 36*f*
Acromioclavicular joint 60
    arthritis, tests for 70
    stability 51
    tenderness 70
Adalimumab 241
Adam's test 211*f*, 212
Adduction 61, 62*f*, 130, 132, 133*f*
    deformity 130
Adductor 265*f*
    magnus tendon 148
    pollicis 261, 262*f*
        Froment's sign foor 262*f*
    tubercle 148
Adson's test 220, 229*f*
Advanced trauma life support 18
    care 21*fc*
Alcohol intake, chronic 240
Allen's test 112
Allergies 9, 183
Allis sign 136
Amiodarone 241

Ample history 20*b*
Amputation 284
    atraumatic 284
    complications of 288
    forequarter 289
    hindquarter 289
    indications for 283
    near-total 25, 26*f*
    principles of 287
    stump 283
        clinical evaluation of 283
        examination of 289
    traumatic 29, 284
Anatomical snuffbox 96, 107*f*, 108
Anconeus triangle 78, 83, 83*f*
    palpation of 86
Ankle 40, 180, 181*b*, 185, 188
    anterior joint line, anterior aspect of 189*f*
    clonus 227
    dorsiflexion 221*f*
    examination proforma 196
    joint 191, 191*f*
        anterior 190*f*
        bony ankylosis of 15*f*
        clinical evaluation of 178
        space, normal 15*f*
    lateral ligaments of 178
    ligament complex, lateral 178*f*
    major ligaments of 178
    medial ligament of 179
    neutral position of 191*f*
    plantar flexion 195*f*, 268*f*
        absence of 195*f*
    posterior aspect of 190*f*
    primary function of 179
    sprain 198
    stability, tests for 193
    surgical anatomy of 178
Ankylosing spondylitis 41, 46, 209, 232
Ankylosis 14
    fibrous 14
Annular ligament 77
Anterior cord syndrome 235, 235*f*

Anterior hip joint line 128
    location of 128*f*
Anterior horn 201
    cell 5*f*, 201
Anterior joint line 60*f*
    palpation technique of 60*f*
Anterior primary rami
    dorsal division of 263
    ventral division of 264
Anterior superior iliac spine 131*f*
    position of 126
Anticonvulsants 241
Antimicrobials 240
Antiretroviral drugs 241
Apley's compression test 171
Apley's distraction test 171
Apley's grinding test 170, 171
Apley's test 172*f*
Aponeurosis 97
Apprehension test 64, 64*f*, 172*f*
Arachonodactyly 38
Arch
    exaggeration of 194*f*
    functions of 179
Arm
    external rotation of 64*f*
    internal rotation of 66*f*
    length measurement 63*f*
Arterial blood gas 21
Arterial Doppler 28
Artery, ulnar 112
Arthritis
    classification of 39*fc*
    glenohumeral 56
    gouty 198
    inflammatory 1, 40, 103
    mutilans 47, 106
    tests for 142
Arthropathy 45
    enteropathic 47
    hemophilic 49
    neuropathic 39
    psoriatic 47
    reactive 47
Arthroscopic appearance 175*f*
Atrophy 229

Index

Attitude 11, 23, 32, 42, 55, 71, 82, 103, 125, 155, 185, 210, 241, 277, 285
Auscultation 27, 304
Autoimmune diseases 238, 240
Autonomic nervous system 200, 202
  examination 246
Avascular necrosis 144, 145*f*
Axilla 297
Axillary nerve 245, 250, 251*t*
  paralysis, features of 251
Axonotmesis 236

B

Babinski sign 227
Baker's cyst 42, 42*f*, 158*f*, 296
  ruptured 155
Ballottement test 159
Barlow test 138, 139*f*
Bechterew's disease 46
Beighton score 60, 161
Belly press test 69, 69*f*
Below-elbow stump 286
Below-knee
  amputation stump 285*f*
  prosthesis 285*f*
  stump 286
Benediction sign 257, 259
Biceps 252
  bulk, loss of 83
  tendon 51
    pathology 64, 69, 71
Bicipital tendinitis 69
Bigelow ligament 120
Blackberry thumb 112
Bladder 228
Blood test 36
Blue sclera 37*f*
Body
  coronal plane of 61
  dermatome of 224*f*
  external rotation of 172*f*
  internal rotation of 172*f*
Bone 5*f*, 7, 158
  acute injury of 18
  length of 34, 300, 304
  lesion, metastatic 275
  metastasis 275
  multiple 277
  pain 275
  shortening of 300
  tumors 272, 273*b*, 275, 276, 280
    benign 273*t*
    classification of 272, 272*fc*
    evaluation of 272
    malignant 273*t*, 276

Bony
  ankylosis 14, 15*f*
  crepitus 25, 34
  erosion 46*f*
  irregularity 34, 43, 303
  landmarks 15
  mass, abnormal 86
  points 78
  swellings, multiple 297
Book test 262*f*
Bortezomib 240
Bouchard node 42, 106*f*
Boutonnière deformity 106
Bowel status 228
Boxer's muscle 250
Brachial plexus 244
  posterior cord of 252
Brachialis 252
  assessment 252*f*
Brachioradialis, tests for 254*f*
Bragard's test 221
Brain 5*f*
Breast carcinoma 240
Brittle bone disease 36
Broadened heel 187
Brodie's abscess 36, 303
Brown-Sequard syndrome 234
Bruise 23
Bryant's triangle, measurement of 135, 135*f*
Burning sensation 284
Bursae around knee 151
Bursitis
  retrocalcaneal 183, 188*f*, 198
  subacromial 62, 64

C

Café-au-lait spots 213, 213*f*, 297
Calcaneofibular ligament 183, 194
Calcaneum 190
  fracture, malunited 187*f*
Calcific tendinitis 53, 56, 75, 75*f*
Calf 185, 187
  muscle, wasting of 126, 126*f*, 127, 127*f*, 133, 136, 162
Capitellum 76
Caplan's syndrome 45
Capsular contractures 7
Capsulitis, adhesive 72
Carbamazepine 241
Cardiovascular drugs 240
Carpal tunnel syndrome 45, 102, 111, 118
  signs of 111*f*
  tests for 111
Carrying angle 82, 88
  measurement 89*f*

Cascade sign 106
Cauda equina 200*f*
  syndrome 235
Cavus foot 184*f*
Cell wall 47
Central cord syndrome 233, 234*f*
Central nervous system 243
Cerebellar
  ataxia gait 295
  disorders 291
Cerebral palsy 291
Cerebrovascular accident 291
  episode of 295
Cervical rib 219, 230*f*
  prominent subcutaneous 230*f*
Cervical spine 53, 71, 205
  anteroposterior X-ray 230*f*
  extension 216*f*
  flexion 216*f*
  lateral rotation 216*f*
  movement 214
    assessment of 216*f*
  prominent spinous process of 215*f*
  right lateral flexion 216*f*
Cervical spondylosis 209
Charcot's arthropathy 40, 48, 49*f*, 184, 313
Charcot's foot 48, 189*f*, 199, 283
Charcot-Marie-tooth disease 241, 291
Chemotherapeutic agents 240
Cheralgia paraesthetica 271
Chest
  expansion 219
  pain 55
Chondromalacia 177*f*
  patella 154, 176
Chondromatosis, synovial 39
Chopart's amputation 288
Chopart's joint 180
Cisplatin 240
Clarke's test 161, 161*f*
Claudication
  neurogenic 207*t*
  vascular 207*t*
Clavicle 60
Claw hand 106, 241*f*, 242
Clonus 227
Clubfoot 197
Codman's triangle 281, 281*f*
Cold abscess 213
Colles' fracture 2
  malunited 116
Compartment syndrome 29
Complex regional pain syndrome 98, 104, 116

Compression test 27, 172f
Compressive symptoms 298
Computed tomography scan 21, 28
Connective tissue disorders 1, 240
Contralateral limb 27
  examination of 304
  measurement of 304
Contusion 23
Conus medullaris syndrome 200f, 235
Coracoid process 60
Coronal plane deformity 155
  assessment 130, 131
Corticospinal tract 234f, 235
  anterior 201, 202
  lateral 201, 202, 234
Coxa valga 291
Coxa vara 144, 291
Cozen's test 89, 90f
  reverse 90, 90f
Cranial nerves 223
Crepitus 8, 162
Crohn's disease 47
Cross-chest adduction test 70, 70f
Cruciate ligament, anterior 148, 149, 151, 173
Cubital fossa 89
  regional lymph nodes of 91
Cubital tunnel syndrome 271
Cubitus
  recurvatum 83f
  valgus 80, 82, 82f, 93
  varus 80, 82, 82f, 93
Cuff arthropathy 56
Cytomegalovirus 240

D

Daily living, activities of 8, 154, 182, 240, 275
De Quervain's tenosynovitis 100, 102, 111, 112f, 115
  tests for 112
Dead tissues 311f
Death, causes of 18
Deep peroneal nerve 193, 245, 265-267
Deep tendon 246
  reflex 227
Deep vein thrombosis
  Homan's sign for 195
  Moses sign for 195
Deformity 7, 12, 22, 23, 31, 41, 42, 80, 101, 104, 105, 123, 129, 131, 155, 182, 207, 213, 241, 274
  alignment of 32
  angular 298, 300
  assessment 129
  principles of 13

calcaneus 187
  pre-existing 15
  rotational 127, 131
  sagittal plane 83, 156
  spasmodic 7
  structural 7
Degloving injury 24
Deltoid 251
  middle penna, tests for 251f
Dermatome 223
Diabetes mellitus 48, 55
Dial test 170
Dimple over lumbosacral junction 213f
Dinner fork deformity 105f
Disability, causes of 18
Disarticulation 289b
Disc herniation, stages of 231f
Discoid meniscus 174
Dislocations 29, 56
  traumatic 54
Distal femur
  fracture of 26f
  lateral view of 281f
  osteosarcoma of 281f
  soap-bubble appearance of 281f
Distal interphalangeal joints 101
Distal radioulnar joint 95, 100, 106, 108, 114
Distal thigh, swelling of 297f
Distraction test 172f
Diurnal variation 100, 122
Dizziness 208
Docetaxel 240
Dorsal aspect, extrinsic muscles of 99
Dorsal extensor compartments 96f
Dorsal interosseous muscle 262f
Dorsal ramus 236
Dorsal spine 205
  kyphotic deformities of 211b
  left lateral rotation of 217f
  movement 216
  right lateral rotation of 217f
Dorsalcolumn tract 201
Dorsiflexion 109f, 191
Dorsolumbar spine, scoliosis of 211f
Drawer test
  anterior 64, 165, 165f, 193, 194f
  posterior 167, 168f
Drop arm test 66
Dupuytren's contracture 103, 105f, 115, 115f
Durkan's median nerve compression test 111
Dysplasia, developmental 1, 124, 138, 143, 143f, 291

E

Edema 276
Eichhoff test 112, 112f
Elbow 101
  bony
    anatomy of 76f
    stabilizer of 76
  clinical diagnostic snippets 81t
  contralateral 81
  examination proforma 92
  flexion movement 14
  instability 89
    tests for 90
  joint 77, 86, 87
    clinical evaluation of 76
  lateral condyle of 76
  ligament of 77f
  movements 87f
  myositis ossificans of 93f
  pain, causes of 79t
  progressive deformity of 80
  sinus over back of 85
  stabilizing structures 77
Electrocardiogram 21
Electrolyte imbalance 291
Elevated arm test 220
Ely's test 137, 139, 139f, 142
Empty can test 66, 67f
Endoneurium 236
Epicondyle, lateral 76, 77, 84f, 149, 159
Epicondylitis, lateral 94
Epileptics 55
Epineurium 236
Epiphyses 297
Equinus deformity 187
Etanercept 241
Ethambutol 240
Eversion 192
Ewing's sarcoma 1, 275, 282, 296
  fibular 282f
Exacerbation 123
Exostoses, multiple 276
Extension 61
  lurch 293
Extensor carpi
  radialis
    brevis 96, 97
    longus 96, 97, 254f
  ulnaris 97, 100, 254f
Extensor digiti minimi 97
Extensor digitorum 96, 97
  communis 254, 254f
  longus 181, 267
  tests for 268f
Extensor hallucis longus 181, 267
  tests for 268f

Index

Extensor indices 96, 97
Extensor lag 162, 163b
Extensor pollicis
  brevis 96, 97
  longus 96, 97, 254, 254f
Extensor retinaculum 96, 96f
  six compartments of 97t
External rotation lag test 67

F
Facet joints 203
Fairbank's apprehension test 172
Fascia, deep 15
Fascial contractures 7
Fascicle 236
Fasciculus
  cuneatus 201, 202, 234
  gracilis 201, 202, 234
Felon 98
Felty's syndrome 45
Femoral condyle 147
  lateral 148, 149, 159
Femoral head
  blood supply of 121f
  vascularity of 120
Femoral nerve 245, 263
  paralysis of 264
  stretch test 222, 222f
Femoroacetabular impingement 145
Femoroacetabular lesion, types of 145f
Femur component, measurement of 135f
Fibrotic scar 311
Fibula, common peroneal nerve over neck of 161
Figure-of-four test 222, 222f
Finger 105
  drop 242
  joint 110
    flex 117f
  pulp, infection of 107
Finkelstein test 112
First carpometacarpal joint 108
  arthritis, tests for 112
Fixed flexion deformity, presence of 162
Flatfoot 194
  congenital 197
Flesche test 215
Flexion 61, 63f, 87
  deformity 12, 80, 130f, 153, 157f
  lateral 215, 218, 218f
  movement 162, 163f
Flexor carpi
  radialis 97, 255
    tests for 257f
  ulnaris 97, 100, 248, 260, 261
    tests for 262f
Flexor digiti minimi 260
Flexor digitorum
  longus 181
  profundus 99, 248, 255, 258
    test 257
  superficialis 99, 255, 258
    test 257, 259b
Flexor hallucis longus 181
Flexor pollicis
  brevis 99, 248, 260
  longus 99, 255
    tests for 257f
Flexor
  retinaculum 95
  retinaculum attachment, anatomy of 96f
Fluid
  synovial 160f
  thrill 302
Foot 180, 181b
  ankle, major extrinsic muscles of 180, 181t
  arches of 179, 180f
  bone of 178t
  borders of 189
  dorsum of 191
  drop 242, 270
  joint, clinical evaluation of 178
  ligaments of 179
  major ligaments of 178
  primary function of 179
  retinaculum of 179
  sensory
    assessment of 193
    innervation of 193f, 265f
  size of 185, 189
  surgical anatomy of 178
Footwear, inspection of 11
Forearm
  length 63
    measurement 63f
  sinus over back of 85
Forefoot 185
Forward bending method 217
Fovea 108
  sign 113
Foveal tenderness 113f
Fracture 98
  acute 27
  blisters 23, 24f
  intra-articular 28
  metacarpal 107f
  open 22b, 25, 28
  pathological 21, 49f
  periarticular 28
  presence of 303
  scaphoid 102
Froment's sign 262f
Frozen shoulder 56, 72
Fulcrum issues 141
Full can test 66, 67f
Functional scoliosis 212, 212f
  obliteration of 212f
Functional spinal unit 204
Fungation 277

G
Gaenslen's test 223, 223f
Gagey's hyperabduction 64
Gait 11, 32, 42, 125, 155, 185, 210, 277, 279, 285, 290
  analysis 291
  antalgic 292, 293f
  ataxic 295
  cerebellar ataxia 295
  circumduction 295
  clinical evaluation of 290
  coxalgic 292, 293f
  cycle 290, 290f
  disturbance 291
    etiology of 290
  festinant 294, 294f
  functional 285
  gluteus maximus 293, 293f
  hemiplegic 295
  high-stepping 292
  knock knee 294, 294f
  patterns 209, 292
    abnormal 31
  phases of 290
  rocking horse 293
  scissoring 293, 294f
  sensory ataxia 295
  stomping 295
  Trendelenburg 292, 293f
Galeazzi test 136, 136f
Ganglion 115, 296
Gap, palpation of 25
Gastrocnemius 268
  lateral head of 149
  medial head of 148
  muscle, tests for 268f, 269f
  tubercle 148
Genu recurvatum 12f, 153, 157f
Genu valgum 42, 153, 156, 156f, 164
  severe 294f
Genu varum 42, 153, 155, 156, 156f, 164
  bilateral 38f
Gerber's lift-off test 68, 68f
Gerdy's tubercle 149
Giant cell tumor 1, 280

Index

Glasgow come scale 20*t*
Glenohumeral joint 51
   arthritis 74
   functional anatomy of 50
Glenohumeral ligament
   anterior inferior 51
   middle 51
   superior 51
Glenoid 50
Glomus tumor 119, 119*f*
Gluteal muscle wasting 127
Golfer's elbow 81, 94
   special tests for 89
   tests for 90
Goniometer, static limb of 134*f*
Gout 48, 80, 183, 296
   acute 48
   chronic 48
Granulation 311*f*
   tissue 33*f*
Greater trochanter
   level of 126, 127
   palpation of 128
Grind test 112
Groin 297
Growth disturbance 298
Gunstock deformity 93
Gustilo-Anderson classification 26*t*
Guyon's canal 271
   compression 271

H

Haglund's bump 183, 188*f*
Haglund's deformity 198
Hair
   loss 104*f*
   over lumbar spine, tuft of 213*f*
Hallux valgus, bilateral 185*f*
Hallux varus 185*f*
Hamstrings 151
   tests for 267*f*
Hand 100*b*
   deformities 100*b*
   function, assessment of 110
   to knee gait 294*f*
   clinical evaluation of 95
   dorsal aspect of 104
   extrinsic muscles of 97, 99*t*
   intrinsic muscles of 97, 99*t*
   ligament of 98
   muscles of 98
   surgical anatomy of 97
   dominance 2, 11, 54
Hansen's disease 48, 240, 271
Hawkins sign 66*f*
Hawkins test 71
Hawkins-Kennedy test 66

Healing, method of 305
Heberden's node 42, 106*f*
Heel
   status 127
   valgus 187*f*
   varus 187*f*
Hematoma, subungual 107
Hemipelvectomy, external 289
Hemophilia
   genetics of 49
   types of 49
Hindfoot 185, 187
   varus 187
Hip 40, 295
   abduction
      deformity, measurement of 131*f*
      ROM, measurement of 134*f*
   abductor mechanism of 140*f*
   adduction 265*f*
   arthritis
      primary 124
      secondary 124
   attitude of 128
   avascular necrosis of 144
   clinical diagnostic snippets 124*t*
   contralateral 142
   developmental dysplasia of 1, 124, 138, 143, 291
   diseases 141
   disorders 125*t*
   examination proforma 142
   extension 132, 223*f*
   flexion 132, 264*f*
   flexor
      strength assessment 264
      tests for 264*f*
   impingement, tests for 139, 140*f*, 142
   joint 120, 121*f*, 122*b*
      clinical evaluation of 120
      ligament of 121*f*
      line, anterior 128
   movement 132*f*, 133*f*
   pain, bilateral 122
   primary osteoarthrosis of 145
   rotations 132
   septic arthritis of 124
   stability 137
      tests for 137
   tuberculosis of 42, 124, 143
   unilateral fixed flexion deformity of 130*f*
Homan's sign 195
Homunculus 201
Hornblower's sign 67, 68*f*, 251, 251*f*
Horse shoe shape swelling 42*f*, 157*f*

Humeral head, proximal migration of 73*f*
Humeroradial articulation 76
Humeroulnar articulation 76
Humerus
   chondrosarcoma of 300*f*
   fracture non-union of lateral condyle of 93
   head of 51
   malunited supracondylar fracture of 93
Hyaluronic acid injection 176
Hyperextension 162
Hypertrophied synovium 161
Hypertrophy 83
Hyperuricemia 183
Hypothenar eminence 99

I

Immunosuppressive 241
Impingement
   syndrome 62
   test 71, 139
Index finger, malrotation of 107*f*
Infection
   acute 98, 152
   chronic 98
Inferior articular facet 204
Inferior end plate 204
Inflammation
   acute 4
   chronic 4
Infliximab 241
Infraspinatus
   muscle wasting of 58*f*
   tear 67
   tendon, tests for 68*f*
Inguinal ligament, mid-point of 128*f*
Injury
   direct 21
   iatrogenic 239
   mechanism of 80, 118
   penetrating 26
   traumatic 239
Instability 41, 153
   feeling of 32
Intercondylar ridge 148
Intermalleolar distance 164
Interosseous nerve, anterior 257
Interphalangeal joint 98, 109, 180
Interstyloid distance 110*f*
   measurement of 110*f*
Intertrochanteric femur, malunited 291
Intervertebral disc 203, 204
   prolapse 229, 231, 244

Intrinsic minus hand 106
Inversion 192
  talar tilt test 194, 194f

J
Jack's test 194, 194f
Jendrassik maneuver 227
Jerk test 64, 65f
Jersey's finger 102, 118
Jobe's supraspinatus test 66
Joint 5f, 18, 30
  above and below 28, 34
    examination of 11, 16, 70, 91, 140, 173
  ankylosed 14
  degeneration, progressive 49
  diseases 43
  instability of 7
  involvement, types of 40
  large 40
  line 158
    anterior 60f
    posterior 61f
    tenderness 159
  movement 279, 289
    normal 5f
  neuropathic 40, 199
  patellofemoral 147
  pathological 39
  proximal 101
  radiocapitellar 83f
  radiocarpal 86, 87, 87b, 88f, 95
  reaction force 140
  sternoclavicular 60
  stiffness of 31
  synovitis 98
  tuberculosis of 42, 44
  types of 51, 77, 97, 120, 150, 180
  weight-bearing 40

K
Keloid 307t
Keratoconjunctivitis sicca 45
Kidney disease, chronic 240
Klippel-Feil syndrome 58, 212f
Knee 40, 45
  attitude of 128
  clinical diagnostic snippets of 154t
  ecchymotic contuse skin over medial aspect of 24f
  examination proforma 173
  extensor
    strength assessment 264
    tests for 264f
  hyperextension 156
  instability 174
  joint 146, 151, 151b, 160b
    anatomy of 146f
    clinical evaluation of 146
    deformity of 12f
    function of 146
    normal hyaline cartilage of 176f
    surgical anatomy of 146
  lateral side 149f
    stabilizers of 149
  ligament of 147, 150t
  medial side 148f
    stabilizers of 148
  pathology 153b
  physiological locking of 147
  plain X-ray of 281f
  primary osteoarthrosis of 175
  stiffness 17
Kyphosis 12
  angular 211f
  round-back 211f

L
Labral pathologies 56
Labrum 50
Lacerated wound over
  cubital fossa 24f
  forefoot 24f
Laceration 23
Lachman test 165, 166f
  modified 166, 166f
Lasegue test 221, 221f
  reverse 222
Lateral collateral ligament 149, 151, 159, 170f
  complex 77, 77f
  stability 90, 169
Lateral cord syndrome 234, 234f
Lateral horn 201
Lateral meniscus 149
  anterior horn of 148, 149
  McMurray for 171
  posterior horn of 149
Lateral tibial
  condyle 281f
  plateau 148, 149, 159
Lateral ulnar collateral
  ligament 77
Leg
  anterior compartment of 267
  lateral compartment of 267
  posterior compartment of 268
Legg-Calve-Perthes disease 143
Less prominent arch 194f
Ligament 5f, 50, 97, 203
  anterior longitudinal 204
  anterolateral 149
  contractures 7
  extra-articular 15
  injury 98, 154
  intermeniscal 148, 149
  laxity 161
  popliteofibular 149
  posterior oblique 148, 149
  syndesmotic 179
Ligamentum
  flavum 204
  teres 121f
Limb 16
  alignment of 32
  attitude of 279
  chronic scarred 300f
  circumference of 304
  contralateral 27
  distal part of 34
  girth of 279
  length 7, 15, 43, 134, 162, 243
    discrepancy 13, 16, 16b, 23, 31, 33, 83, 88, 123, 127, 153, 157, 291
    measurement of 27, 133
  lower 213, 295
  major vascular injury of 29
  measurement of 15, 279
  neurological status of 313
  shortening of 7
  state of 284
  traumatic amputations of 29
  upper 213, 247, 287, 295
Limp 5, 123, 291
  painless 123
Linezolid 240
Lipoma 296, 302
  multiple 297
Lisfranc's amputation stump 288, 288f
Lisfranc's joint 180
Liver disease, chronic 240
Lobstein syndrome 36
Locking 7, 41, 153
Long bone disease 30
Long thoracic nerve 250, 250f
  palsy 250f
  features of 250
Looser's zone 233
Lower limb 213, 295
  amputee 287
  attitude 125f
  nerves, examination of 263
  neurovascular examination of 164
  rotational deformity of 127
  sensory innervation of 244f
Lower motor neuron lesion 226t

Index

Lumbar
  canal stenosis 232
  intervertebral disc 209
  lordosis 127, 129, 130*f*
    attenuated 211
    exaggerated 128*f*, 130*f*
  spinal canal stenosis 209
  spine 205, 219
    extension 217, 218*f*
    flexibility 217
    flexion 217
    forward flexion 218*f*
    movement 217, 218*f*
    lateral flexion of 218, 218*f*
    limited movements of 219*b*
Lumbosacral nerve root compression, special tests for 220
Lumbosacral spine, sagittal section of 200*f*
Lunate 108
Lung 45
  pleural effusion of 276
Lyme's disease 240
Lymph node 34, 297, 305, 309
  assessment 279
  biopsy 248
  draining stump, examination of 289
  enlargement 276
  examination 11, 17, 70, 113, 140, 142, 173, 195, 228, 247, 279

M

Madelung deformity 118, 119*f*
Magnetic resonance imaging 28
Malignancy, primitive neuroectodermal tumor group of 282
Mallet finger 102, 117, 118*f*
Malunion 35
Mangled extremity 24
Manus valgus deformity 105*f*
March fracture 191
Marfan's syndrome 38
Marie-Strumpell disease 46
Marjolin's ulcer 311
  over leg 311*f*
Massive transfusion protocol 22
McMurray test 170, 171*f*
Medial ankle ligament complex 179*f*
Medial arch collapse 189*f*
Medial collateral ligament 148, 151, 159, 170*f*
  complex 77, 77*f*
  stability 90
    tests for 168
Medial epicondyle 76, 77, 84*f*, 148, 159

Medial epicondylitis 90, 94
Medial femoral condyle 148, 159, 161
Medial longitudinal arch, flexibility of 194
Medial meniscus 148, 149
  anterior horn of 149
  McMurray for 170
  posterior horn of 149
Medial patellofemoral ligament 148, 150
Medial plantar nerves 193
Medial retinaculum 179
Medial tibial plateau 148, 149, 159
Median nerve 108, 111, 245, 255, 255*t*
  injury signs, summary of 259
  palsy, features of 256
  sensory 255
Meningocele over lumbosacral spine 214*f*
Meningomyelocele 48
Meniscal tear 170, 174
Menisci 149
  function of 150
Meniscus
  lateral 149
  test 173
Mental function, higher 223
Meralgia paraesthetica 271
Mesoneurium 236
Metacarpophalangeal joints 98, 109
Metastasis 305
  bone 275
  evidence of 276
Midfoot 185
Minor's elbow 94
Monoarticular exacerbation 45
Mononeuritis multiplex 45
Mononeuropathy 238, 238*b*
Morant-Baker cyst 155
Morel-Lavallée lesion 24, 25*f*
Morning stiffness 123
Morrant-Baker's cyst 176
Morton's neuroma 184, 191, 199
Moses sign 195
Motion
  around elbow, range of 88*b*
  restriction of 207
Motor 250, 252
  assessment 193
  ataxia 291
  examination 225, 243, 246
  functions assessment 255
  march 238, 243
    phenomena 247
  power 287
    examination 246*b*
  tract 202

Movements 11, 13, 27, 34, 51, 61, 77, 86, 109, 120, 131, 150, 161, 191, 192, 205, 243, 279, 289, 304
  abnormal 246
  difficulty in 53, 101, 153
  involuntary 226
  loss of 41
  normal range of 62*b*, 87*b*
  painful 62
  range of 109, 110
Mulder's click 191
Multiple abrasions over
  arm 24*f*
  forearm 24*f*
Multiple swelling 297
  over forehead 297*f*
Muscle 5*f*, 97, 251
  around
    elbow joint 78
    hip joint 120, 121*t*
    knee joint 151, 151*t*
    shoulder 51
    wrist joint 97*t*
  bulk 246
    arm circumference for 63
    forearm circumference for 63
  contracture 137
    tests for 139, 142
  girth 34
  interosseous 105*f*
  popliteus 147
  power of 226*b*, 246
  spasm 229
  spastic 295
  tendon
    complex 15
    contractures 7
  tone of 246
  wasting 13, 33, 42, 58, 58*f*, 83, 104, 156, 213, 241, 243, 286, 300
Muscular dystrophies 291
Musculocutaneous nerve 251, 252, 252*t*
  paralysis, features of 252
Myeloma, multiple 240, 275
Myositis ossificans 81, 93*f*

N

Nail changes 107, 242
Nailbeds 109
Napoleon test 69
Narath vascular sign 138
Neck 58, 101, 212
  normal appearance of 58*f*
  pain 54

Index

Necrosis
  idiopathic avascular 124
  secondary avascular 124
Neer's sign 65, 65f, 71
Neighboring joint 300
  swelling 304
Neoplasia 4
Nerve
  compression 298
  infections of 240
  injury 270
    chronic 241
    classification of 236
    types of 238t
  recovery, clinical signs of 243, 247
  root 5f, 200
    affection 224b
    compression 209
    level disorder 244
    structure of 237f
  subscapular 247
Nervous system 203t
Neurapraxia 236
Neurilemmal sheath 236
Neuroblastoma 275
Neurofibromatosis 297f
Neurological diseases 291
Neurological examination 223, 229, 243
Neuroma, presence of 287
Neuromuscular junction 5f, 237f
Neuromusculoskeletal pathway 5f
Neuropathy 313
  compressive 78, 238
  entrapment 45
Neurotmesis 236
Neurovascular compression 305
Neurovascular examination 11, 16, 27, 71, 136, 142, 173, 193, 279
Night cries 40
Nodules 45
Non-healing ulcer over heel 188f, 311f
Nonsteroidal anti-inflammatory drugs 176
Nonunion 35
Numbness 80, 101, 182
Nursemaid's elbow 93

O

O'Brien test 69, 70f
O'Donoghue triad 166
OA knee, typical 44
Obturator nerve 245, 264
  tests for 265f
Occiput-wall distance test 215
Ochsner's clasping sign 259, 259f
Ok sign 257
Olecranon 83f, 84f
  bursa 94, 94f
  position of 83, 84
  process, palpation of 85
Onion-peel appearance, typical 282f
Open fracture 22b, 25, 28
  Gustilo-Anderson classification of 26t
Opera hand 47
Opponens
  digiti minimi 260
  pollicis 248, 256
  tests for 258f
Orthopedics 1, 10b
  semergencies, trauma-related 28
Orthosis 11
Ortolani test 139, 139f
Osgood-Schlatter disease 177, 177f
Osteitis deformans 38
Osteoarthritis 43, 175, 176f
  glenohumeral 56
  primary 46f, 106f, 145, 155
Osteoarthrosis
  carpometacarpal 42
  degenerative 39
  post-traumatic 122
  primary degenerative 43
Osteochondritis dissecans 39
Osteochondroma 280
  femur, X-ray of 280f
Osteoclastoma 280
Osteogenesis imperfecta 36, 37f
Osteology 50, 97, 120, 146, 178, 200
Osteomalacia 37, 233
Osteomyelitis
  acute 300
  chronic 36, 303
  tubercular 36
Osteopenia 46f
Osteophytes 46f
  humeral 74f
  lack of 46f
Osteoporosis 38, 233
Osteoporotic vertebral body fractures 209
Osteosarcoma 1, 275, 280, 281f, 296

P

Paclitaxel 240
Paget's disease 38
Pain 3, 22, 31, 40, 53, 54, 79, 98, 122, 152, 152b, 181, 206, 274, 284, 297
  bone 275
  cardiac origin 55
  character of 31, 40, 122, 207
  chest 55
  first rule out cervical causes of 56
  mechanical 3, 40, 152
  mild 3
  moderate 3
  moderate-to-severe 98
  nature of 100, 206
  onset of 31, 122, 206
  radiation of 122, 206
  referred 122
  severity of 122
  site of 206
  throbbing 297
  timing of 3, 53, 206
Painful arc syndrome 74, 74f
Palm 99
Palmar
  aponeurosis 98
  fascia 105f
    contractures of 104
  flexion 90f, 109f
  interossei 99, 261
  tendon palpation 108
Palpate popliteal fossa 161
Paralysis, delayed onset 239
Paraolecranon fossa 84, 84f
Paraspinal spasm 213, 214
Parasympathetic nervous system 204
Paresthesia 287
Parkinson's disease 291
Paronychia 98, 107
Pars interarticularis 232f
Passive stretch pain 27
Patella 147, 148
  dislocation 1
  grind test 161f
  instability 154
  orientation 126
  stability 173
Patellar cartilage
  fibrillation of 176
  fraying of 176
Patellar clonus 227
Patellar tap 159, 160f
Patellar tendon 168f
  over proximal tibia 159f
Patte's test 67, 251, 251f
Pelvis 27, 130, 276
  examination of 228, 287
  fracture 25f
  level of 229
  squared 130
Pen test 257
  positive 260
Periarthritis shoulder 72

Index

Pericardial effusion 28
Perineurium 236
Peripheral nerve 5f
  affections 291
  autonomous zone of 245b
  basic unit of 236
  clinical evaluation of 236
  examination 248
    proforma 270
  function of 236
  injury 291
  surgical anatomy of 236
Peripheral nervous system 243
  formation of 237f
Perkin's method 131
Peroneal nerve injury 270
Peroneus brevis 181
Peroneus longus 181
  tests for 268f
Perthes' disease 1, 39, 122, 124, 143
Pes
  anserinus bursitis 158f
  cavus 186f
  planus 186, 186f, 197
Phalen's sign 111
  reverse 111
Phantom limb sensation 284
Phenobarbitone 241
Phenytoin 241
Piano key
  sign 113f
  test 113
Pirogoff amputation 289
Pivot shift test 166, 167f
  reverse 170
Plantar
  fasciitis 183, 197
  flexion 191, 191f
  nerves, lateral 193
Platelet rich plasma 176
Pleural effusion 45, 276
Podagra 198f
Pointing finger 242
Pointing index sign 257, 259, 259f, 260
Policeman's tip hand 242
Poliomyelitis 240, 291
Polyneuropathy 238, 238b
Polytrauma 18
  clinical evaluation of 18
  concepts of 18
  summary of 21fc
Popeye sign 57, 57f
  reverse 83
Popliteal fossa 42f, 127, 150, 157f, 176
  examination of 157

Posterior column tract 201
Posterior cord syndrome 235, 235f
Posterior cruciate ligament 147-149, 151, 173
  stability tests for 167
Posterior horn 201
Posterior inferior glenohumeral ligament 51
Posterior instability, tests for 64
Posterior interosseous nerve 97
  palsy, features of 254
Posterior joint line 61f
  palpation technique of 61f
Posterior stability test 173
Posterior superior iliac spine 218, 229
  level of 127
Posterolateral corner, stability of 173
Posteromedial corner, stability of 173
Preacher's hand 259
Prepatellar bursa 158f
Pressure
  effects 300
  temporary 239
Pronators 255
Prosthesis 11
  examination of 287, 289
  fitting of 284
Proximal forearm 24f
Pseudo-ankylosis 14
Pseudoarthrosis 37
  congenital 37, 37f
Pseudo-coxalgia 143
Pseudogout 48, 80
Psoriasis 106, 106b, 106f
Pulled elbow 93
Pulp changes 107
Pulses, peripheral 28
Pyogenic tenosynovitis 98

Q

Q-angle 150, 162
Quadriceps 151
  active test 168, 169f
  angle 150
  weakness 294, 294f

R

Radial artery 96
Radial collateral ligament 77
Radial deviation 105f, 109f
Radial head 76
  palpation of 85, 86f
Radial nerve 111, 245, 252, 253t
  autonomous zone of 253f
  function assessment of 253
  injury 254
  summary of 255

paralysis
  features of 254
  low 254
  sensory innervation 96
Radial styloid process 108
Radiation 4, 53, 122, 206
Radioulnar joint, superior 76f, 77
Radius, distal end of 108
Ranvier node 238
Raynaud's phenomena 107
Rectus femoris contracture 139, 139f
Recurvatum 12, 12f
  knee 156
Red flag sign 27
Reflex 226, 246, 287
  superficial 226
  sympathetic dystrophy 116
Regimental badge sign 251f
Regional lymph node 313
  examination of 304
Reiter's syndrome 47
Renal failure 48
Renal phosphate wasting 37
Resisted external rotation test 67
Rest pain 3, 40, 152
Retinaculum
  around wrist 95
  peroneal 179
Rheumatoid 1, 80
  arthritis 1, 41, 46f, 103, 106, 106b, 106f
  nodule over extensor 299f
  wrist, typical deformity of 105f
Rhizomelic dwarfism 36, 36f
Rhomberg sign positive 295
Rickets 37, 38f
  hypocalcemic 37
  hypophosphatemic 37
  renal 37
Road traffic accident 17
Rocker bottom foot 188f
Roos test 220, 220f
Root compression 219
Rotator cuff 50
  arthropathy 73, 73f
  integrity signs 71
  tear 54, 56, 64, 73
    tests for 66
  tendinopathy 56, 72

S

Sacroiliac joint, special tests for 222
Sacroiliitis 219
Sag sign 167f
  modified 167, 168f
  posterior 167
Saphenous nerve 193, 245, 265

Index

Sausage-shaped digit 106
Scaphoid tubercle 107*f*
Scapula 58, 212
   inferior angle of 215*f*
   level of inferior angle of 58
   shape of 58
   winging of 59, 242
Scapular plane 61
Scar 34, 85, 86, 214, 241, 242, 242*f*, 277
   clinical evaluation of 296
   contractures 7
   examination of 305
   hypertrophic 307*t*
   inspection of 305
   mobility of 306
   palpation of 306
Scarf test 70
Scarpa's triangle 126, 127
   anatomy of 126*b*
   content of 126*b*
Scarring, pathological 306
Schober's method, modified 217
Schober's test 218*f*
Sciatic nerve 265, 266, 266*t*
   injury 270
   palsy, features of 266
Sclerosis 49*f*, 211, 211*f*
Scoliosis 12, 211*f*
   functional 212, 212*f*
Segmental length 15, 164*f*
Senile kyphosis 209
Sensation 8
Sensory 250, 252
   ataxia 291
   deficits 287
   examination 223, 243
      method of 245*b*
   innervation around knee 151
   loss 256, 261
   neuropathies 241
   tracts 201
Septic arthritis, acute 44
Serratus anterior 250*f*
   function of 250
Shoulder 101
   abduction of 74*f*
   anterior dislocation of 57*f*
   appearance 58*f*
   clinical diagnostic snippets 56*t*
   contour 56
   dislocation 1
   examination proforma 71
   girdle
      muscles 248*fc*
      seven nerves around 247
   instability, tests for 64

joint 51*f*, 62*b*, 62*f*
   anatomy of 51*f*
   clinical evaluation of 50
   line 60
   lateral aspect of 59*f*
   level of 57, 127, 229
   normal appearance of 58*f*
   pain 54
   pathologies 53*b*
   posterior aspect of 59*f*
   recurrent dislocation 56
   rotators of 54
   subluxation of 54
Simian hand 256*f*
Single spinal nerve 223
Sinus 31, 34, 86, 214, 277, 286, 297, 297*f*
   absence of 286
   clinical evaluation of 296
   discharging 6
   examination of 286, 307
   presence of 33
Skin 7, 15, 185
   breakdown, presence of 306
   changes 104*f*
   condition 228
   glistening 277
   loss 24
   over joint 42
   overlying limb 33
   pinchability 278
   stretched 277
   surrounding scar 306
Slap tear test 71
Slipped capital femoral epiphysis 1, 124, 144, 144*f*
Soft tissue 5*f*, 158, 159*f*, 230, 286
   crepitus 27
   landmarks 86, 86*b*, 158*b*
   laxity 60
   pathway 5
   planes 27
Sole 185, 188
   palpation of 191*f*
Soleus 268
   muscle, tests for 268*f*
Sound ankylosis 15
Specific nerve palsy 242*b*
Speed's test 69, 70*f*
Spider fingers 38
Spina bifida 313
   aperta 213
Spinal accessory nerve 248, 249*f*, 249*t*
   paralysis, features of 249
   site 242*f*
   supplies 248

Spinal artery
   anterior 201, 202, 235
   posterior 201, 202, 235
Spinal cord 5*f*, 200, 201, 201*f*, 202, 204*f*, 224*b*
   arterial supply of 202*f*
   blood supply of 202
   cross-section of 5*f*, 201*f*
   hemisection of 234
   sensory tracts 225*t*
   surgical anatomy of 200
   upper 248
Spinal ligaments 203
Spine 27, 58, 126, 127, 287
   alignment of 210, 214, 229
   clinical diagnostic snippets of 209*t*
   curvature of 203
   examination proforma 229
   functions of 205
   mobility of 203
   normal appearance of 58*f*
   osteology of 200
   pathology 206*b*
   red flags of 208
   surgical anatomy of 200
   tenderness 214
   tuberculosis of 209, 230
Spinothalamic tract
   anterior 201
   lateral 201, 234, 235
Spinous process, direct palpation of 215*f*
Spondylitis 231
Spondyloarthropathy
   Gustilo-Anderson classification of 46
   seronegative 46, 206, 209
Spondylolisthesis 232, 232*f*
Spondylolysis 232, 232*f*
Spondylosis, degenerative 231
Sports injuries 1
Sprengel shoulder 59*f*
Spurling test 219, 219*f*
Stability tests 71, 142, 173
Static valgus stress test 90, 91*f*
Static varus stress test 90, 91*f*
Sternocleidomastoid 248, 249, 249*f*
Steroid, intra-articular 176
Stiff hip 291
Stiff joint 6*b*, 14
Stiffness 31, 80
   loss of 41
Straight leg raising test 220, 221*f*
Stroke test 160*f*
Student's elbow 94

Stump 284
  inspection of 285, 289
  measurement of 289
  palpation of 286
  swelling of 286
  vascularity of 287
Styloid process 108, 109f, 110, 110f
Subscapularis tear 68
Subtalar joint 192, 268f
  inversion-eversion, assessment of 192f
Sudeck's osteodystrophy 116
Sudomotor function 246
Superficial peroneal nerve 193, 245, 265-267
Superficial radial nerve 96, 244
Superior articular facet 204
Superior labrum anterior posterior tear, tests for 69
Supplies serratus anterior muscle 250
Supracondylar fracture malunion 81
Supracondylar ridges, palpation of 85
Supraspinatus 51
  muscle wasting of 58f
  tear 66
  tendon, tests for 67f
Sural nerve 193, 245, 265
Swan-neck deformity 106
Swelling 4, 22, 23, 31, 33, 40, 42, 54, 57, 80, 83-85, 100, 104, 107, 108, 152, 156, 158, 182, 189f, 208, 213, 214, 274, 296, 298, 302, 302b, 303, 303f
  around heel 188
  benign 296, 305t
  bony 302
  causes of 126
  chronic 31
  clinical evaluation of 296
  consistency of 278f
  differential diagnosis of 299t
  diffuse 101
  distal 242, 278
  examination of 296
  extent of 278f
  inflammatory 296
  intra-articular 4, 302
  large diaphyseal 282f
  local 242
    examination of 298
  location of 274
  lying over artery 301
  malignant 296, 305t
  multiple 297

palpation of 86
plane of 278, 302, 302b
pulsatile 301, 302f
specific characteristics 301
submuscular 302
supramuscular 302
Swing phase 290
Swinging upper extremity 78
Syme's amputation stump 288, 288f
Sympathetic nervous system 202, 204
Syndactyly 118f
Syndesmosis 189f
Synovial hypertrophy 43, 152, 160
  palpation of 161f
Syringomyelia 48
Systemic lupus erythematosus 45, 106

T
Tabes dorsalis 48
Tailors bunion 186
Talar body 192
Talipes equinovarus, congenital 183, 291
Tall stature 38
Talofibular ligament, anterior 183, 189f
Tardy ulnar nerve palsy 81, 263, 263b
Tarsal tunnel syndrome 190, 271
Telescopy test 137, 137f
Tenderness 33, 43, 59, 108, 128, 129, 158, 189, 278, 278f, 301
  around wrist 107
  bony 25, 35, 36
  over stump 286
  retropatellar 161
Tendinopathy, chronic 98
Tendinosis 183
Tendo-achilles 181, 190
  tendon, integrity of 195
Tendon 5f
  peroneal 190
  popliteus 149
  superficial 246
Tennis elbow 81, 89, 94
  special tests for 80
Tenosynovitis, inflammatory 98
Teres minor 251
  tests for 67
Thalidomide 240
Thenar
  eminence 99
  muscles 256f
Thessaly test 170, 171, 172f

Thigh
  muscle, wasting of 127f, 133, 136, 162
  wasting, measurement of 137f
Thomas hip flexion test 129, 130f
  rationale of 129
Thompson-Simmond test 195, 195f
Thoracic outlet syndrome 219, 220f, 230
Thoracolumbar outflow 202
Three ligaments stabilize hip joint 120
Thromboangiitis obliterans 313
Thumb
  abduction 257
  movements 110f
Thyroid dysfunction 55
Tibia
  anterior pull of 165f
  congenital pseudoarthrosis of 37
  lower end 189f
  pagetic bowing of 38f
  proximal 26f
Tibial component, measurement of 135f
Tibial condyles 147
Tibial nerve 190, 245, 265, 266, 268
Tibial plateau 149f
Tibial tuberosity 164f
  prominence of bilateral 177f
Tibialis anterior 181, 267, 269
  tests for 267f
Tibialis posterior 181, 190, 269
  insufficiency 183
  tendinitis 198
  tests for 269f
Tibiofemoral compartment 147
Tight plaster cast 239
Tinel's sign 238, 243, 247
Tingling 80, 101, 182, 284
Tissue, subcutaneous 15
Toe
  deformities 186b
  gangrene of 312f
Tone 225
Torticollis 12, 210f
Trabaculae crossing joint 15f
Transverse ligament 121f
Trapezius 249, 249f
  muscle 248
Trauma 4
  accidents
    high-velocity of 22
    low-velocity of 22
  acute 152
  characteristic of 98

Index

episode, elaboration of 79
  force of 21
  mechanism of 21
  velocity of 21
Trendelenburg test 137, 138, 138f, 140
  positive 138
  prerequisites for 138
  standard 138
Triangular fibrocartilage complex 95, 95f, 100, 114
  injury, tests for 113, 113f
Triceps, tests for 254f
Trigger finger 102, 116
Trochanteric region 126
Trochlea 76
  lateral half of 76
Tuberculosis 42, 44, 98, 124, 143, 209, 230
Tuberosity, humeral 51f
Tumor 119, 296
  benign 273, 275t
  bone 272, 273b, 275, 276, 280
  examination proforma 279
  inspection of 279
  malignant 273, 275t
  pressure symptoms of 275
  secondary metastatic 298
Typical nutritional deficiency rickets 37

U

Ulcer 33, 34, 86, 286
  chronic non-healing 311f
  clinical evaluation of 296
  edge, types of 312f
  examination of 286, 309
  neuropathic 313
  over toe 312f
Ulna, distal end of 108
Ulnar claw hand, classic 260f
Ulnar collateral ligament complex 77
Ulnar deviation 109f
Ulnar nerve 86, 108, 111, 245, 248, 255f, 260, 261f
  autonomous zone of 260f

near
  elbow, higher-level lesion of 263
  wrist, lower level lesion of 263
palsy
  features of 261
  high 261
  low 261
  signs 263
  site 242f
Ulnar paradox 263, 263b
Ulnar styloid process 89, 108
Unilateral flexion deformity, tests for 129
Unsound ankylosis 15
Upper limb 213, 247, 287, 295
  length measurement 63f, 89f
  measurement of 63
  muscles 248fc
  neurovascular examination of 64, 89, 111
  sensory innervation of 244f
Upper motor neuron lesion 226t
Urethral sphincter
  external 203, 204
  internal 203, 204
Urinary bladder 203, 203t
  innervation 204f

V

Valgus 12, 12f
  angulation 187f
  deformity 46f, 187
  stress 171f
  indicates direction of 91f
  test 168, 169, 169b, 170f
Varus 12, 12f
  deformity 33f, 46f
  stress 91f, 170f
  test 169, 170b, 170f
Vascular compression 298
Vasculitis 45
Vasomotor function 246
Veins, dilated 277
Venous ulcer 312f
  over lateral malleolus 309f
Ventral ramus 236

Vertical talus, congenital 183
Vinca alkaloids 240
Vitamin
  B12 deficiency 291
  deficiency 240, 291
Volkmann's ischemic contracture 117, 117f
Volkmann's sign 117, 117f
Vrolik disease 36

W

Walking aids, use of 123
Wall push-up test 250f
Wallerian degeneration 236, 238
Wallerian regeneration 236, 238, 247
Wartenberg syndrome 271
Weakness 31, 54, 101
Well-leg raising test 222
Windswept deformity 42
Wound
  open 22
  puncture 23, 25f
Wrist 100b, 104, 242
  attempted dorsiflexion of 117f
  clinical evaluation of 95
  drop 241f, 242
  ganglion 102
    over dorsum of 105f, 299f
  hand
    clinical diagnostic snippets 102t
    examination proforma 114
  joint 109, 109b
    line 108
    surgical anatomy of 95
  ligament of 95
  osteology of 95
  pain, causes of 100t
  radial deviation of 105f
  volar
    subluxation of 105f
    surface of 108f

Y

Yersinia 47